CRACK THE
CORE EXAM
CASE COMPANION

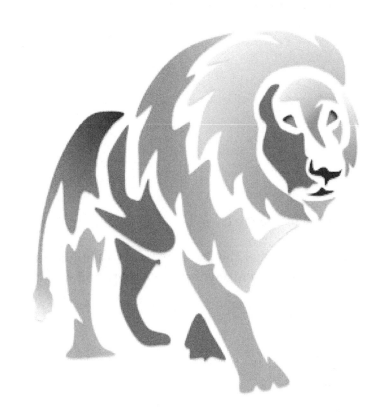

PROMETHEUS LIONHART, M.D.

Crack the Core Exam - Case Companion

First Ed. - Version 2.1 (July 2016)

Disclaimer:

Readers are advised - this book is **NOT to be used for clinical decision making**. Human error does occur, and it is your responsibility to double check all facts provided. To the fullest extent of the law, the Author assumes no responsibility for any injury and/or damage to persons or property arising out or related to any use of the material contained in this book.

Copyright © 2015 by Prometheus Lionhart,

All rights reserved - Under International and Pan-American Copyright Conventions. This book, or parts thereof, may not be reproduced in any form without permission from the Author.

Published by: Prometheus Lionhart

Title ID: 5260855

ISBN-13: 978-1507810859

Cover design, texts, and illustrations: copyright © 2015 by Prometheus Lionhart

Cover Art modified from Licensed Art — Nathapol HPS/Shutterstock.com

Part 1: "Aunt Minnie's" - 125 Cases

- Neuro (Cases 1-19)
- MSK (Cases 20 - 43)
- Cardiac (Cases 44 - 53)
- Thoracic (Cases 54- 59)
- GI (Cases 60 - 70)
- GU (Cases 71 - 75)
- GYN (Cases 76 - 79)
- Nukes (Cases 80 - 83)
- Reproductive (Cases 84- 86 , 91- 92)
- Peds (Cases 89 - 90, 93 - 100)
- Mammo (Cases 101 - 103)
- Vascular / IR (Cases 104 - 108)
- Physics (Cases 109 - 125)
- Non-Interpretive Skillz (Cases 126-130)

Concentrated Reviews of:
- Phakomatoses (pg 19-20)
- The Sinus (pg 25-26)
- Cord Tumors (pg 41-42)
- Arthritis (pg 59-60)
- Knee Meniscus (pg 79-80)
- Cardiac MRI (pg 109-110)
- Congenital Heart (pg 119-120)
- Cystic Renal Disease (pg 161-162)
- Dementia Imaging (pg 181-182)
- Uterine Malformations (pg 203-204)
- Peds Age & Syndrome (pg 221-222)

Part 2: "This vs That" - 50 Cases

- Neuro (Cases 1-12)
- MSK (Cases 13 - 15)
- Thoracic (Cases 16 - 19)
- GI (Cases 21 - 24, 26)
- GYN / Reproductive (Case 25, 27)
- Peds (Cases 28- 33)
- Nukes (Cases 34 - 42)
- Mammo (Cases 43 - 45)
- Vascular / IR (Cases 46- 50)

Part 3: "Anatomy" - 30 Cases

- Neuro (Cases 1 - 11)
- Vascular / Angiograms (Cases 12 - 19)
- Cardiac (Cases 20 - 21)
- Abdomen US / Prostate MR (Cases 22 - 23)
- MSK - (Cases 24 - 27)
- Nukes Mystery Whole Body Scans (Cases 28 - 30)

Disclaimer:

Readers are advised - this book is **NOT to be used for clinical decision making**. Human error does occur, and it is your responsibility to double check all facts provided. To the fullest extent of the law, the Author assumes no responsibility for any injury and/or damage to persons or property arising out or related to any use of the material contained in this book.

FATE RARELY CALLS UPON US AT A MOMENT OF OUR CHOOSING

Optimus Prime

AUNT MINNIE'S

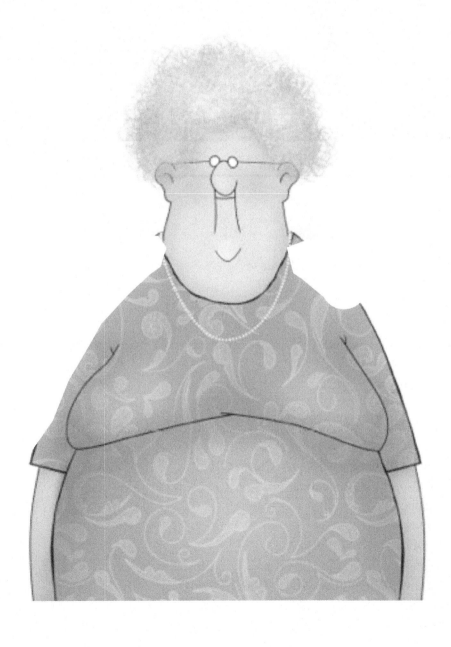

Case 1 - 31 year old Female

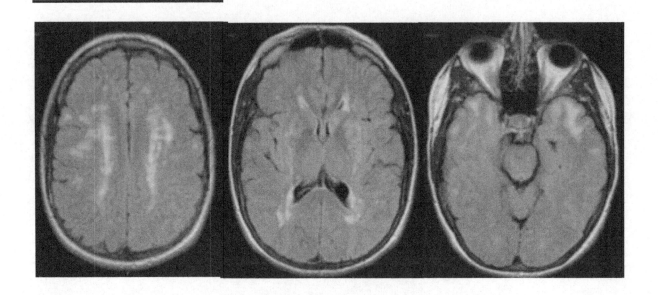

1. What is the Dx?
A. Rasmussen Encephalitis
B. Chronic Ischemic White Matter Disease
C. PRES
D. CADASIL

2. What is the "Classic History" ?
A. Gelastic Seizures
B. Precocious Puberty
C. Migraines
D. Ascending Paralysis

3. White matter involvement where is "Classic" ?
A. It classically spares white matter
B. Temporal Lobes
C. Parietal Lobes
D. Occipital Lobes

4. Sparing of the white matter where is "Classic" ?
A. Frontal Lobes
B. Temporal Lobes
C. Parietal Lobes
D. Occipital Lobes

Case 1 - CADASIL

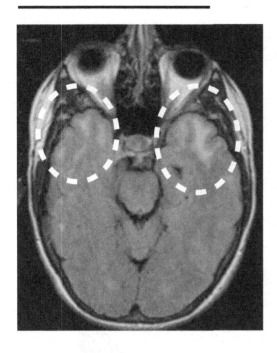

1. What is the Dx?
A. Rasmussen Encephalitis
B. Chronic Ischemic White Matter Disease
C. PRES
D. CADASIL

2. What is the "Classic History" ?
A. Gelastic Seizures
B. Precocious Puberty
C. Migraines
D. Ascending Paralysis

3. White matter involvement where is "Classic" ?
A. It classically spares white matter
B. Temporal Lobes
C. Parietal Lobes
D. Occipital Lobes

4. Sparing of the white matter where is "Classic" ?
A. Frontal Lobes
B. Temporal Lobes
C. Parietal Lobes
D. Occipital Lobes

CADASIL

Cerebral Autosomal Dominant Arteriopathy with Subcortical Infarcts and Leukoencephalopathy).

Essential Trivia:

- It's an inherited condition (hence the name). It typically presents between age 30-40.

- The history of migraines (sometimes with aura) is classic. Depression and focal neurologic defects can also occur. For the purpose of multiple choice, I'd go with migraine.

- Lots of things involve the frontal white matter. However, involvement of the temporal white matter - especially when severe in a 30 year old should make you say CADASIL.

- The other classic finding is relative sparing of the occipital subcortical white matter and U-Fibers.

- The MRA is usually normal, with minimal if any atherosclerosis.

Case 2 - Developmental Delay

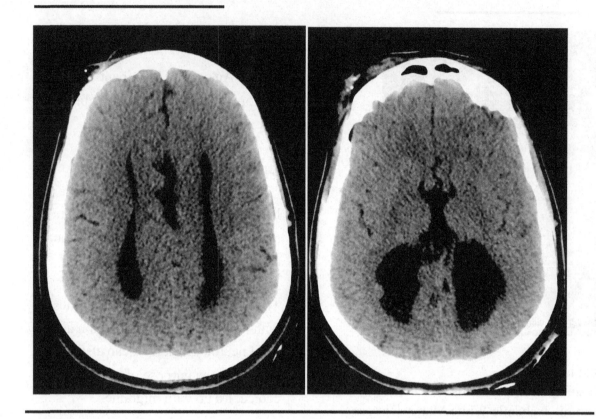

1. What is the diagnosis ?
A. Looks normal to me
B. Polymicrogyria
C. Hydranencephaly
D. Schizencephaly
E. Agenesis of the corpus callosum

2. What part of the corpus callosum forms first ?
A. Genu
B. Splenium
C. Body
D. Rostrum

3. What condition(s) are classically associated with agenesis of the Corpus Callosum ?
A. Intracranial Lipoma
B. Hydrocephalus (Colpocephaly)
C. Chiari II Malformations
D. Dandy Walker Spectrum
E. All of the above

Case 2 - Agenesis of the Corpus Callosum

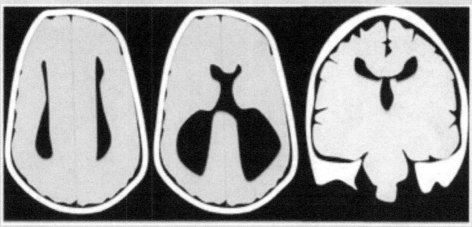

The 3 Classic Looks
(Notice the Sagittal is not among them - that makes it too obvious)

Wide Spaced Vertical Ventricles | Colpocephaly | Steer Horn Appearance on Coronal

1. What is the diagnosis?
A. Looks normal to me
B. Polymicrogyria
C. Hydranencephaly
D. Schizencephaly
E. Agenesis of the corpus callosum

2. What part of the corpus callosum forms first?
A. Genu
B. Splenium
C. Body
D. Rostrum

3. What condition(s) are classically associated with agenesis of the Corpus Callosum ?
A. Intracranial Lipoma
B. Hydrocephalus (Colpocephaly)
C. Chiari II Malformations
D. Dandy Walker Spectrum
E. All of the above

Essential Trivia:

- There are 3 classic ways to show this (as above)

- There are tons of associations. The ones I would know are: Colpocephaly (30%), Intracranial Lipoma (10%), Dandy Walker (11%), Chiari II (7%), Holoprosencephaly, and Fetal EtOH syndrome.

- The C.C. forms front to back then Rostrum last.

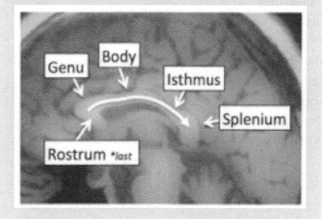

Aunt Minnie 4

Case 3 - Ataxia and Sleep Apnea

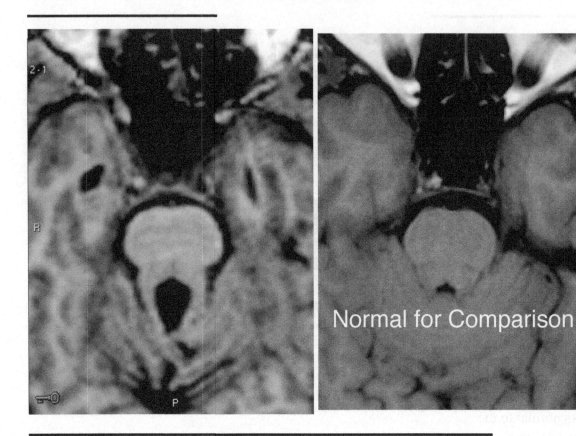

1. What is the diagnosis?
A. Normal
B. Chiari II Malformation
C. Dandy Walker Spectrum
D. Joubert Syndrome

2. What is the buzzword ?
A. Prominent Vermis
B. Eye of the Tiger Sign
C. Panda Sign
D. Molar Tooth Sign

3. What is the most common association
A. Retinal Dysplasia
B. Aortic Aneurysm
C. Medulloblastoma
D. Syndactyly

Case 3 - Joubert Syndrome

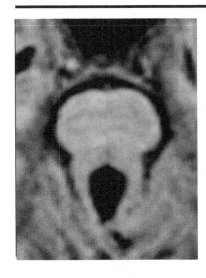
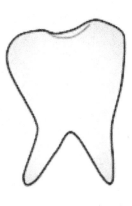

1. What is the diagnosis?
A. Normal
B. Chiari II Malformation
C. Dandy Walker Spectrum
D. Joubert Syndrome

2. What is the buzzword?
A. Prominent Vermis
B. Eye of the Tiger Sign
C. Panda Sign
D. Molar Tooth Sign

3. What is the most common association
A. Retinal Dysplasia
B. Aortic Aneurysm
C. Medulloblastoma
D. Syndactyly

Joubert Syndrome

Also known as vermian aplasia or molar tooth midbrain-hindbrain malformation.

Essential Trivia:

- This is an inherited condition (AR)

- A lack of normal decussation of superior cerebellar peduncular fiber tracts leads to enlargement of the peduncles. All this together makes the midbrain look like a **molar tooth**.

- There are several associations that are worth knowing:
  • Retinal Dysplasia (occurs in 50% of cases)
  • Multicystic dysplastic kidney (occurs in 30% of cases)
  • Polydactyly (occurs in 15% of cases)

Case 4- Notorious Drunk, Now with quadriplegia

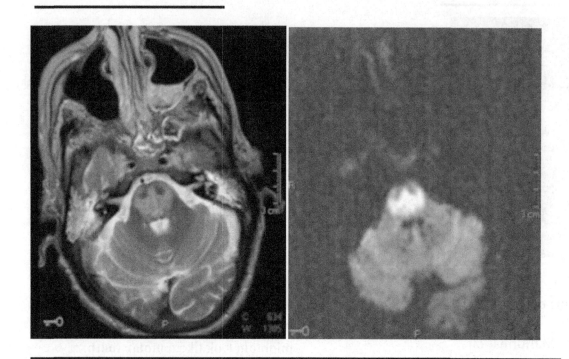

1. What is the diagnosis?
A. Pontine Glioma
B. Marchiafava-Bignami
C. Wernicke encephalopathy
D. Central pontine myelinolysis

2. What is the pathophysiology?
A. Rapid correction of Thiamine
B. Rapid correction of Na+
C. Correction of Na+ was too slow
D. Autoimmune Demyelination

3. What is the earliest sign?
A. Restricted diffusion in the lower pons
B. T2 Hypointensity
C. Homogeneous Contrast Enhancement
D. Blooming on Gradient

Case 4 - Central pontine myelinolysis (CPM)

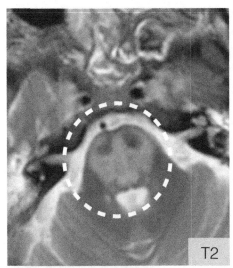
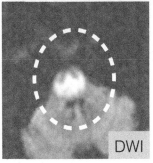

1. What is the diagnosis?
A. Pontine Glioma
B. Marchiafava-Bignami
C. Wernicke encephalopathy
D. Central pontine myelinolysis

2. What is the pathophysiology?
A. Rapid correction of Thiamine
B. Rapid correction of Na+
C. Correction of Na+ was too slow
D. Autoimmune Demyelination

3. What is the earliest sign?
A. Restricted diffusion in the lower pons
B. T2 Hypointensity
C. Homogeneous Contrast Enhancement
D. Blooming on Gradient

CPM

This is an acute demyelination of the white matter tracts of the pons. It's seen in the setting of acute osmotic changes, classically described with the rapid correction of hyponatremia

Essential Trivia:

- The classic history is a chronic alcoholic (nursing home patient or transplant patient), who had a rapidly corrected Na+. He/She felt much better after the correction, then returns to the ED **3 days later** with spastic quadriparesis and pseudobulbar palsy (hyperactive gag reflex, and dysarthria).

- The first sign is restricted diffusion in the lower Pons.

- Low signal on T1 and high signal on T2 in the same region (lower pons) may not show up for two weeks.

- It can enhance like an acute MS plaque (but doesn't have to).

- Peripheral fibers are classically spared.

Case 5- History Withheld

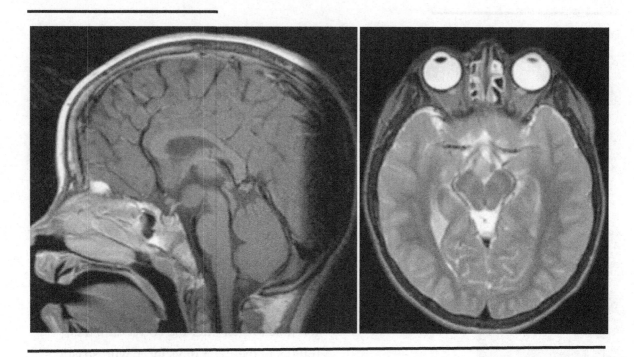

1. What is the diagnosis?
A. Pituitary Adenoma
B. Teratoma
C. Glioma
D. Tuber Cinereum Hamartoma

2. What is the classic history?
A. Infertility
B. Sudden Death
C. Gelastic seizures
D. Grand mal seizures

3. What the hell is this "tuber cinereum" ?
A. It's part of the pituitary
B. It's part of the optic chiasm
C. It's part of the mammillary bodies
D. It's part of the hypothalamus

Case 5 - Tuber Cinereum Hamartoma

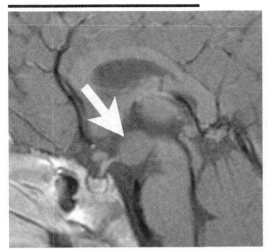

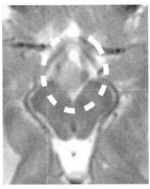

1. What is the diagnosis?
A. Pituitary Adenoma
B. Teratoma
C. Glioma
D. Tuber Cinereum Hamartoma

2. What is the classic history?
A. Infertility
B. Sudden Death
C. Gelastic seizures
D. Grand mal seizures

3. What the hell is this "tuber cinereum"?
A. It's part of the pituitary
B. It's part of the optic chiasm
C. It's part of the mammillary bodies
D. It's part of the hypothalamus

> **Tuber Cinereum Hamartoma**
>
> A hamartoma located within a specific location of the hypothalamus
>
> *Essential Trivia:*
>
> - The location is very typical. This is a true Aunt Minnie.
>
> - In addition to the characteristic location, this thing should be iso-intense to cortex on T1 with no enhancement.
>
> - The most testable trivia regarding these things is the classic clinical history. There are actually two classic clinical stories:
>   • Gelastic (laughing) seizures
>   • Precocious Puberty
>
> - The tuber cinereum is the part of the hypothalamus located between the optic chiasm and the mammillary bodies.

Case 6 - Altered Mental Status

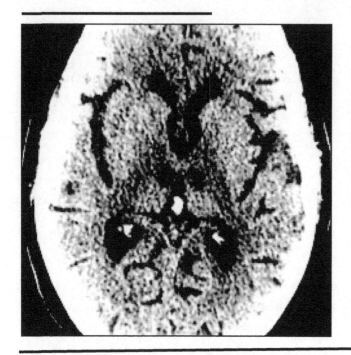
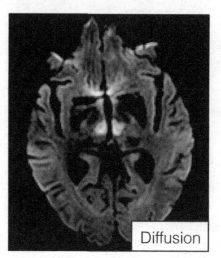

1. What is the diagnosis?
A. MCA infarct
B. ACA infarct
C. Artery of Heubner Infarct
D. Artery of Percheron infarct

2. Which of the follow could also be included in the differential for bilateral thalamic Hypodensities on CT?
A. Wernicke-Korsakoff
B. Internal Cerebral Vein Thrombosis
C. Top of the Basilar Syndrome
D. All of the Above

3. The Artery of Percheron arises from _____, and supplies _____ ?
A. Bilateral PCAs, Unilateral Thalamus
B. Unilateral PCA, Unilateral Thalamus
C. Bilateral PCAs, Bilateral Thalamus + Midbrain
D. Unilateral PCA, Bilateral Thalamus + Midbrain

Case 6- Artery of Percheron Infarct

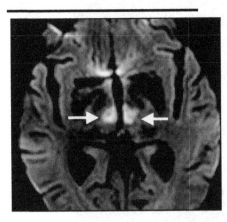
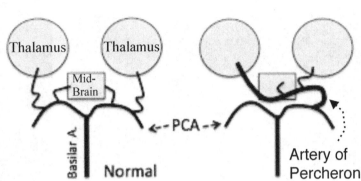

1. What is the diagnosis?
A. MCA infarct
B. ACA infarct
C. Artery of Heubner Infarct
D. Artery of Percheron infarct

2. Which of the follow could also be included in the differential for bilateral thalamic Hypodensities on CT?
A. Wernicke-Korsakoff
B. Internal Cerebral Vein Thrombosis
C. Top of the Basilar Syndrome
D. All of the Above

3. The Artery of Percheron arises from _____, and supplies _____?
A. Bilateral PCAs, Unilateral Thalamus
B. Unilateral PCA, Unilateral Thalamus
C. Bilateral PCAs, Bilateral Thalamus + Midbrain
D. Unilateral PCA, Bilateral Thalamus + Midbrain

Artery of Percheron Infarct

The artery of Percheron is a rare vascular variant, in which a single common trunk arises from one of the PCAs to supply both thalami and the midbrain.

Essential Trivia:

- This is a unique example of a unilateral blood vessel supplying structures on both sides of the midbrain.

- Occlusion of the Artery of Percheron will cause a bilateral infarction of the thalamus and a "V-Shaped" infarct of the rostral midbrain.

- On CT, occlusion of the bilateral cerebral veins, occlusion of the tip of the basilar artery, or even Wernickes can give a similar appearance.

Case 7- History Withheld

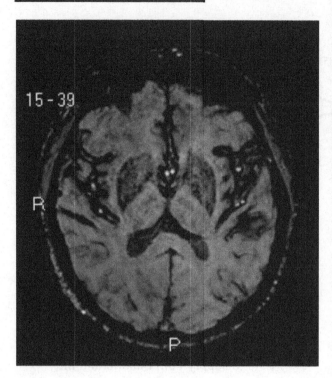
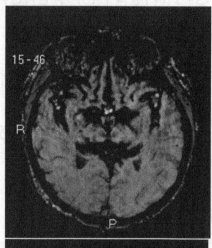
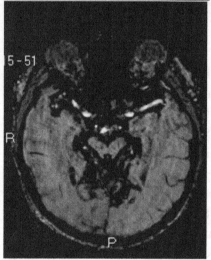

1. What is the Diagnosis?
A. Looks normal to me
B. Superficial Siderosis
C. Cavernoma(s)
D. Leptomeningeal Spread of CA (or infection)

2. What is the classic presentation?
A. Seizure
B. Thunderclap Headache
C. Gelastic Seizures
D. Sensorineural Hearing Loss

3. What is the classic history?
A. AVM or Aneurysm
B. Down Syndrome
C. NF -2
D. Pituitary Teratoma

4. What is the "next step" ?
A. PET CT
B. CT with Perfusion
C. Conventional Angiogram
D. No further imaging needed.

Case 7- Superficial siderosis

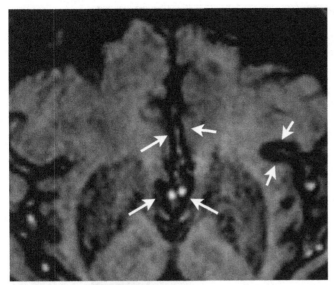

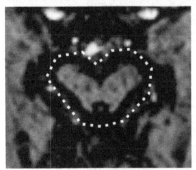

Superficial Siderosis

Deposition of hemosiderin along the leptomeninges.

Essential Trivia:

- The etiology is typically recurrent or extensive subarachnoid hemorrhage. This can be from any cause; trauma, bleeding brain tumor, AVM, or aneurysm.

- If you are forced into a "next step" situation, you would want to look for the cause of bleeding. Angiogram (conventional or CTA) would be the answer I would choose.

- Sensorineural hearing low is found in 95% of patients, and is the most common clinical presentation. It is typically bilateral and gradual in onset.

- The second most common symptom (found in 88% of cases) is ataxia.

1. What is the Diagnosis?
A. Looks normal to me
B. Superficial Siderosis
C. Cavernoma(s)
D. Leptomeningeal Spread of CA (or infection)

2. What is the classic presentation?
A. Seizure
B. Thunderclap Headache
C. Gelastic Seizures
D. Sensorineural Hearing Loss

3. What is the classic history?
A. AVM or Aneurysm
B. Down Syndrome
C. NF -2
D. Pituitary Teratoma

4. What is the "next step" ?
A. PET CT
B. CT with Perfusion
C. Conventional Angiogram
D. No further imaging needed.

Case 8 - History Withheld

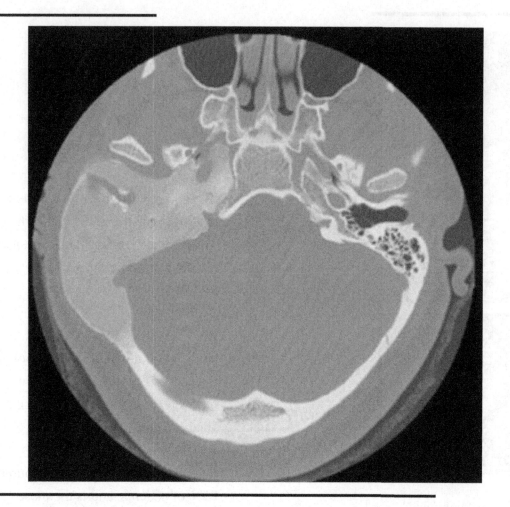

1. What is the diagnosis?
A. Chondrosarcoma
B. Osteosarcoma
C. Fibrous Dysplasia
D. Mets (breast or lung)

2. Fibrous Dysplasia vs Pagets ?
A. Fibrous Dysplasia involves the inner table
B. Pagets involves the inner table
C. Fibrous Dysplasia never crosses sutures
D. Fibrous Dysplasia spares the sinuses

3. What if this patient had "cafe au lait" spots?
A. Mazabraud Syndrome
B. McCune-Albright Syndrome
C. Jaffe–Campanacci Syndrome
D. Rhinophyma

4. What if this patient had intramuscular myxomas ?
A. Mazabraud Syndrome
B. McCune-Albright Syndrome
C. Jaffe–Campanacci Syndrome
D. Rhinophyma

Case 8 - Fibrous Dysplasia

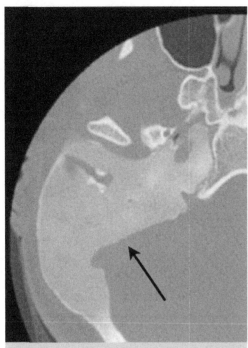

Expanded Ground Glass Matrix

Fibrous Dysplasia

Benign tumor like process, that occurs as a result of screwed up osteoblastic function. The result is the progressive replacement of normal bone with immature woven bone.

Essential Trivia:

- *"Leontiasis Ossea"* or "Lion Face" is the historic term used for craniofacial F.D.

- "Ground Glass" is the classic buzzword.

- Pagets is the primary DDx. The difference is that F.D. spares the inner table, and Pagets classically involves it.

- *McCune Albright Syndrome:* precocious puberty + 'cafe au lait' spots + polyostotic fibrous dysplasia

- *Mazabraud Syndrome:* polyostotic fibrous dysplasia + multiple soft tissue myxomas (usually in large muscle groups). This has an increased risk of malignant transformation

1. What is the diagnosis?
A. Chondrosarcoma
B. Osteosarcoma
C. Fibrous Dysplasia
D. Mets (breast or lung)

2. Fibrous Dysplasia vs Pagets ?
A. Fibrous Dysplasia involves the inner table
B. Pagets involves the inner table
C. Fibrous Dysplasia never crosses sutures
D. Fibrous Dysplasia spares the sinuses

3. What if this patient had "cafe au lait" spots?
A. Mazabraud Syndrome
B. McCune-Albright Syndrome
C. Jaffe–Campanacci Syndrome
D. Rhinophyma

4. What if this patient had intramuscular myxomas ?
A. Mazabraud Syndrome
B. McCune-Albright Syndrome
C. Jaffe–Campanacci Syndrome
D. Rhinophyma

Case 9 - Headache

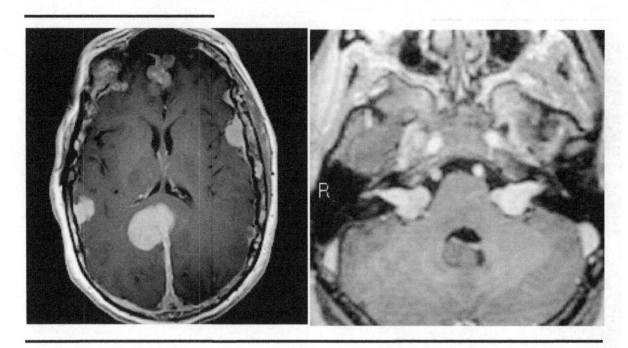

1. What is the diagnosis?
A. Von Hippel Lindau
B. NF-1
C. NF-2
D. Tuberous Sclerosis

2. Unlike NF-1, NF-2 is NOT associated with?
A. Schwannomas
B. Meningiomas
C. Ependymomas
D. Neurofibromas

3. Which of the following is associated with NF-1?
A. Bilateral Vestibular Schwannomas
B. Giant Cell Tumors of the Humerus
C. Lateral Thoracic Meningocele
D. Cardiac Rhabdomyomas

4. NF-1 Patients get Optic Nerve Gliomas, these are typically ____ ?
A. Higher Grade than those that occur sporadically
B. Lower Grade than those that occur sporadically
C. Equal Grade compared to those that occur sporadically
D. NF-1 Patients never get optic nerve gliomas

Aunt Minnie 17

Case 9 - NF-2

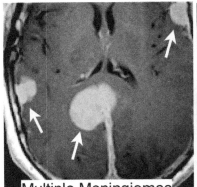
Multiple Meningiomas

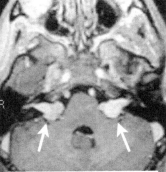
Bilateral Schwannomas

1. What is the diagnosis?
A. Von Hippel Lindau
B. NF-1
C. NF-2
D. Tuberous Sclerosis

2. Unlike NF-1, NF-2 is NOT associated with?
A. Schwannomas
B. Meningiomas
C. Ependymomas
D. Neurofibromas

3. Which of the following is associated with NF-1?
A. Bilateral Vestibular Schwannomas
B. Giant Cell Tumors of the Humerus
C. Lateral Thoracic Meningocele
D. Cardiac Rhabdomyomas

4. NF-1 Patients get Optic Nerve Gliomas, these are typically ____?
A. Higher Grade than those that occur sporadically
B. Lower Grade than those that occur sporadically
C. Equal Grade compared to those that occur sporadically
D. NF-1 Patients never get optic nerve gliomas

NF-2

Rare Autosomal Dominant Neurocutaneous Disorder.

Essential Trivia:

- *"MISME"* - Multiple Inherited Schwannomas Meningiomas and Ependymomas

- Neurofibromas are NOT part of the NF-2 spectrum, making the name a misnomer.

- The finding of a meningioma in a child should raise the question of NF-2.

- Ependymomas associated with NF-2 are typically spinal (not intracranial).

- Schwannomas associated with the NF-2 usually involve the vestibular branch of CN8.

THE OTHER PHAKOMATOSES - ESSENTIAL TRIVIA

NF-1

There are multiple associations that are testable including:
- Sphenoid Wing Dsyplasia
- Plexiform Neurofibromas
- Bad Scoliosis
- Renal Vascular Hypertension
- Lateral Thoracic Meningioceles***
- Pseudoarthrosis of the Fibula

The optic nerve gliomas seen with NF-1 are typically WHO Grade 1 JPAs. The optic nerve gliomas seen in the wild are typically WHO Grade 4 GBMs (which fucking destroy you).

TUBEROUS SCLEROSIS

- *In the Brain* - Think Cortical Tubers, Subependymal Tubers, and Subependymal Giant Cell Astrocytomas (SGCA).

- *Renal AMLs* - Tend to be large, multiple and bilateral

- *Lungs* - Lymphangioleiomyomatosis (LAM). Thin walled cysts + Chylous Pleural Effusions.

- *Cardiac Rhabdomyomas* - Typically involve the ventricular septum, and nearly all occur before 1 year of age.

VON HIPPEL LINDAU

- *In the Brain* - Think Hemangioblastomas (cyst and nodule), and Endolymphatic sac tumors (temporal bone thing, more on this later).

- *In the Abdomen* -
    - Think "Lots of Cysts." Cysts in the kidneys, cysts in the liver, simple cysts in the pancreas, Serous "Cyst"adenomas in Pancreas.
    - Then some tumors too: Pheochromocytomas, and Bilateral Clear Cell RCCs.

Cowden Syndrome

- Bowel Hamartoma + **BREAST CANCER** + <u>Lhermitte Duclos</u> (Dysplastic Cerebellar Gangliocytoma).

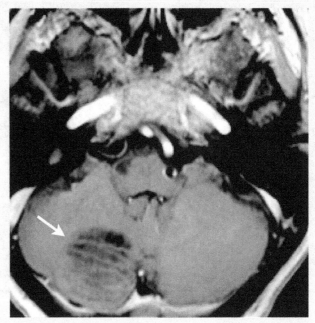

- *Lhermie Dulcos* - Striated non-enhancing cerebellar tumor, that does NOT cross the midline.

Gorlin Syndrome

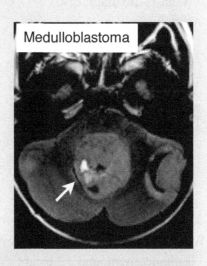

Medulloblastoma

This one has tons of features, but the ones I would remember are:

Multiple Odontogenic Cysts + Massive Falx Cerebri Calcifications + Medulloblastoma

The reason there is any clinical utility to knowing this at all is that when they get radiation for their medulloblastoma they develop LOTS OF BASAL CELLS

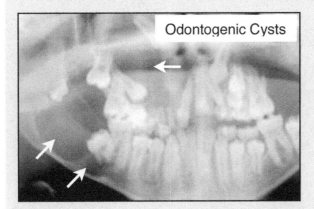

Odontogenic Cysts

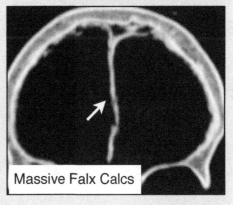

Massive Falx Calcs

Case 10 - Stuffy Nose

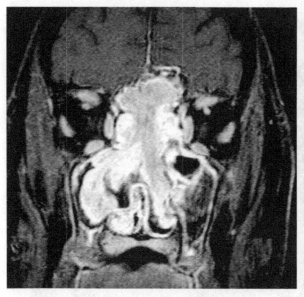
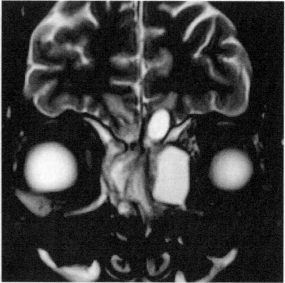

1. What is the diagnosis?
A. SNUC
B. Inverting Papiloma
C. Fungal Sinusitis
D. Esthesioneuroblastoma

2. This cancer originates from ?
A. The submucosal cells of the sinonasal tract
B. The middle turbinate
C. The olfactory cells
D. The osseous maxilla

3. What is the classic finding (s) for the tumor?
A. Enhancement, and T2 bright
B. Bony destruction, and T2 bright
C. Peritumoral cysts, and "Dumbbell" appearance
D. Large Mass without MIBG uptake

4. The typical age for this tumor is?
A. < 20
B. Bimodal: 20s and 50s
C. Always > 60
D. It's random, can occur at any age.

Case 10 - Esthesioneuroblastoma

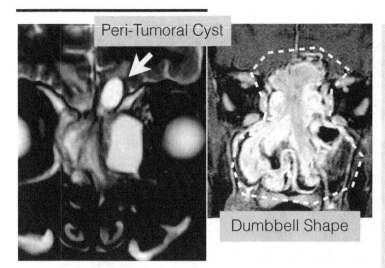

1. What is the diagnosis?
A. SNUC
B. Inverting Papiloma
C. Fungal Sinusitis
D. Esthesioneuroblastoma

2. This cancer originates from ?
A. The submucosal cells of the sinonasal tract
B. The middle turbinate
C. The olfactory cells
D. The osseous maxilla

3. What is the classic finding (s) for the tumor?
A. Enhancement, and T2 bright
B. Bony destruction, and T2 bright
C. Peritumoral cysts, and "Dumbbell" appearance
D. Large Mass without MIBG uptake

4. The typical age for this tumor is?
A. < 20
B. Bimodal: 20s and 50s
C. Always > 60
D. It's random, can occur at any age.

Esthesioneuroblastoma

Essentially a neuroblastoma of the olfactory cells.

Essential Trivia:

- Has a bimodal distribution- occurs 20s and 50s

- Starts growing at the cribriform plate then (usually) grows down and up, waisting in the middle. This creates a dumbbell appearance.

- The characteristic finding is peritumoral cysts at the top. If they want a single diagnosis they have to show you this (otherwise it's a squamous cell - which is more common).

- They enhance avidly (duh, they are tumors).

- They take up MIBG, because they are basically a neuroblastoma.

Case 11 - Stuffy Nose

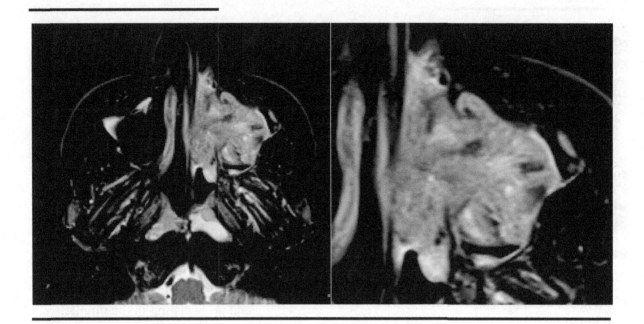

1. What is the diagnosis?
A. SNUC
B. Inverting Papilloma
C. Fungal Sinusitis
D. Esthesioneuroblastoma

2. What is the classic finding (s) for the tumor?
A. The superior turbinate
B. The middle turbinate
C. The cribriform plate
D. The nasal septum

3. What is classic "buzzword" finding?
A. Peritumoral Cysts
B. Light bulb bright T1
C. Panda Sign
D. Cerebriform pattern

4. Hidden within 10-15% of inverting papillomas is?
A. A piece of chewing gum
B. That crayon you stuck up there in 1st Grade
C. A squamous cell cancer
D. A fungal ball

Case 11 - Inverting Papilloma

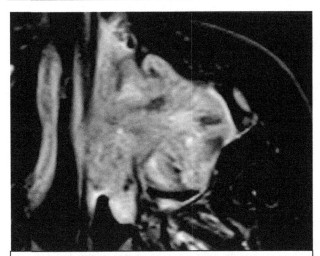

"Cerebriform pattern" of alternating high and low signal

1. What is the diagnosis?
A. SNUC
B. Inverting Papilloma
C. Fungal Sinusitis
D. Esthesioneuroblastoma

2. What is the classic finding (s) for the tumor?
A. The superior turbinate
B. The middle turbinate
C. The cribriform plate
D. The nasal septum

3. What is classic "buzzword" finding?
A. Peritumoral Cysts
B. Light bulb bright T1
C. Panda Sign
D. Cerebriform pattern

4. Hidden within 10-15% of inverting papillomas is?
A. A piece of chewing gum
B. That crayon you stuck up there in 1st Grade
C. A squamous cell cancer
D. A fungal ball

Inverting Papilloma

This is a benign sinonasal tumor, with distinctive imaging features (making it testable).

Essential Trivia:

- The most testable fact (probably) is the 10-15% conversion to squamous cell CA.

- The typical location is the lateral wall of the nasal cavity, *associated with the middle turbinate.*

- On MRI - They have the classic **"cerebriform pattern"** of *alternating high and low signal (supposedly looks like cortical gyrations).* This is seen on both T2 and T1+C. The sign is pretty good, found in at least 50% of these, and fairly unique to the tumor.

- On CT - These look like lobulated masses *containing fragments of destroyed bone.*

- When I say *"frequent local recurrence despite adequate resection"*, you say **Schneiderian CA**. This is a rare form of malignancy that has histology indistinguishable from the usual inverting papilloma.

The Sinus - Essential Trivia

Fungal Sinusitis

There are 4 types of fungal sinusitis: Allergic, non-invasive, acute invasive, and chronic invasive. Allergic and Invasive are the most likely tested.

Allergic - The most common. This occurs as an IgE response to fungal antigens. Tends to affect all the sinuses at the same time. Mucin (which contains concentrated protein, fungal elements, and heavy metals) results in a **hyper dense look on CT and a DARK look on both T1 and T2**. This *mimics a pneumatized sinus*. Trying to get you to call a fungus laden sinus as pneumatized sinus on MRI is the oldest trick in the book.

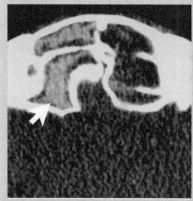 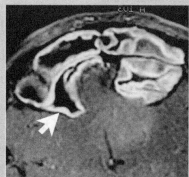 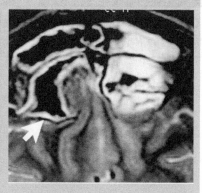

Dark on Both T1 and T2

Angio-Invasive - Think about Mucor eating the diabetic dudes face off.

Essential trivia

- CT best for bony change. MRI best for intracrainal or orbital spread.

-The *"black turbinate sign"* - an ischemic (non enhancing) middle turbinate mucosa is an early indicator of invasive fungal.

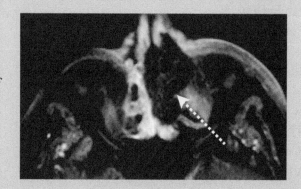

Juvenile Nasopharyngeal Angiofibroma

Benign but locally aggressive vascular tumor.

ALWAYS seen in MALES around age of 15-20.

Bloody nose is the classic history, but can also come in with chronic ear infections from eustachian tube blockage.

Testable Point = Arise in the Sphenopalatine Foramen

Testable Point = Classically extend into the Pterygopalatine Fossa

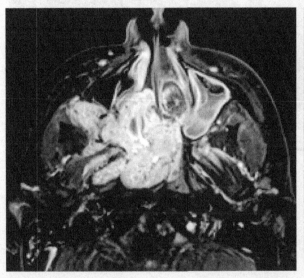
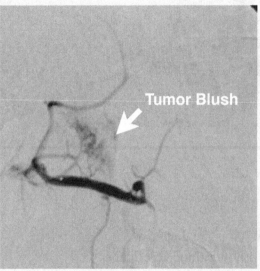

Sinus Tumor Essential Trivia Blitz

Inverting Papilloma = 10-15% Harbor a Squamous Cell CA

Inverting Papilloma = Cerebriform Pattern

Esthesioneuroblastoma = Dumbbell Shaped with Peritumoral Cysts

Esthesioneuroblastoma = MIBG Avid

Squamous Cell CA = Most Common Sinonasal Malignancy

SNUC = Monster Squamous Cell CA

CASE 12 - HISTORY WITHHELD

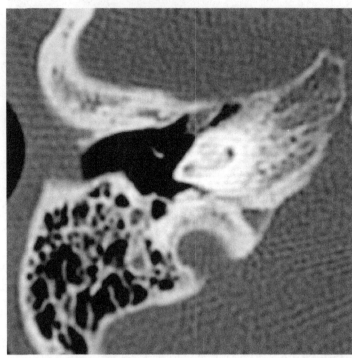
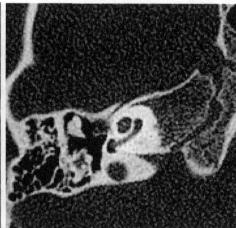
Normal for Comparison

1. What is the diagnosis?
A. Labyrinthine Ossificans
B. Otosclerosis
C. Gusher Syndrome
D. Wide Vestibular Aqueduct

2. What is the classic history?
A. Childhood meningitis
B. History of MS
C. Progressive conductive hearing loss
D. Aneurysm repair 3 months ago

3. This condition has what surgical implication?
A. Requires a transmastoid approach to repair
B. Requires both sides be performed on the same day
C. Increases the risk of ACA territory intact
D. May complicate or preclude cochlear implantation

CASE 12 - LABYRINTHINE OSSIFICANS

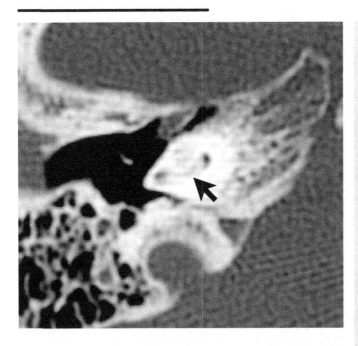

1. What is the diagnosis?
A. Labyrinthine Ossificans
B. Otosclerosis
C. Gusher Syndrome
D. Wide Vestibular Aqueduct

2. What is the classic history?
A. Childhood meningitis
B. History of MS
C. Progressive conductive hearing loss
D. Aneurysm repair 3 months ago

3. This condition has what surgical implication?
A. Requires a transmastoid approach to repair
B. Requires both sides be performed on the same day
C. Increases the risk of ACA territory intact
D. May complicate or preclude cochlear implantation

Labyrinthine Ossificans

Fibroblasts from prior infection (or inflammation) lead to a pathologic ossification of the normally fluid filled spaces of the bony labyrinth.

Essential Trivia:

- Bacterial meningitis is the most common acquired cause

- Usually associated with severe sensorineural hearing loss

- The other major symptom with this is vertigo (this is one of the "dead ear" vertigo causes).

- The earliest changes are typically seen in the basal turn of the cochlea and scala tympani

- Osseous destruction at the round window niche makes placement of the cochlear implant difficult *(the further into the cochlear turns you can put the electrode the better they do).*

Case 13 - Headache

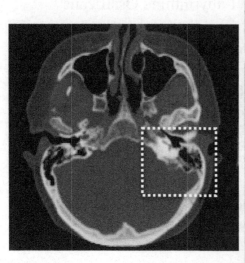
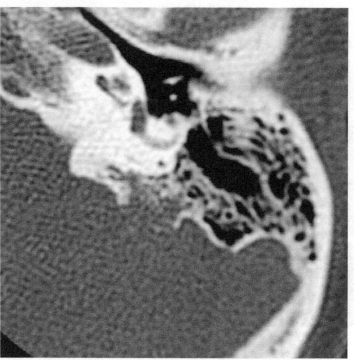

1. What is the diagnosis?
A. Dehiscent Jugular Bulb
B. Paraganglioma (jugulare)
C. Wide Vestibular Aquaduct
D. Endolymphatic Sac Tumor

2. This diagnosis is found in what syndrome?
A. Tuberous Sclerosis
B. NF-1
C. NF-2
D. Von Hippel Lindau

3. What is classic for the diagnosis?
A. The location
B. Enhancement patterns
C. Bony Destruction
D. It's totally non-specific

CASE 13 - ENDOLYMPHATIC SAC TUMOR

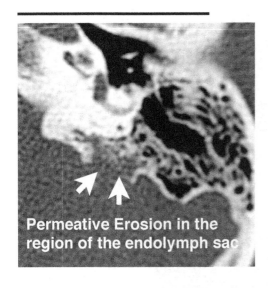

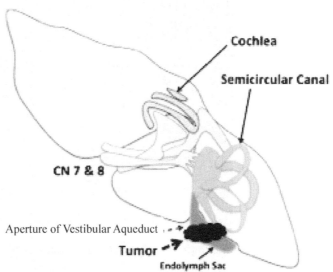

1. What is the diagnosis?
A. Dehiscent Jugular Bulb
B. Paraganglioma (jugulare)
C. Wide Vestibular Aqueduct
D. Endolymphatic Sac Tumor

2. This diagnosis is found in what syndrome?
A. Tuberous Sclerosis
B. NF-1
C. NF-2
D. Von Hippel Lindau

3. What is classic for the diagnosis?
A. The location
B. Enhancement patterns
C. Bony Destruction
D. It's totally non-specific

Endolymphatic Sac Tumor

Rare locally invasive tumor of the endolymph sac. It doesn't metastasize, but does locally invade and cause hearing loss.

Essential Trivia:

- The location is very typical (the region of the endolymph sac).

- The boney erosion pattern is sometimes called "moth-eaten"

- Highly associated with VHL (about 15% of VHLers have them)

Case 14 - History Withheld

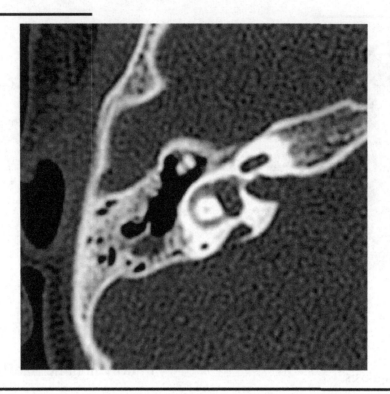

1. What is the diagnosis ?
   A. Dehiscent Jugular Bulb
   B. Paraganglioma (jugulare)
   C. Wide Vestibular Aqueduct
   D. Endolymphatic Sac Tumor

2. What is the classic history ?
   A. Childhood meningitis
   B. History of MS
   C. Conductive hearing loss
   D. Sensorineural hearing loss

3. How often is this finding bilateral ?
   A. Never
   B. Always
   C. Usually
   D. Rarely

4. This is associated with absence of the "?" 90% of the time
   A. Bony Modiolus
   B. Scutum
   C. Lenticular Process
   D. Tympanic Membrane

Case 14 - Large Vestibular Aqueduct Syndrome

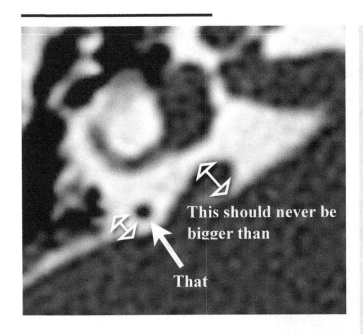

1. What is the diagnosis ?
A. Dehiscent Jugular Bulb
B. Paraganglioma (jugulare)
C. Wide Vestibular Aqueduct
D. Endolymphatic Sac Tumor

2. What is the classic history ?
A. Childhood meningitis
B. History of MS
C. Conductive hearing loss
D. Sensorineural hearing loss

3. How often is this finding bilateral ?
A. Never
B. Always
C. Usually
D. Rarely

4. This is associated with absence of the "?" 90% of the time
A. Bony Modiolus
B. Scutum
C. Lenticular Process
D. Tympanic Membrane

Large Vestibular Aqueduct Syndrome (LVAS)

Possibly resulting from reflux of fluid from the endolymph sac into the inner ear, this is a very common cause of sensorineural hearing loss.

Essential Trivia:

- You aren't born deaf. It's progressive.

- As a helpful rule, if the Vestibular Aqueduct is larger than the posterior semicircular canal (or facial nerve canal) then they have LVAS

- It is usually bilateral (50-90%)

- LVAS is often associated with other malformations - the most common of which is absence of the bony modiolus (seen in 90%).

Extra Credit: **Mondini Abnormality**
- Abnormal Cochlea (missing a turn)
- Enlarged Vestibule, but normal SCC
- Enlarged Vestibular Aquaduct

Case 15 - History Withheld

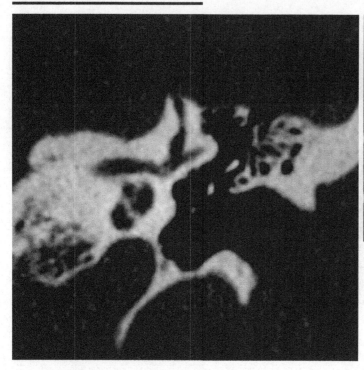
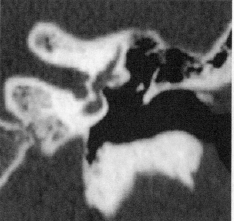

Normal for Comparison

1. What is the diagnosis?
A. Dehiscent Jugular Bulb
B. Paraganglioma (jugulare)
C. Wide Vestibular Aqueduct
D. Superior semicircular canal dehiscence

2. What is the classic symptom for this syndrome?
A. Noise induced vertigo
B. Motion induced nausea
C. Noise induced nausea
D. Motion induced vertigo

3. Is this finding always associated with symptoms?
A. Yes
B. No

Case 15 - Superior semicircular canal dehiscence syndrome

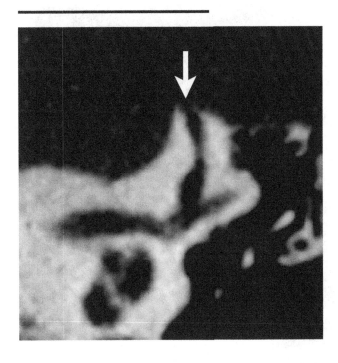

1. What is the diagnosis?
A. Dehiscent Jugular Bulb
B. Paraganglioma (jugulare)
C. Wide Vestibular Aqueduct
D. **Superior semicircular canal dehiscence**

2. What is the classic symptom for this syndrome?
A. **Noise induced vertigo**
B. Motion induced nausea
C. Noise induced nausea
D. Motion induced vertigo

3. Is this finding always associated with symptoms?
A. Yes
B. **No**

Superior Semicircular Canal Dehiscence Syndrome

Clinical syndrome associated with absence of the bony covering of the superior semicircular canal

Essential Trivia:

- The bony covering of the SSC is absent in about 10% of the general population.

- The classic symptom is a noise induced vertigo "Tullio Phenomenon." This was originally described in pigeons after a mad scientist drilled holes in their heads.

- Tullio also created a "Pigeon-Rat" by sewing the back of a pigeon to the back of a rat.

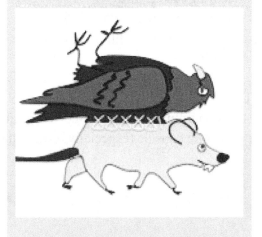

Aunt Minnie 34

Case 16 - History Withheld

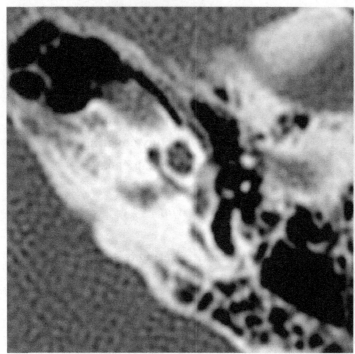
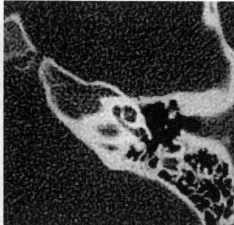

Normal for Comparison

1. What is the diagnosis?
A. Otosclerosis (Otospongiosis)
B. Dehiscent Jugular Bulb
C. Paraganglioma (jugulare)
D. Wide Vestibular Aqueduct

2. What is the typical history?
A. Hearing loss at birth
B. Hearing loss in childhood (5-10)
C. Hearing loss in adulthood (40s)
D. Vertigo

3. The most common location of the lesion is?
A. The margin of the oval window (fissula ante fenestram)
B. The otic capsule (especially around the cochlea)

Case 16 - Otosclerosis (Otospongiosis)

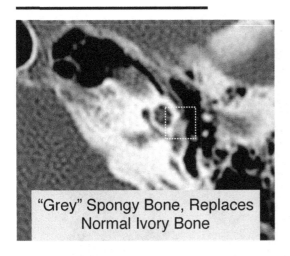

"Grey" Spongy Bone, Replaces Normal Ivory Bone

1. What is the diagnosis?
A. Otoscleroris (Otospongiosis)
B. Dehiscent Jugular Bulb
C. Paraganglioma (jugulare)
D. Wide Vestibular Aqueduct

2. What is the typical history?
A. Hearing loss at birth
B. Hearing loss in childhood (5-10)
C. Hearing loss in adulthood (40s)
D. Vertigo

3. The most common location of the lesion is?
A. The margin of the oval window (fissula ante fenestram)
B. The otic capsule (especially around the cochlea)

Otospongiosis (Fenestral)

Idiopathic disorder of the bony labyrinth in which the dense, ivory like endochondral bone is replaced with a spongy irregular haversian bone (deafness follows).

Essential Trivia:

- It's usually seen in white women in their 40s.

- If you catch it early you can prevent their deafness. If you miss it, I'm sure the jury will understand. "Let him off judge… he's doing his best."

- It might get worse with pregnancy

- There are two types:
  - *Fenestral* (most common) - targets the anterior margin of the oval window (fissula ante fenestram), more conductive hearing loss

  - *Retrofenestral* (less common) - targets the otic capsule around the cochlea, causes a more sensorineural hearing loss.

Case 17 - Vision Problems (Age 3)

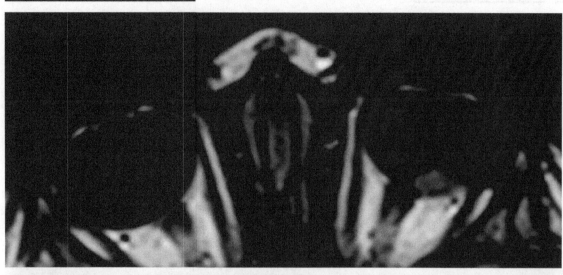

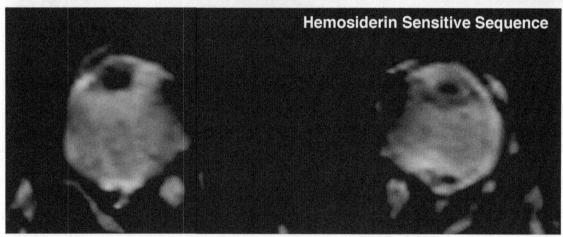

Hemosiderin Sensitive Sequence

1. What is the diagnosis?
   A. Phthisis Bulbi
   B. Retinoblastoma
   C. Orbital Rhabdomyosarcoma
   D. PHPV

2. Children are also at increased risk of?
   A. Osteosarcoma
   B. Fibrous Dysplasia
   C. Ewing Sarcoma
   D. Aneurysmal Bone Cysts

3. What is this "trilateral retinoblastoma" ?
   A. Retinoblastoma in both eyes + cerebellum
   B. Retinoblastoma in both eyes + CSF mets
   C. Retinoblastoma in both eyes + optic chiasm
   D. Retinoblastoma in both eyes + pinealoblastoma

Case 17 - Retinoblastoma

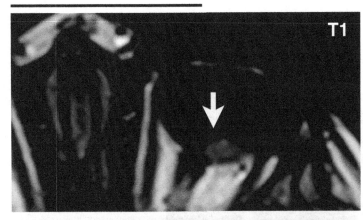

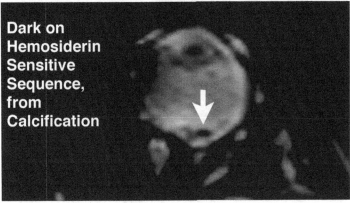

Dark on Hemosiderin Sensitive Sequence, from Calcification

1. What is the diagnosis?
A. Phthisis Bulbi
B. Retinoblastoma
C. Orbital Rhabdomyosarcoma
D. PHPV

2. Children are also at increased risk of?
A. Osteosarcoma
B. Fibrous Dysplasia
C. Ewing Sarcoma
D. Aneurysmal Bone Cysts

3. What is this "trilateral retinoblastoma" ?
A. Retinoblastoma in both eyes + cerebellum
B. Retinoblastoma in both eyes + CSF mets
C. Retinoblastoma in both eyes + optic chiasm
D. Retinoblastoma in both eyes + pinealoblastoma

Retinoblastoma

The most common intraocular neoplasm of childhood.

Essential Trivia:

- These usually occur around 18 months of age, and nearly always occur before age 5.

- There is an association with a bad RB suppressor gene, which also affects osteosarcoma patients.

- On CT think about a **calcified intraoccular mass, in a kid**, with a normal sized globe.

- For the purpose of multiple choice tests any mass in the globe of a kid is probably RB, especially if shown on gradient (for the blooming).

- It's bilateral about 30% of the time, and can also be "trilateral" with development of a pinealoblastoma about 3 years after the ocular lesions form.

- DDx:
  - **Coats** - Not usually calcified.
  - **Persistent Hyperplastic Primary Vitreous (PHPV)** = small globe
  - **Retinopathy of prematurity** = small globe

Case 18 - Back Pain

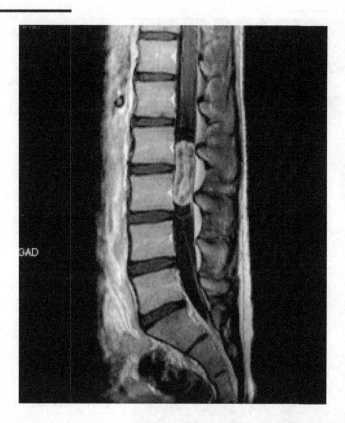

1. What is the diagnosis?
A. Neurofibroma
B. Schwannoma
C. Myxopapillary Ependymoma
D. Hemangioblastoma

2. Is this location typical for this tumor?
A. Yup
B. Nope

3. Compared to the normal ependymomas, the myxopapilaries do what?
A. Are found in the cervical cord more
B. Are found in the thoracic cord more
C. Tend to bleed more
D. Present under the age of 20

Case 18 - Myxopapillary ependymoma

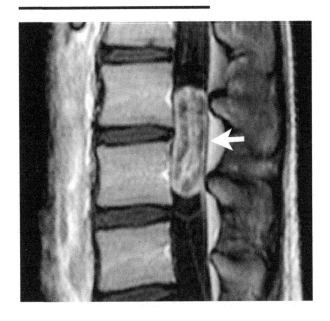

1. What is the diagnosis?
A. Neurofibroma
B. Schwannoma
C. Myxopapillary Ependymoma
D. Hemangioblastoma

2. Is this location typical for this tumor?
A. Yup
B. Nope

3. Compared to the normal ependymomas, the myxopapilaries do what?
A. Are found in the cervical cord more
B. Are found in the thoracic cord more
C. Tend to bleed more
D. Present under the age of 20

Myxopapillary Ependymoma

The most common primary cord tumor of the lower spinal cord

Essential Trivia:

- This form is almost exclusively seen in the conus and film (95%)

- More than 50% of all tumors of the film terminal and conus medullaries are myxopapillary ependymomas.

- They have a tendency to bleed, even more so than the intramedullary type

- They tend to occur in the 40s-50s.

- They can usually be excised completely, but if they extend into the subarachnoid space and/or surround the roots of the cauda equina then they are a huge pain in the ass to get rid of.

Cord Tumors - Essential Trivia

Tumors are grouped based on location.

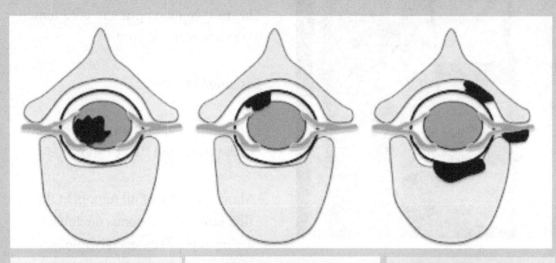

Intramedullary DDx:
- Astrocytoma
- Ependymoma
- Hemangioblastoma

Extramedullary - Intradural DDx:
- Schwannoma
- Meningioma
- Neurofibroma

Extradural DDx:
- Disc Disease
- Bone Tumors
- Mets
- Lymphoma
- Epidermoid Cysts

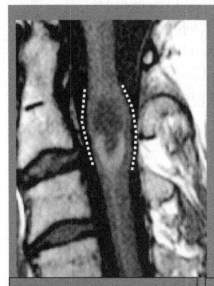

Intramedullary
- Expanded Cord
- "Snake ate the Mouse"
- This was an Ependymoma

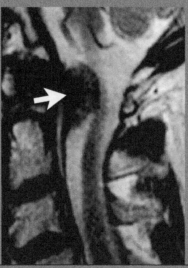

Extrameduallary Intradural
- "Marble under the Rug" or "Mouse in the house, with the Snake"
- This was a meningioma

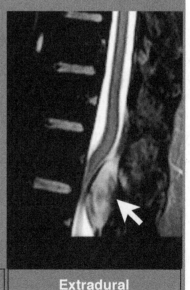

Extradural
- Note the Displaced CSF
- This was an epidermoid cyst

Intramedullary Trivia

Astrocytoma:

- Most common intramedullary tumor in child (2nd most common in adults).

- Heterogenous Enhancement

- Eccentric Cord (they arise from astrocytic cells)

- They bleed less

Ependymoma

- More common in adults (2nd most common in kids)

- Homogenous enhancement

- Central Cord (they arise from ependymal cells)

- Hemosiderin Cap (dark)

- They bleed more.

- They syrinx more

Hemangioblastoma

- 30% have Von Hippel Lindau

- Typical in thoracic cord

- Lot of edema

- Adjacent serpiginous areas of signal void (draining veins) are typical

Extramedullary- Intra Dural Trivia

Schwannoma

- Don't envelop the dorsal sensory nerve root. Instead grow asymmetrically next to the nerve.

- Generally Solitary

- NOT associated with NF (in the spine).

- High peripheral T2, with low signal in center "target"

Neurofibroma

- Do envelop the dorsal sensory root

- Generally multiple

- Associated with NF even when single

Meningioma

- Adhere to (but don't originate from) the dura.

- Posterior lateral in thoracic spine. Anterior to cervical spine.

- Enhance homogeneous (more than schwannoma), and slight T2 bright (less than schwannoma).

- F > M

Case 19 - Butt Dimple

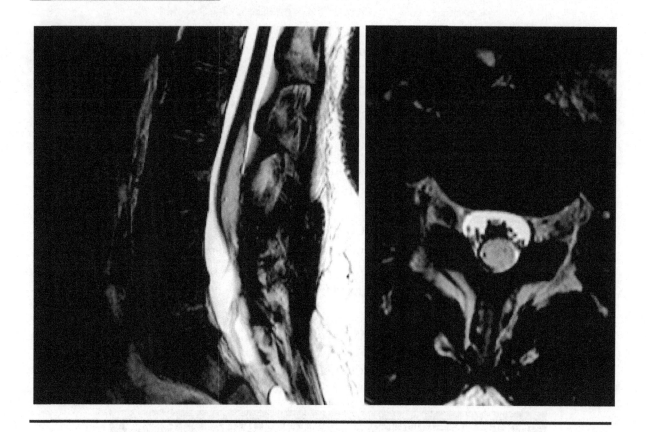

1. What is the diagnosis?
A. Lipoma
B. Tethered Cord with Lipoma
C. Terminal Ventricle
D. Tabes Dorsalis

2. The cord is considered low lying when the tip of the conus is below?
A. T12
B. L1
C. L2
D. L3

3. Fat associated with the film terminal is?
A. Always bad and associated with horrible things
B. Never bad and often a sign of good luck (buy a lottery ticket!)
C. Usually an incidental finding (seen about 5% of time), but sometimes associated with cord tethering.

Case 19 - Tethered Cord with Lipoma

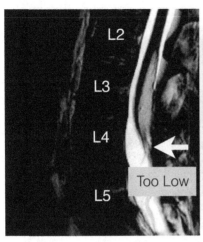
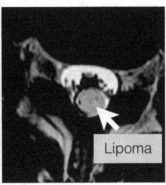

1. What is the diagnosis?
A. Lipoma
B. Tethered Cord with Lipoma
C. Terminal Ventricle
D. Tabes Dorsalis

2. The cord is considered low lying when the tip of the conus is below (in an adult) ?
A. T12
B. L1
C. L2
D. L3

3. Fat associated with the film terminal is?
A. Always bad and associated with horrible things
B. Never bad and often a sign of good luck (buy a lottery ticket!)
C. Usually an incidental finding (seen about 5% of time), but sometimes associated with cord tethering.

Tethered Cord with Lipoma

Abnormal spinal cord attachment that can lead to neurologic symptoms from stretching of the cord.

Essential Trivia:

- The spinal column grows faster than the cord, so if the cord is tethered by an abnormal attachment it can / will get stretched.

- A lipoma of the filum terminale is common (usually incidental) but is associated with a tethered cord.

- Tethered cord is closely linked to spina bifida.

- Normally the conus should NOT be lower than L2-L3 (L1-L2 in adults). Any cord below L3 is suspect.

- With regard to screening, just remember that **low sacral dimples** (< 2.5cm from the anus) **don't need to be screened**. Pretty much everything else does.

Case 20 - New Mom with Wrist Pain

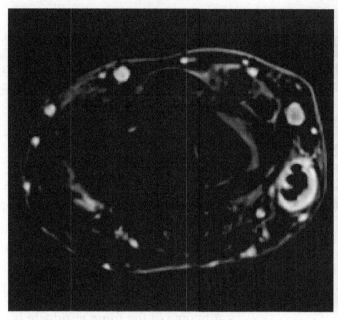
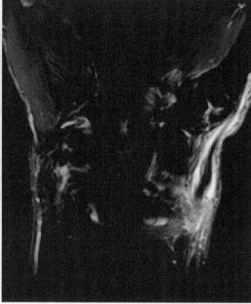

1. What is the diagnosis?
A. De Quervain's Tenosynovitis
B. Mycobacterial Infection
C. Intersection Syndrome
D. Drummer's Wrist

2. What tendon(s) are involved?
A. Extensor Carpi Radialis (Brevis & Longus)
B. Extensor Digiti Minimi
C. Extensor Carpi Ulnaris
D. Extensor Pollicis Brevis and Abductor Pollicis Longus

3. What extensor compartment is involved?
A. 1
B. 2
C. 3
D. 7

Case 20 - De Quervain's Tenosynovitis

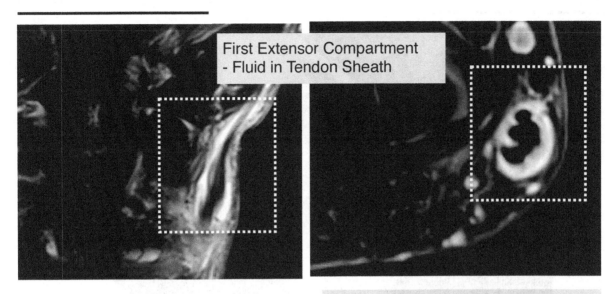

1. What is the diagnosis?
A. De Quervain's Tenosynovitis
B. Mycobacterial Infection
C. Intersection Syndrome
D. Drummer's Wrist

2. What tendon(s) are involved?
A. Extensor Carpi Radialis (Brevis & Longus)
B. Extensor Digiti Minimi
C. Extensor Carpi Ulnaris
D. Extensor Pollicis Brevis and Abductor Pollicis Longus

3. What extensor compartment is involved?
A. 1
B. 2
C. 3
D. 7

De Quervain's Tenosynovitis

An overuse tendinopathy classically seen in mothers and childcare worker's afflicted with the terrible task of lifting infants

Essential Trivia:

- The EPB and APL are involved (first compartment)

- The ortho test is the "positive Finkelstein test" - pain with passive ulnar deviation.

- Tenosynovitis is pretty nonspecific (fluid in the tendon sheath, and peritendinous edema / enhancement). The location is classic.

- First Compartment = De Quervains
- 2nd Compartment = Intersection Syndrome ** *overuse tendinopathy seen in rowers*

Case 21 - Pain

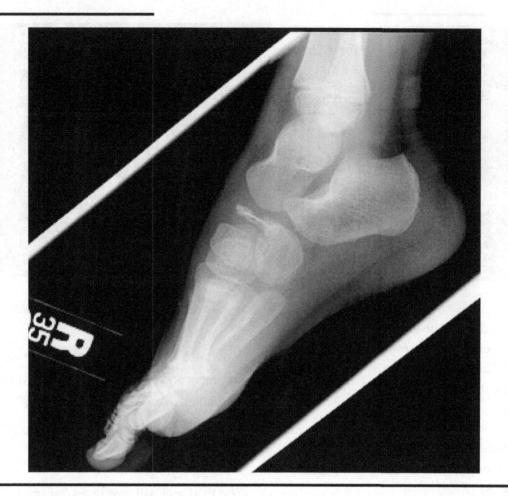

1. What is the diagnosis?
A. Sever's Disease
B. Kohler Disease
C. Panner's Disease
D. Diaz Disease

2. What is the typical age for this to occur?
A. Adults (30s-40s)
B. Elderly (60s-80s)
C. Teenagers
D. Young School Age (4-8)

3. What is the mechanism here?
A. It's post traumatic (jumping)
B. It's AVN - maybe from a vascular insult
C. It's secondary to infection

Case 21 - Kohlers

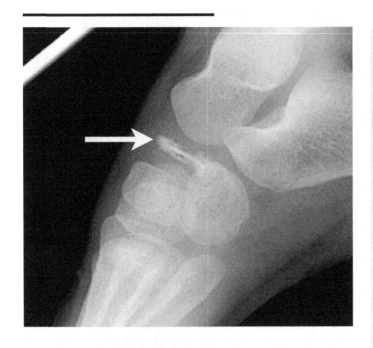

1. What is the diagnosis?
A. Sever's Disease
B. Kohler Disease
C. Panner's Disease
D. Diaz Disease

2. What is the typical age for this to occur?
A. Adults (30s-40s)
B. Elderly (60s-80s)
C. Teenagers
D. Young School Age (4-8)

3. What is the mechanism here?
A. It's post traumatic (jumping)
B. It's AVN - maybe from a vascular insult
C. It's secondary to infection

Kohlers

This is an AVN of the navicular bone, causing a wafer-like appearance. This belongs to a group of things called "osteochondroses."

Essential Trivia:
- You see this in kids (4-8 years old).

- Believe it or not with treatment (rest and / or cast), this gets better and goes back to normal.

- Osteochondroses - These are a group of conditions (usually seen in childhood) that are characterized by involvement of the epiphysis, or apophysis with findings of collapse, sclerosis, and fragmentation – suggesting osteonecrosis.

- Other Notable Osteochondroses:
- **Freiberg** - Second Metatarsal Head, seen in Adolescent Girls
- **Severs** - Calcaneal Apophysis - maybe a normal "growing pain"
- **Panners** - Capitellum of school age throwers
- **Perthes** - Femoral Head - white kids school age (4-8)
- **Kienbock** - Carpal Lunate - associated with ulnar negative variance

Case 22 - Pain

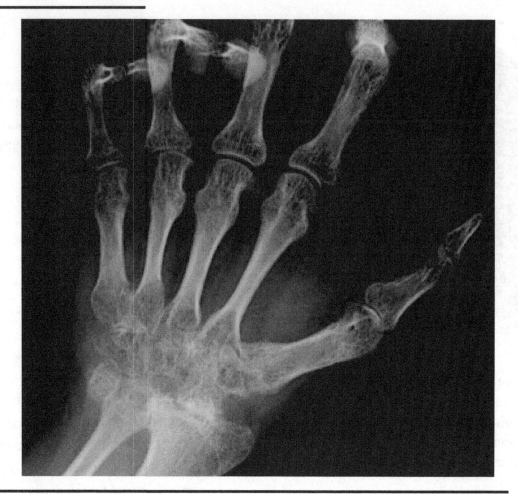

1. What is the diagnosis?
A. Klippel-Feil Syndrome
B. Juvenile Rheumatoid Arthritis
C. Panner's Disease
D. Ankylosing Spondylitis

2. What makes this different than the adult variety?
A. It favors the carpals
B. It has symmetric joint space narrowing
C. It causes ankylosis
D. RF factor is usually negative

3. When it occurs in teenagers, it favors?
A. Boys
B. Girls
C. It has no gender bias

Case 22 - Juvenile rheumatoid arthritis (JRA)

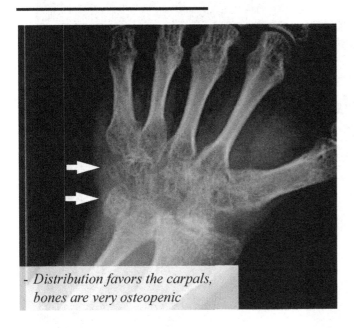

- Distribution favors the carpals, bones are very osteopenic

1. What is the diagnosis?
A. Klippel-Feil Syndrome
B. Juvenile Rheumatoid Arthritis
C. Panner's Disease
D. Ankylosing Spondylitis

2. What makes this different than the adult variety?
A. It favors the carpals
B. It has symmetric joint space narrowing
C. It causes ankylosis
D. RF factor is usually negative

3. When it occurs in teenagers, it favors?
A. Boys
B. Girls
C. It has no gender bias

JRA

Inflammatory Arthritis (> 6 weeks) PLUS Growing Skeleton (< 16 years old)

Essential Trivia:
- It's usually seronegative -*RF lab test is negative* (like 85%)

- It usually affects females, except when it occurs acutely under the age of 5 "*Stills Disease*" - then it's M=F

- The knee is the most common involved (ankle is #2, wrist is #3)

- Characteristic findings are
  - osteopenia,
  - uniform joint space narrowing,
  - bony ankylosis

Case 23 - Pain

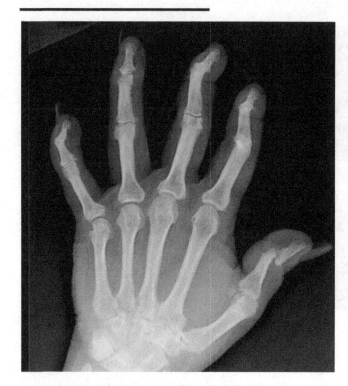
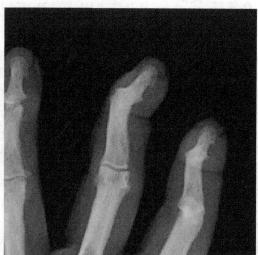
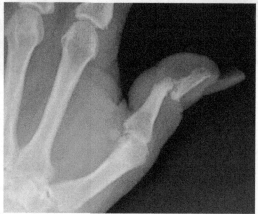

1. What is the diagnosis?
A. Psoriatic Arthritis
B. Juvenile Rheumatoid Arthritis
C. Osteoarthritis
D. Ankylosing Spondylitis

2. The distribution in the hands typically ?
A. Favors the carpals
B. Favors the MCP Joint
C. Favors the IP Joints
D. Mainly just targets the DRUJ

3. The SI joint involvement is usually?
A. Unilateral
B. Bilateral - Symmetric
C. Bilateral - Asymmetric

Case 23 - Psoriatic Arthritis

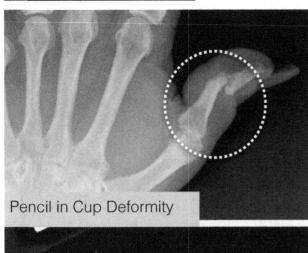

Pencil in Cup Deformity

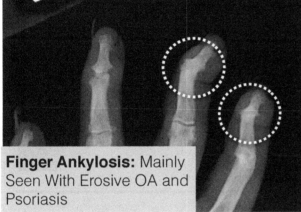

Finger Ankylosis: Mainly Seen With Erosive OA and Psoriasis

1. What is the diagnosis?
A. Psoriatic Arthritis
B. Juvenile Rheumatoid Arthritis
C. Osteoarthritis
D. Ankylosing Spondylitis

2. The distribution in the hands typically?
A. Favors the carpals
B. Favors the MCP Joint
C. Favors the IP Joints
D. Mainly just targets the DRUJ

3. The SI joint involvement is usually?
A. Unilateral
B. Bilateral - Symmetric
C. Bilateral - Asymmetric

Psoriatic Arthritis

Inflammatory Arthritis associated with the gross "yucky" skin of psoriasis.

Essential Trivia:

- This is one of the "seronegative spondyloarthritides." The other 3 are Inflammatory Bowel related (Enteropathic), Reiters (Reactive), and Ankylosing Spondylitis.

- About 30% of psoriasis patients get it - with the skin finding showing up about 10 years earlier.

- Finger nail involvement is very common (85%)

- In general: Erosive change + adjacent bone proliferation with a distal involvement (IP joints more than MCP).

- SI joint involvement is asymmetrical

- There are lots of characteristic buzzwords for this one:

  - "Pencil in Cup" Deformity
  - "Fuzzy Appearance" near affected joint - from bone proliferation
  - "Sausage Digit" - soft tissue swelling
  - "Ivory Phalanx" - Sclerotic looking big toe

Case 24 - Pain

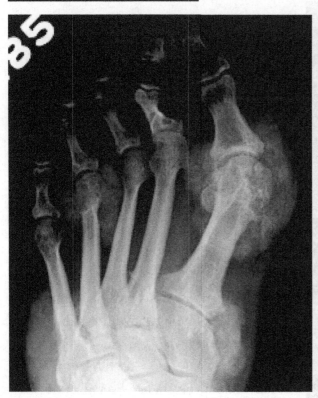
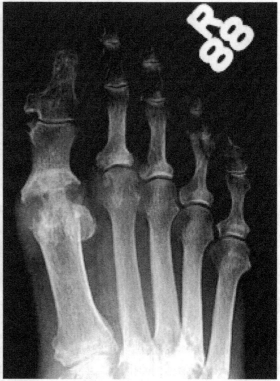

1. What is the diagnosis?
A. Psoriatic Arthritis
B. Gout
C. Osteoarthritis
D. Ankylosing Spondylitis

2. This disease "NEVER" ?
A. Involves the knee
B. Causes erosions
C. Causes joint space narrowing
D. Has sclerotic margins

3. This modern technique can be used to accurately diagnose Gout
A. MRI Spectroscopy
B. F-18 PET-CT
C. Dual Energy CT

Case 24 - The Gout

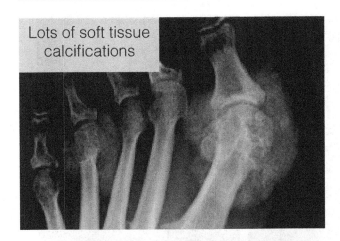

Lots of soft tissue calcifications

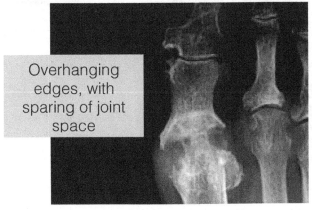

Overhanging edges, with sparing of joint space

1. What is the diagnosis?
A. Psoriatic Arthritis
B. Gout
C. Osteoarthritis
D. Ankylosing Spondylitis

2. This disease "NEVER" ?
A. Involves the knee
B. Causes erosions
C. Causes joint space narrowing
D. Has sclerotic margins

3. This modern technique can be used to accurately diagnose Gout
A. MRI Spectroscopy
B. F-18 PET-CT
C. Dual Energy CT

The Gout

Crystal arthropathy (monosodium urate). Causes well defined erosions with sclerotic margins and the classic "overhanging edges."

Essential Trivia:

- It does not happen (usually) in men younger than 30, and in women prior to menopause.

- Often targets the big toe first "Podagra"

- *Radiologic Buzzwords / Findings:'*

- Well marginated eccentric erosions, with "overhanging edges"
- Erosions appear "punched out" - with sclerotic margins
- "NEVER" causes joint space narrowing — until it does - with end stage forms of the disease

- Using Dual energy CT can be done by using 80 and 140 kVp energies plus a material decomposition algorithm to identify uric acid.

Case 25 - Pain

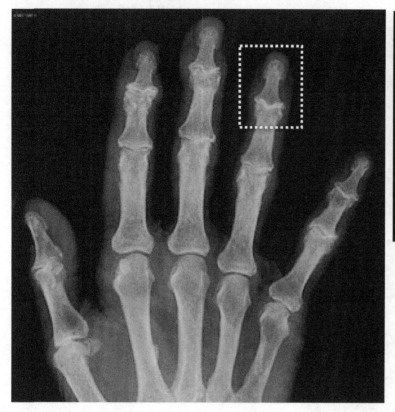
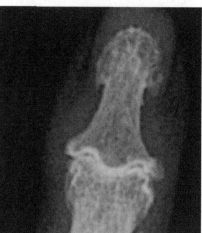

1. What is the diagnosis?
A. Psoriatic Arthritis
B. Gout
C. Osteoarthritis
D. Erosive Osteoarthritis

2. The typical demographic for this group is
A. Young Men
E. Young Women
F. Old Men
G. Old (Postmenopausal) Women

3. The classic finding for this diagnosis is?
A. Marginal Erosions
B. Central Subchondral Erosions
C. Fusiform Soft Tissue Swelling
D. Osteopenia

Case 25 - Erosive Osteoarthritis

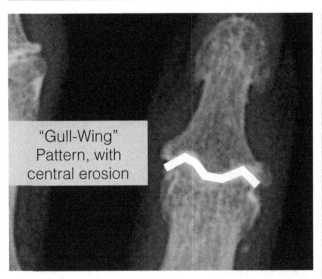

"Gull-Wing" Pattern, with central erosion

1. What is the diagnosis?
A. Psoriatic Arthritis
B. Gout
C. Osteoarthritis
D. Erosive Osteoarthritis

2. The typical demographic for this group is
A. Young Men
E. Young Women
F. Old Men
G. Old (Postmenopausal) Women

3. The classic finding for this diagnosis is?
A. Marginal Erosions
B. Central Subchondral Erosions
C. Fusiform Soft Tissue Swelling
D. Osteopenia

Erosive Osteoarthritis

This is a subtype of osteoarthritis that includes an erosive / inflammatory component.

Essential Trivia:

- For the purpose of multiple choice this only occurs in postmenopausal females

- The hand is the most commonly involved body part (hip and knee are rarely involved).

- Onset is typically more rapid than the conventional OA

- *Radiologic Buzzwords / Findings:*

• Central subchondral erosions - **"gull-wing"** - this is the "Classic Feature"
• Joint Ankylosis
• Diffuse cartilage space loss

- *Why is this not RA?*

• The distribution favors the DIP, PIP, and First CMC —- unlike RA which is more carpals and MCP
• Typically RF Negative
• Erosions are more central (RA has more marginal)

Case 26 - Pain

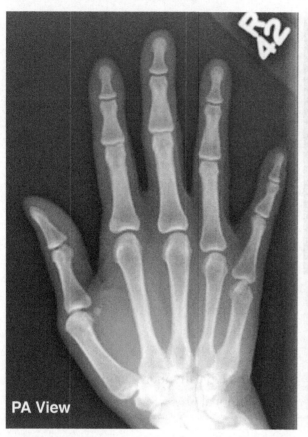
PA View

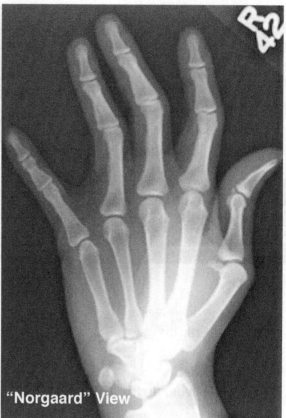
"Norgaard" View

1. What is the diagnosis?
A. Psoriatic Arthritis
B. Lupus
C. Osteoarthritis
D. Rheumatoid Arthritis

2. A mimic for this diagnosis is?
A. Reactive (Reiters) Arthritis
E. Jaccoud's Arthritis
F. Erosive O.A.
G. Hemochromatosis

3. The classic finding for this diagnosis is?
A. Deformation with Erosions
B. Deformation without Erosions
C. Fusiform Soft Tissue Swelling
D. First CMC Osteophyte Formation

Case 26 - SLE (Lupus) Arthritis

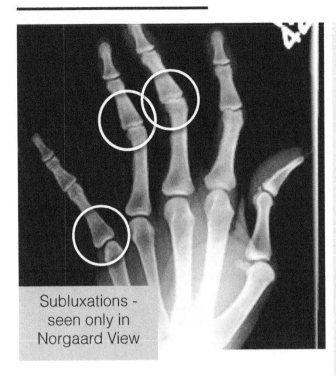

Subluxations - seen only in Norgaard View

1. What is the diagnosis?
A. Psoriatic Arthritis
B. Lupus
C. Osteoarthritis
D. Rheumatoid Arthritis

2. A mimic for this diagnosis is?
A. Reactive (Reiters) Arthritis
E. Jaccoud's Arthritis
F. Erosive O.A.
G. Hemochromatosis

3. The classic finding for this diagnosis is?
A. Deformation with Erosions
B. Deformation without Erosions
C. Fusiform Soft Tissue Swelling
D. First CMC Osteophyte Formation

SLE Arthritis

Arthritis seen with Lupus is common (up to 80% of patients).

Essential Trivia:

- The classic feature is a deforming arthritis without erosions

- The finding of "reversing subluxations" is the classic way to show this. Hands flat against the film in the PA reduce the subluxation, which then reoccur in the ball catcher (Norgaard) view.

- The main mimic is "Jaccoud Arthropathy" causes a similar reversing subluxation - usually ulnar sided. The only thing to know is that it occurs post rheumatic fever.

- Lupus patients are at an increased risk of tendon rupture and AVN with steroid therapy.

- *Radiologic Buzzwords / Findings:*

- Symmetric Polyarthritis involving the hands and knees
- It's non erosive
- Nonspecific periarticular osteopenia
- Correctable Subluxations - usually ulnar sided.

Arthritis - Essential Trivia

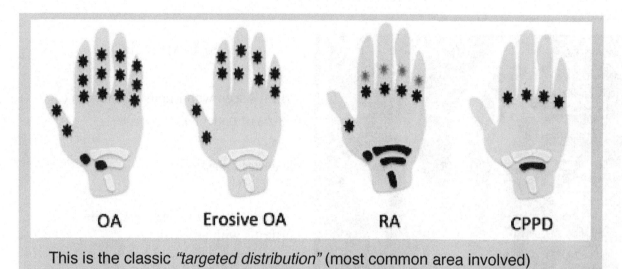

This is the classic *"targeted distribution"* (most common area involved)

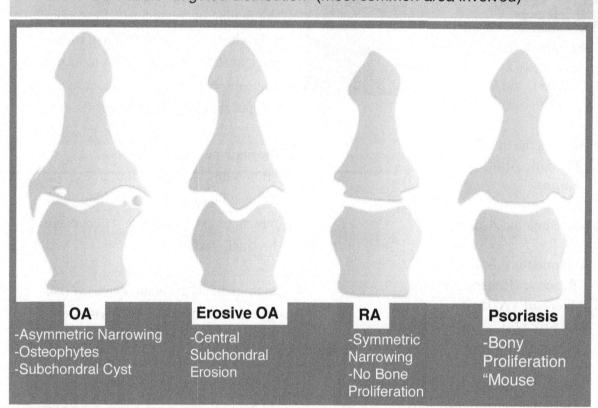

OA
- Asymmetric Narrowing
- Osteophytes
- Subchondral Cyst

Erosive OA
- Central Subchondral Erosion

RA
- Symmetric Narrowing
- No Bone Proliferation

Psoriasis
- Bony Proliferation "Mouse"

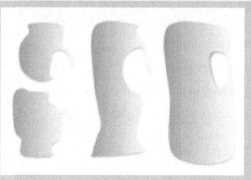

The Gout

This is the classic - "over hanging edge", and "punched out lesions."

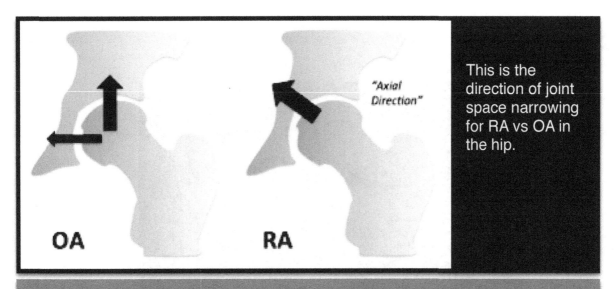

Hyperparathyroidism

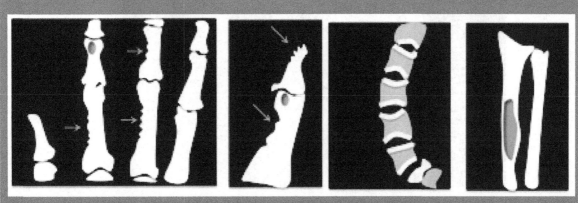

Subperiosteal Resorption, Tuft Resorption | Rugger | Brown Tumor

SI Joints

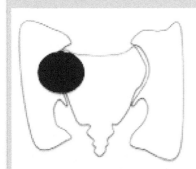
Unilateral = Infection

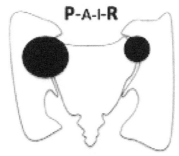
Asymmetric = Psoriasis, Reiters

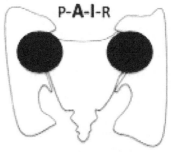
Symmetric = Inflammatory Bowel, AS

Case 27 - Pain

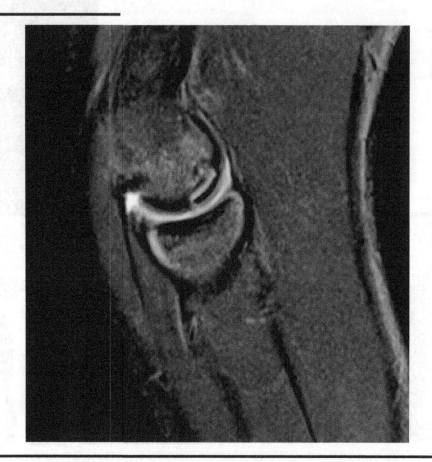

1. The most common location for this type of lesion is?
A. Femoral Condyle
B. Talus
C. Capitellum of Elbow
D. Rib

2. The most important goal of MRI with a lesion such as this is to?
A. Determine the location of the lesion
B. Determine if the lesion is solitary or multiple
C. Determine the size of the lesion
D. Determine the stability of the lesion

3. Stable vs Unstable is denoted by?
A. Cartilage Injury = Unstable
B. Subchondral Edema = Unstable
C. High Signal around fragment = Unstable
D. T2 Dark Signal within the fragment = Unstable

Case 27 - Osteochondral Lesion

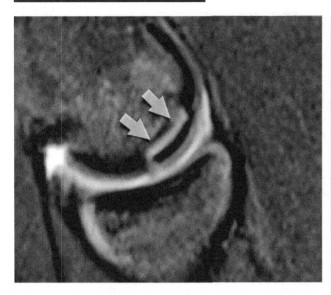

1. The most common location for this type of lesion is?
A. **Femoral Condyle**
B. Talus
C. Capitellum of Elbow
D. Rib

2. The most important goal of MRI with a lesion such as this is to?
A. Determine the location of the lesion
B. Determine if the lesion is solitary or multiple
C. Determine the size of the lesion
D. **Determine the stability of the lesion**

3. Stable vs Unstable is denoted by?
A. Cartilage Injury = Unstable
B. Subchondral Edema = Unstable
C. **High Signal around fragment = Unstable**
D. T2 Dark Signal within the fragment = Unstable

Osteochondral Lesion

Injury to both articular cartilage and bone, though to be secondary to repetitive trauma. In the elbow, it's usually from gymnastics or throwing. The typical age is a young teenager.

Essential Trivia:

- The most common location is the medial femoral condyle, (second most common is the talar dome, third most common is the anterolateral capitellum).

- MRI is obtained to tell if the lesion is stable or not.

- Under cutting of T2 high signal around the fragment defines it as unstable (by MRI)

- The *"pseudodefect"* of the capitellum is the most common pitfall. This occurs by the sharp change in angle on coronal images around the posterior lateral edge (remember this OCL is usually anterior not posterior).

- *"Panner's Disease"* is an osteochondrosis (AVN) of the capitellum. It occurs in a **younger** age (5-10), is self limiting, and **does NOT have loose bodies**.

Case 28 - Pain

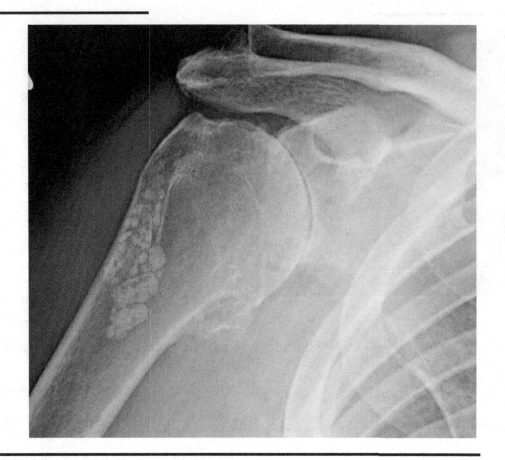

1. What is the diagnosis?
A. Pigmented Nodular Synovitis
B. Synovial Chondromatosis
C. Lipoma Arborescens
D. Hemophilia

2. What factors favor primary type over secondary type?
A. Severe degenerative changes
B. History of trauma
C. Loose bodies are different sizes
D. Loose bodies are similar sizes

3. Is the primary form a malignant cancer?
A. Yup - get the saw ready
B. Nope - won't need to amputate this time

Case 28 - Synovial Chondromatosis

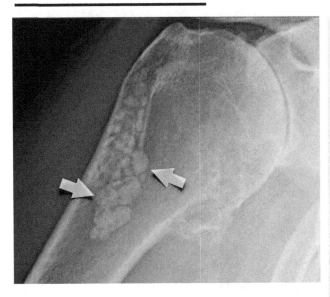

1. What is the diagnosis?
A. Pigmented Nodular Synovitis
B. Synovial Chondromatosis
C. Lipoma Arborescens
D. Hemophilia

2. What factors favor primary type over secondary type?
A. Severe degenerative changes
B. History of trauma
C. Loose bodies are different sizes
D. Loose bodies are similar sizes

3. Is the primary form a cancer?
A. Yup - get the saw ready
B. Nope - won't need to amputate this time

Synovial Chondromatosis

Disorder with multiple intra-articular cartilaginous loose bodies. There are two distinct subtypes.

Essential Trivia:

- *Primary Type* - Self limiting neoplastic process in which the synovium of a single joint goes bananas and starts proliferating into chondroid nodules. These flake off into the joint and are bathed in the synovial fluid - which makes them grow big. The key is they are usually all the same size.

- *Secondary Type* - This is associated with trauma, or bad OA. You get cartilage knocked off which gets bathed by synovial fluid and starts to grow. The loose bodies are different sizes in a background of bad degenerative change.

- Treatment between primary and secondary types is different. Both get the loose bodies removed, but sometimes surgeons will do a synovectomy in the primary type (local recurrence rates are quoted between 3-23%).

- Seen more commonly in bigger joints (shoulders and knees), but can occur in any joint (even the TMJ).

Case 29- Pain

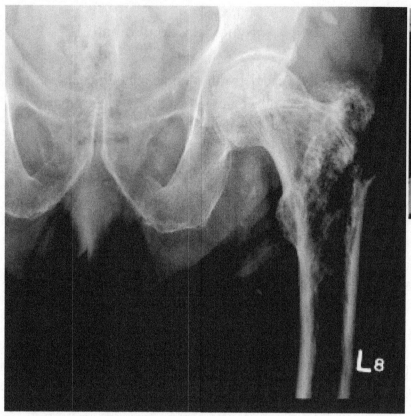
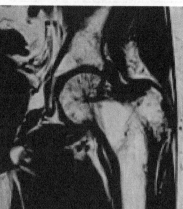

1. What is the diagnosis?
A. AVN of the femoral head
B. Multiple Myeloma
C. Pagets
D. Giant Cell Tumor

2. What is the most common location
A. Femoral Condyle
B. Talus
C. Skull
D. Pelvis

3. What is the major concern?
A. Soft tissue involvement
B. Progression to ankylosis
C. Malignant Transformation
D. High Risk of Osteomyelitis

4. In diffuse disease what bone is most likely to be spared?
A. The fibula
B. The tibia
C. The skull
D. The spine

Case 29 - Pagets

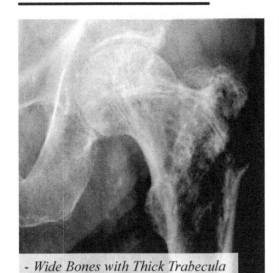

- *Wide Bones with Thick Trabecula*

1. What is the diagnosis?
A. AVN of the femoral head
B. Multiple Myeloma
C. Pagets
D. Giant Cell Tumor

2. What is the most common location
A. Femoral Condyle
B. Talus
C. Skull
D. Pelvis

3. What is the major concern?
A. Soft tissue involvement
B. Progression to ankylosis
C. Malignant Transformation
D. High Risk of Osteomyelitis

4. In diffuse disease what bone is most likely to be spared?
A. The fibula
B. The tibia
C. The skull
D. The spine

Pagets

Poorly understood, relatively common (4% at 40, 8% at 80) chronic disease of bone formation.

Essential Trivia:

- *"Wide Bones with Thick Trabecula"* (nothing else really does that).

- *Complications:* Deafness (actually pretty common), spinal stenosis, stress fracture, CHF (high output), secondary hyperparathyroidism (10%)

- *"Most feared complication"* = secondary osteosarcoma - high grade and a mother fucker

- *Skull* - Large areas of osteolysis in the Frontal and Occipital Bones "Osteoporosis Circumscripta", in the lytic phase. The skull will look "cotton wool" in the mixed phase. Both inner and outer table (favors the inner table).

- *Spine* - Cortical Thickening can cause a "picture frame sign" (same as osteopetrosis). Also can give you an ivory vertebral body.

- *Pelvis* - Most common bone involved. "Always" involves the iliopectineal line on the pelvic brim.

- *Long Bones* - Advancing margin of lucency from one end to the other is the so called "blade of grass" or "flame." Will often spare the fibula.

Case 30 - Pain

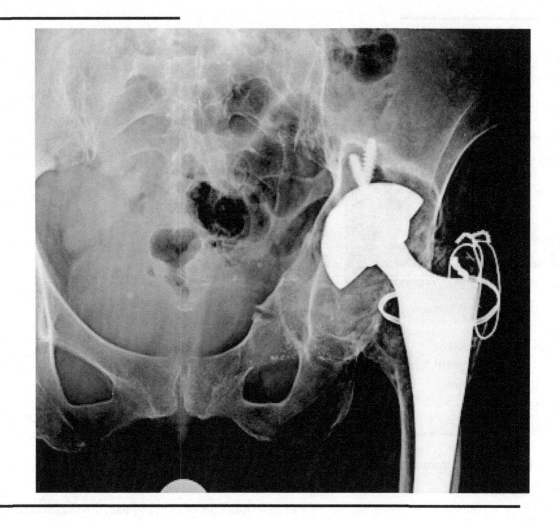

1. What is the diagnosis?
A. Chordoma
B. Pagets
C. Particle Disease
D. Plasmacytoma

2. A key feature to this diagnosis is?
A. Marked sclerotic border
B. No secondary reaction (no periosteal reaction)
C. Loose bodies of different sizes
D. Associated asymmetric SI joint erosions

3. If the patient has no fever / no white count, MRI of the lytic areas will probably be?
A. T2 Bright
B. T2 Isointense to muscle

Case 30 - Particle Disease

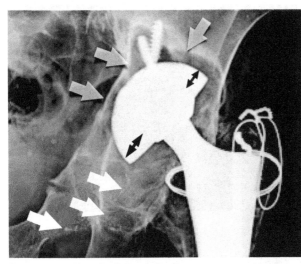

Gray Arrows = Bad Osteolysis
White Arrows = Tiny flecks of particle
Black arrows = Probably some wear / shift lateral

1. What is the diagnosis?
A. Chordoma
B. Pagets
C. Particle Disease
D. Plasmacytoma

2. A key feature to this diagnosis is?
A. Marked sclerotic border
B. No secondary reaction (no periosteal reaction)
C. Loose bodies of different sizes
D. Associated asymmetric SI joint erosions

3. If the patient has no fever / no white count, MRI of the lytic areas will probably be?
A. T2 Bright
B. T2 Isointense to muscle

Particle Disease

Locally aggressive histolytic response to small polyethylene particles shed from the lining

Essential Trivia:

- *Mechanism:* Small particles are shed into the joint fluid and leak into the adjacent bones - often through the screw holes. These particles illicit a sterile inflammatory response which lysis the crap out of the bone. Bones wiggle more, particles spread more.

- Typically occurs between 1-5 years after surgery.

- *Radiologic Buzzwords / Findings:*
 • Aggressive osteolysis around the hardware
 • Often associated with polyethylene wear (but doesn't have to be)
 • The key feature is that there is no secondary bone response (no sclerotic reaction)

- *Why is this not infection?*
 • Clinically won't have fever and/or other signs of infection
 • On MRI - lytic lesions of osteomyelitis tend to be T2 bright. Particle disease lytic lesions are mainly inflammatory and fibrous tissue which is isointense to muscle on T1 and T2

Case 31 - Pain

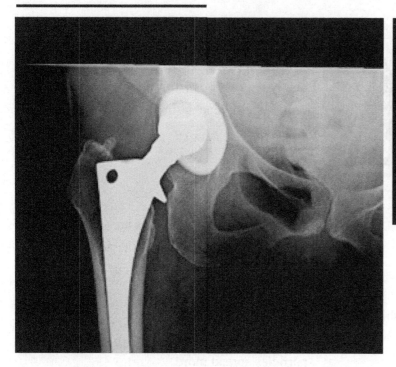
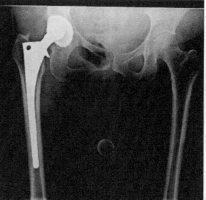

1. What is the diagnosis?
A. Creep
B. Wear
C. Loosening
D. Fracture

2. Shifting of the head inside the cup is considered pathologic when?
A. It's towards the spine
B. It's lateral

3. This finding predisposes to what?
A. Particle disease
B. Infection
C. Myositis Ossificans
D. Heterotopic Ossification

Case 31 - Polyethylene Wear

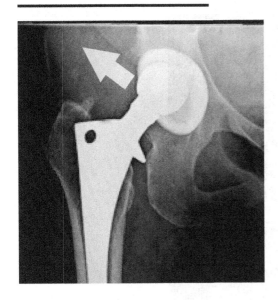

1. What is the diagnosis?
A. Creep
B. Wear
C. Loosening
D. Fracture

2. Shifting of the head inside the cup is considered pathologic when?
A. It's towards the spine
B. It's lateral

3. This finding predisposes to what?
A. Particle disease
B. Infection
C. Myositis Ossificans
D. Heterotopic Ossification

Polyethylene Wear

The prosthetic head should be centered symmetrically within the cup. *Lateral shifting is considered pathologic.*

Essential Trivia:

- Poor Locking of the PE linear in the cup, micro-motion, or abnormal loading can predispose to wear.

- **Creep** = A normal process of mild penetration of the femoral head component into the cup (in the direction of the spine). This occurs in the first 2 years of placement.

• Breaking down of the the PE linear can lead to particle disease (as seen in case 30)

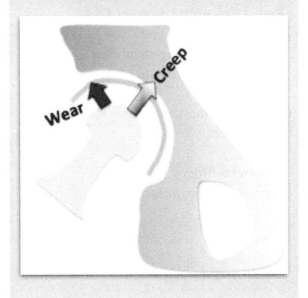

Case 32 - Pain

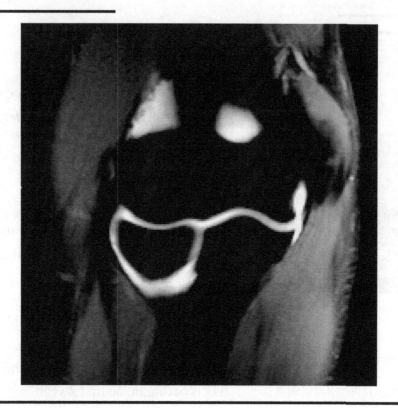

1. What is the diagnosis?
A. Radial Collateral Ligament Tear
B. Annular Ligament Tear
C. Ulnar Collateral Ligament Tear
D. Lateral Ulnar Collateral Ligament Tear

2. This injury is most commonly seen in?
A. Linebackers
B. Kickers
C. Throwers - from valgus stress
D. Throwers - from varus stress

3. Which bundle of the UCL is the "most important" stabilizer?
A. Anterior
B. Posterior
C. Transverse
D. All are equally important

4. Where does the UCL attach?
A. The Sublime Tubercle
B. The Olecranon Fossa
C. The Radial Tuberosity
D. Gerdes Tubercle

Case 32 - Partial Ulnar Collateral Ligament Tear - "The 'T' Sign"

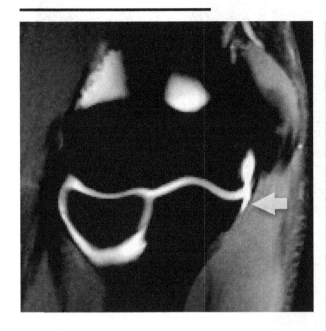

1. What is the diagnosis?
A. Radial Collateral Ligament Tear
B. Annular Ligament Tear
C. Ulnar Collateral Ligament Tear
D. Lateral Ulnar Collateral Ligament Tear

2. This injury is most commonly seen in?
A. Linebackers
B. Kickers
C. Throwers - from valgus stress
D. Throwers - from varus stress

3. Which bundle of the UCL is the "most important" stabilizer?
A. Anterior
B. Posterior
C. Transverse
D. All are equally important

4. Where does the UCL attach?
A. The Sublime Tubercle
B. The Olecranon Fossa
C. The Radial Tuberosity
D. Gerdes Tubercle

Partial UCL Tear "T-Sign"

The Ulnar Collateral Ligament normally attaches firmly to the "sublime tubercle." When it tears, gadolinium will undercut the tubercle creating the appearance of a "T."

Essential Trivia:

- The ulnar collateral ligament consists of 3 bundles (anterior, posterior, and transverse). The anterior one is the most important restraint to the valgus stress seen in throwers.

- Throwers injure 3 main things from valgus overload - the UCL, the common flexor tendons, and the ulnar nerve

- Because the flexor / pronator mass keeps the function of the elbow normal even after a tear of the UCL, it's usually managed with conservative therapy - in the non-athlete.

- For the elite athlete (or for high schooler whose father failed to achieve their own dreams and are trying to live them out through their children), the "Tommy John" reconstruction can be done. Usually the palmaris longus is used as the donor tendon.

Case 33 - Felt a Bump

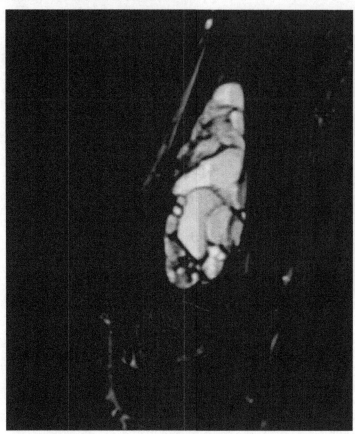
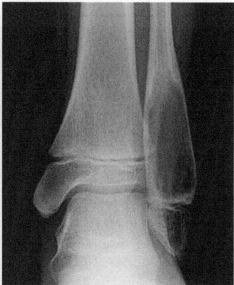

1. What is the diagnosis?
A. Fibrous Dysplasia
B. Pagets
C. Enchondroma
D. Aneurysmal Bone Cyst

2. Up to 40% of the time a secondary ABC is associated with?
A. Osteosarcoma
B. Chondrosarcoma
C. Giant Cell Tumor
D. Bizarre Parosteal Osteochondromatous Proliferation (BPOP)

3. The typical age for the lesion is?
A. > 30
B. < 30
C. No age preference

Case 33 - Aneurysmal Bone Cyst

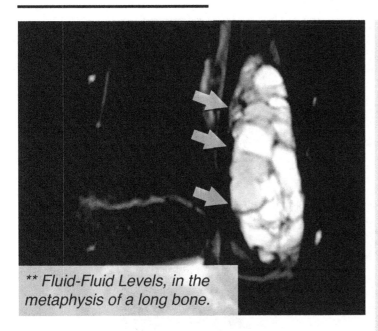

** Fluid-Fluid Levels, in the metaphysis of a long bone.

1. What is the diagnosis?
A. Fibrous Dysplasia
B. Pagets
C. Enchondroma
D. Aneurysmal Bone Cyst

2. Up to 40% of the time a secondary ABC is associated with?
A. Osteosarcoma
B. Chondrosarcoma
C. Giant Cell Tumor
D. Bizarre Parosteal Osteochondromatous Proliferation (BPOP)

3. The typical age for the lesion is?
A. > 30
B. < 30
C. No age preference

Aneurysmal Bone Cyst (ABC):

Aneurysmal bone cysts are aneurysmal lesions of bone with thin-walled, blood-filled spaces (fluid-fluid level on MRI).

Essential Trivia:

- They are typically thought of as either primary or secondary. The secondary ones arise out of another tumor *(classically Giant Cell Tumors)*.

- They can develop after a trauma

- Most Patients are less than 20

- The metaphysis of tibia is the most common location, *(the second most common is the posterior elements)*.

- *DDx for a Fluid-Fluid Level on MRI:*
  - ABC
  - Giant Cell Tumor
  - Telangiectatic Osteosarcoma
  - Simple Bone Cyst (after Fx)

Case 34 - Pain -

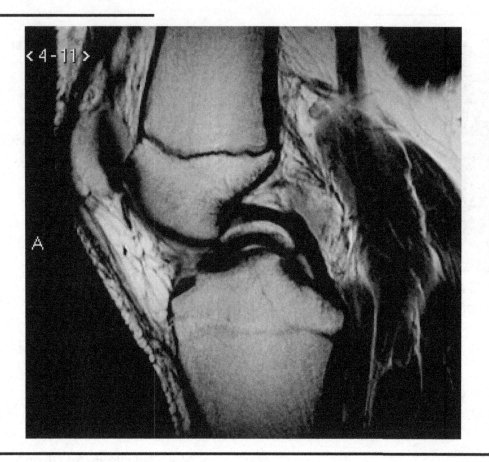

1. What is the diagnosis?
A. ACL Tear
B. PCL Tear
C. MCL Tear
D. Medial Meniscus Tear

2. The *"Double PCL sign"* can only occur with a medial meniscal tear when?
A. The ACL is also torn
B. The ACL is intact
C. The PCL is also torn
D. The MCL is also torn

3. Which sequence is the least sensitive for meniscal tears?
A. T1
B. T2
C. Proton Density (PD)

Case 34 - Bucket Handle Meniscus Tear - "Double PCL"

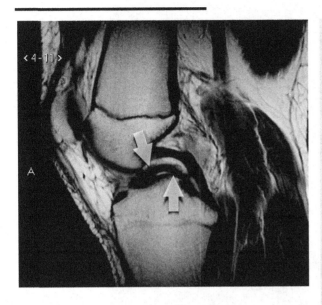

1. What is the diagnosis?
A. ACL Tear
B. PCL Tear
C. MCL Tear
D. Medial Meniscus Tear

2. The *"Double PCL sign"* can only occur with a medial meniscal tear when?
A. The ACL is also torn
B. The ACL is intact
C. The PCL is also torn
D. The MCL is also torn

3. Which sequence is the least sensitive for meniscal tears?
A. T1
B. T2
C. Proton Density (PD)

Bucket Handle Meniscus Tear

The result of a torn inner meniscal segment from a longitudinal or oblique tear "flipping" - most commonly into the intercondylar notch.

Essential Trivia:

- The "double PCL sign", as seen in this case, consists of meniscus flipped into the notch, inferior and parallel to the PCL seen in the same sagittal plane.

- It's more common medially

- It's only seen medially - in the setting of an intact ACL.

- The "Absent Bow Tie Sign" describes the absent meniscal body on two consecutive slices — with false positives seen in children, and small adults.

- A short TE is required to see meniscal tears effectively. Longer TEs miss the differences between an intact meniscus and one that is chewed up. This is why T2 sucks for the meniscus. *Remember T1 and PD have short TE, and T2 has a long TE.*

Case 35 - Pain -

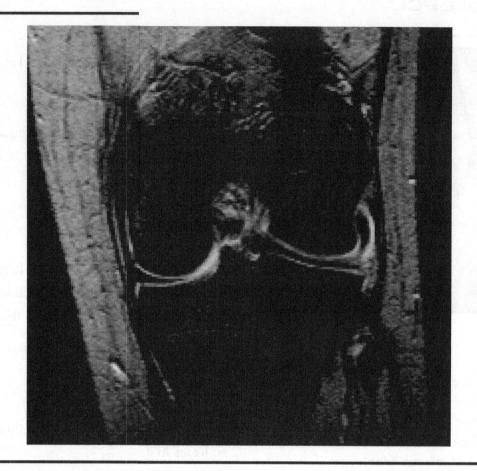

1. What is the diagnosis?
A. Discoid Meniscus
B. Mensical Seperation
C. Parrot Beak Meniscal Tear
D. Flipped Meniscal Fragment (Bucket Handle Tear)

2. Discoid meniscus is most commonly seen on?
A. The Medial Side
B. The Lateral Side
C. Both Sides Equally

3. Which discoid variant has no posterior coronary or capsular attachment?
A. The "Complete"
B. The "Incomplete"
C. The "Wrisberg"
D. The "Humphrey"

Case 35 - Discoid Meniscus

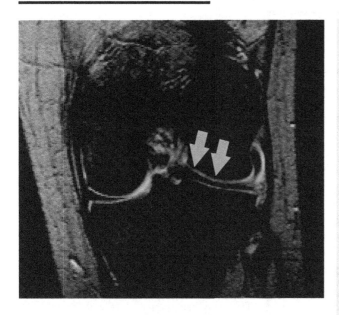

1. What is the diagnosis?
A. Discoid Meniscus
B. Mensical Seperation
C. Parrot Beak Meniscal Tear
D. Flipped Meniscal Fragment (Bucket Handle Tear)

2. Discoid meniscus is most commonly seen on?
A. The Medial Side
B. The Lateral Side
C. Both Sides Equally

3. Which discoid variant has no posterior coronary or capsular attachment?
A. The "Complete"
B. The "Incomplete"
C. The "Wrisberg"
D. The "Humphrey"

Discoid Meniscus

Congenital variant in which the meniscus is nearly disk shaped (instead of "C shaped").

Essential Trivia:

- The diagnosis is suggested by meniscal tissue on 3 contiguous sagittal slices *"too many bow-ties"*, or a meniscal body extending into the intercondylar notch on coronal images (as in this case).

- The discoid meniscus has an increased incidence of tearing.

- The 3 subtypes of discoids are: complete, incomplete, and Wrisberg. The Wrisberg has the most symptoms (snapping sensations), and has no posterior coronary or capsular attachment.

- Discoid meniscus is more common in Asians (Japanese and Koreans) up to 15% - depending on what you read.

Meniscus - Essential Trivia

Medial Meniscus	Lateral Meniscus
Covers 50% of the medial plateau	Covers 70% of the lateral plateau
More "Open" C Shape	More "Closed" C Shape
Posterior Horn is Thicker than Anterior Horn	Anterior Horn = Posterior Horn
Anterior Horn attaches in front of the ACL	Anterior horn has fibers from the ACL extending into it's root. This causes a *"striated"* or *"comb-like"* appearance
Less Mobile - because of peripheral attachments to the deep MCL fibers	Meniscofemoral ligaments *(Wrisberg and Humphrey)* attach to the posterior horn

Vascularity

The vascularity of the meniscus is divided in a "Red Zone" and a "White Zone."

Red Zone – The peripheral 30%. It has good blood flow, and can potentially heal if injured.

White Zone – The inner 70%. It has shitty blood flow, and will not heal.

The percentage of "Red Zone" is more like 50% in kids. This is why they heal their meniscus better than adults.

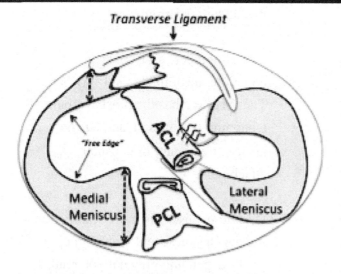

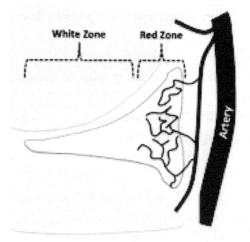

Meniscal Tear in the Setting of ACL Tear:

- Acute ACL Tear – The **Lateral** Meniscus is torn twice as often as the Medial

- Most Meniscal Tears (in the setting of acute ACL injury) are peripheral longitudinal tears of posterior horn of the lateral meniscus

- In the Chronic Setting ("ACL Deficient knee") – increased mobility leads to shear forces of the less mobile posterior horn of the **Medial** meniscus

Diagnosis and Classification of the Tear:

The normal meniscus is dark on all sequences. Criteria for calling a tear is going to be either (a) abnormal signal extending to the meniscal articular surface, or (b) abnormal morphology – *i.e. the triangle looks blunted.*

Tears can be thought of as either (1) vertical , (2) horizontal, or (3) "complex" (both). Horizontal is just plain horizontal. However, vertical is sub-divided into longitudinal, radial, or parrot-beak. The parrot beak is uncommon - forget I mentioned it.

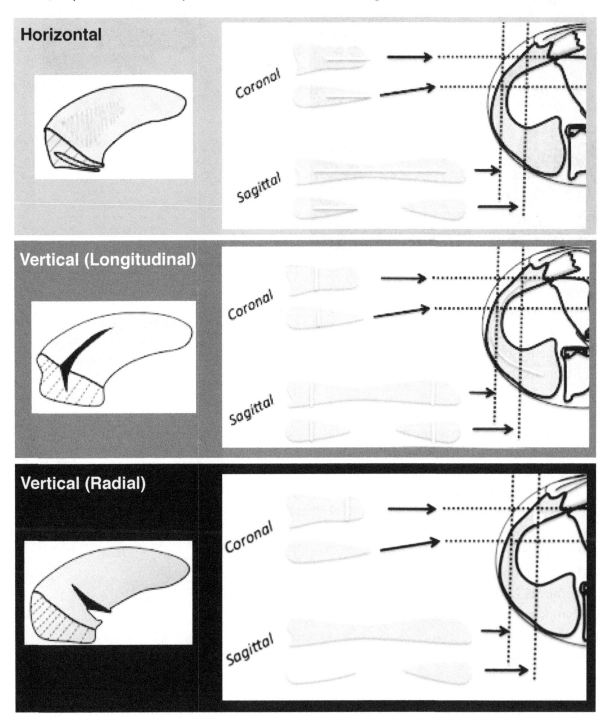

Case 36 - Pain -

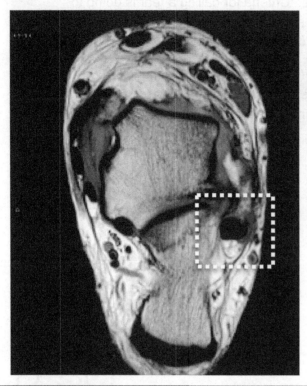
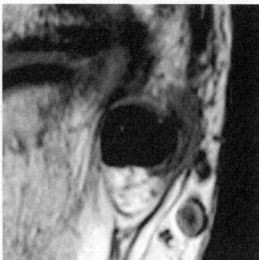

1. What is the diagnosis?
A. Flexor Digitorum Tear
B. Flexor Hallucis Longus Tear
C. Peroneus Longus Tear
D. Peroneus Brevis Tear

2. This injury is associated with?
A. The presence of a peroneus quartus
B. The absence of a peroneus quartus
C. The presence of an accessory navicular
D. The absence of an accessory navicular

3. Avulsion fractures at the base of the 5th Metatarsal involve what tendon?
A. Flexor Digitorum
B. Flexor Hallucis Longus
C. Peroneus Longus
D. Peroneus Brevis

Case 36 - Split Peroneus Brevis

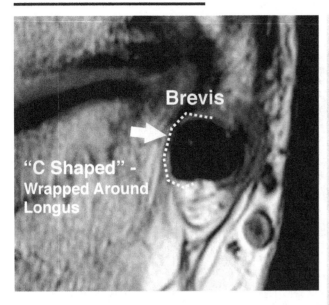

1. What is the diagnosis?
A. Flexor Digitorum Tear
B. Flexor Hallucis Longus Tear
C. Peroneus Longus Tear
D. Peroneus Brevis Tear

2. This injury is associated with?
A. The presence of a peroneus quartus
B. The absence of a peroneus quartus
C. The presence of an accessory navicular
D. The absence of an accessory navicular

3. Avulsion fractures at the base of the 5th Metatarsal involve what tendon?
A. Flexor Digitorum
B. Flexor Hallucis Longus
C. Peroneus Longus
D. Peroneus Brevis

Split Peroneus Brevis

Split tearing of the peroneus brevis is common with inversion injury.

Essential Trivia:

- Things that predispose to tearing of the peroneus brevis include things that crowd the tendon (low lying peroneal muscle body, accessory muscles - most famously the peroneus quartus, and thickening of the calcaneofibular ligament). When you dorsiflex and invert your foot ("twist your ankle") - the tendon gets smashed into the lateral malleolus. Over time it tears.

- Tearing is characteristically in the shape of a "C" or a "boomerang."

- There is an 80% association with lateral ligament tears and split tears of the peroneus brevis. This is why the injury is associated with chronic ankle instability

- Another classic piece of trivia is that the peroneus brevis inserts onto the base of the 5th Metatarsal. When you get an avulsion fracture of the 5th MT *"Dancer's Fracture"* this is the tendon that does the avulsing.

Case 37 - Pain

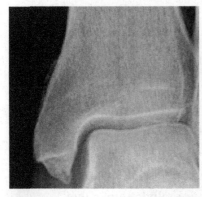
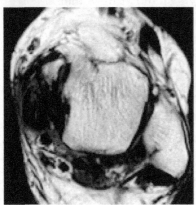
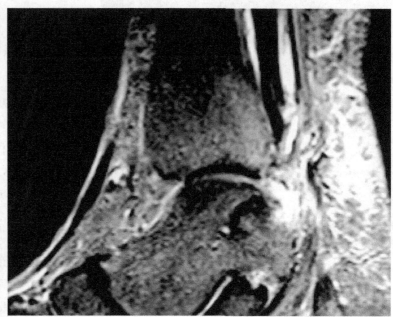

1. What is the diagnosis?
A. Flexor Digitorum Tear
B. Flexor Hallucis Longus Tear
C. Posterior Tibialis Tear
D. Peroneus Longus Tear

2. This injury is associated with?
A. Development of pes planus (flat foot)
B. Development of pes cavus
C. Development of hindfoot varus
D. The absence of an accessory navicular

3. Rupture of this tendon places abnormal stress on which ligament?
A. The Deltoid Ligament
B. The Anterior Talar Fibular Ligament
C. The Posterior Talar fibular Ligament
D. The Spring Ligament (plantar calcaneonavicular)

Case 37 - Tearing of Posterior Tibial Tendon

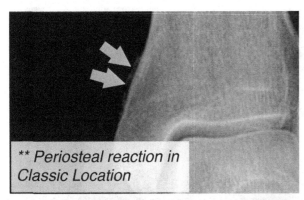

** Periosteal reaction in Classic Location

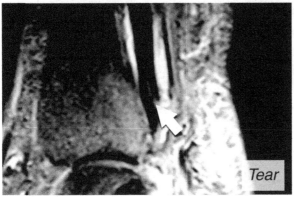

Tear

1. What is the diagnosis?
A. Flexor Digitorum Tear
B. Flexor Hallucis Longus Tear
C. Posterior Tibialis Tear
D. Peroneus Longus Tear

2. This injury is associated with?
A. Development of pes planus (flat foot)
B. Development of pes cavus
C. Development of hindfoot varus
D. The absence of an accessory navicular

3. Rupture of this tendon places abnormal stress on which ligament?
A. The Deltoid Ligament
B. The Anterior Talar Fibular Ligament
C. The Posterior Talar fibular Ligament
D. The Spring Ligament (plantar calcaneonavicular)

Tear of the Posterior Tibial Tendon

This is the most commonly injured medial ankle tendon.

Essential Trivia:

- The posterior tibial tendon is the largest and most medial of the 3 medial ankle tendons (**T**om, **D**ick and **H**arry - or Posterior **T**ibialis, Flexor **D**igitorum, and Flexor **H**allucis Longus)

- Tearing of the tendon is most common at the level of the medial malleolus

- The tendon is a major supporter of the arch. A tear of the tendon can lead to collapse of the longitudinal arch.

- When you have a posterior tibial tendon tear, there is a cascade of events that can occur:
  - (1) PTT Tears
  - (2) Spring Ligament Fails
  - (3) SubTalar Ligaments Fail (causing *Sinus Tarsi Syndrome*).
  - (4) Pt walks on a painful flat foot - and tries to heel strike to avoid pain. This leads to *Plantar Fasciitis*.

- Tearing of the tendon is associated with the presence of an accessory navicular bone or large medial tubercle (cornuate process).

Case 38 - Pain

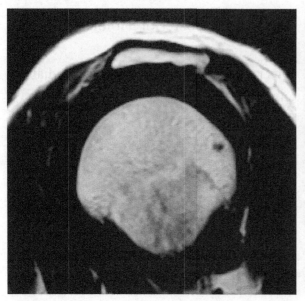 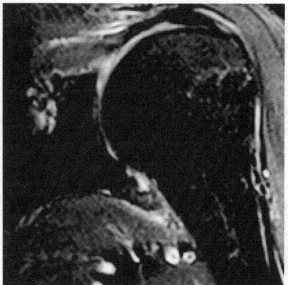

1. What is the diagnosis?
A. Humeral Avulsion of the Glenohumeral Ligament (HAGL)
B. "Perthes" Lesion
C. Adhesive Capsulitis
D. Long Head of Biceps Tear

2. What is the classic diagnostic finding?
A. Thickening of the inferior glenohumeral ligament
B. Absence of the middle glenohumeral ligament
C. Absence of the anterior superior labrum
D. Medial Subluxation of the Long Head of the Biceps

3. What might you expect on arthrography?
A. Increased Joint Capacity (can hold more than 30 cc comfortably)
B. Decreased Joint Capacity (can hold less than 10 cc)
C. Gad in the sub deltoid bursa
D. Gad in the subscapularis muscle

Case 38 - Adhesive Capsulitis

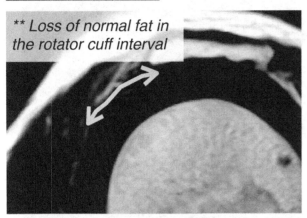
** Loss of normal fat in the rotator cuff interval

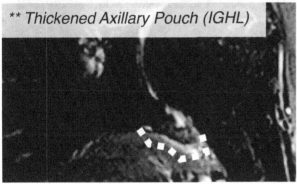
** Thickened Axillary Pouch (IGHL)

1. What is the diagnosis?
A. Humeral Avulsion of the Glenohumeral Ligament (HAGL)
B. "Perthes" Lesion
C. Adhesive Capsulitis
D. Long Head of Biceps Tear

2. What is the classic diagnostic finding?
A. Thickening of the inferior glenohumeral ligament
B. Absence of the middle glenohumeral ligament
C. Absence of the anterior superior labrum
D. Medial Subluxation of the Long Head of the Biceps

3. What might you expect on arthrography?
A. Increased Joint Capacity (can hold more than 30 cc comfortably)
B. Decreased Joint Capacity (can hold less than 10 cc)
C. Gad in the sub deltoid bursa
D. Gad in the subscapularis muscle

Adhesive Capsulitis

"Frozen Shoulder" - Contraction of the joint capsule - often seen after surgery or trauma.

Essential Trivia:

- The clinical buzz phrase is *"Severe glenohumeral limitation to movement without other cause."*

- The diagnosis is traditionally considered a clinical one... until you are asked to make it on a multiple choice test.

- On Arthrography low capacity (less than 10cc) of the joint is a classic sign (it's too stiff to be distended by contrast).

- Classic MRI Findings include:
  - Thickening of the Inferior Glenohumeral Ligament, Capsular Structures, Axillary Pouch,
  - Loss of Fat in the Rotator Cuff Interval

Case 39 - Pain

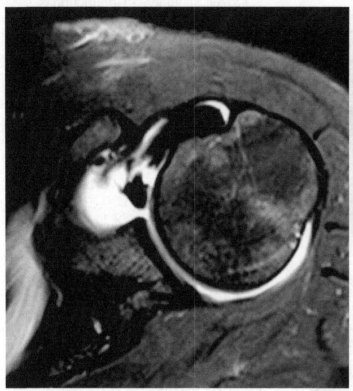
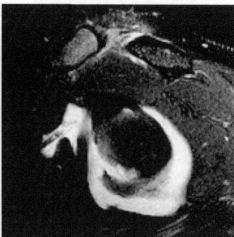

1. What is the diagnosis?
A. Humeral Avulsion of the Glenohumeral Ligament (HAGL)
B. "Perthes" Lesion
C. Anterior Labral Periosteal Sleeve Avulsion (ALPSA)
D. Buford Complex

2. The Buford Complex is?
A. A tearing of the superior labrum seen commonly in throwers
B. A tearing of the posterior labrum seen commonly in swimmers
C. A tearing of the anterior labrum seen in both throwers and swimmers
D. A normal varient

3. What is thickened in the Buford Complex?
A. The anterior band of the inferior glenohumeral ligament
B. The posterior band of the inferior glenohumeral ligament
C. The middle glenohumeral ligament (MGHL)
D. The superior glenohumeral ligament (SGHL)

Case 39 - Buford Complex

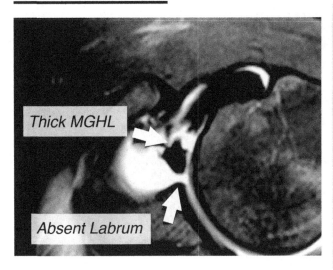

1. What is the diagnosis?
A. Humeral Avulsion of the Glenohumeral Ligament (HAGL)
B. "Perthes" Lesion
C. Anterior Labral Periosteal Sleeve Avulsion (ALPSA)
D. Buford Complex

2. The Buford Complex is?
A. A tearing of the superior labrum seen commonly in throwers
B. A tearing of the posterior labrum seencommonly in swimmers
C. A tearing of the anterior labrum seen in both throwers and swimmers
D. A normal varient

3. What is thickened in the Buford Complex?
A. The anterior band of the inferior glenohumeral ligament
B. The posterior band of the inferior glenohumeral ligament
C. The middle glenohumeral ligament (MGHL)
D. The superior glenohumeral ligament (SGHL)

Buford Complex

Normal variant of the glenoid labrum, seen in about 1.5% of the general population.

Essential Trivia:

- The complex has 3 components:
  - (1) Absent Anterior Superior Labrum,
  - (2) Thickened Middle Glenohumeral Ligament (MGHL), and
  - (3) Origination of the MGHL in a more superior position - at the base of the biceps labrum anchor.

- It's important to recognize, as it can mimic a labrum tear. However, if ortho "repairs" it - that can lead to altered mechanics… and probably a law suit, of which you'll certainly get drawn into (fucking scumbag lawyers).

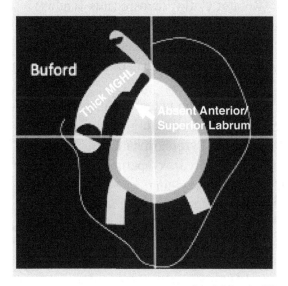

Case 40 - Pain

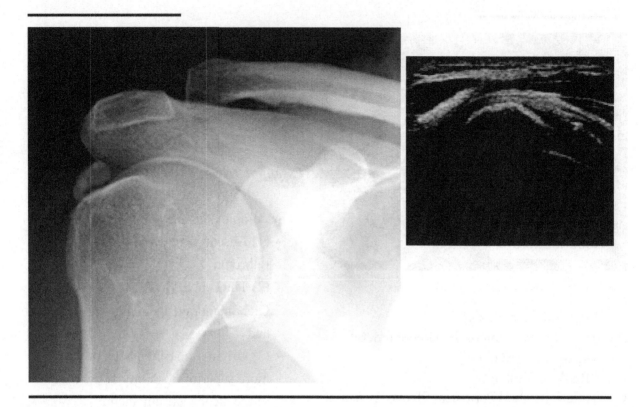

1. What is the diagnosis?
A. Chondrocalcinosis
B. Rotator Cuff Tear
C. Calcium Hydroxyapatite Deposition
D. Uric Acid Deposition

2. The most common location for this diagnosis?
A. Rotator Cuff (Supraspinatus Tendon)
B. Rotator Cuff (Subscapularis Tendon)
C. Knee (Quadriceps Tendon)
D. Shoulder (Long Head of Biceps Tendon)

3. Mineralization within cartilage is most likely?
A. Uric Acid Deposition
B. Calcium Pyrophosphate Dihydrate (CPPD)
C. Calcium Hydroxyapatite Deposition
D. Could be anything…

Case 40 - Calcific Tendonitis

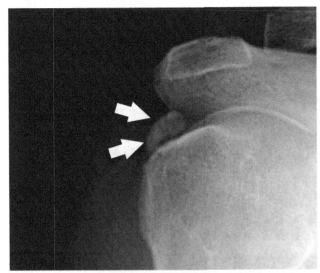

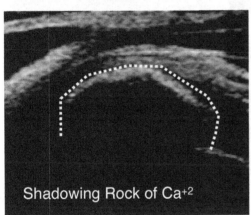

Shadowing Rock of Ca^{+2}

1. What is the diagnosis?
A. Chondrocalcinosis
B. Rotator Cuff Tear
C. Calcium Hydroxyapatite Deposition
D. Uric Acid Deposition

2. The most common location for this diagnosis?
A. Rotator Cuff (Supraspinatus Tendon)
B. Rotator Cuff (Subscapularis Tendon)
C. Knee (Quadriceps Tendon)
D. Shoulder (Long Head of Biceps Tendon)

3. Mineralization within cartilage is most likely?
A. Uric Acid Deposition
B. Calcium Pyrophosphate Dihydrate (CPPD)
C. Calcium Hydroxyapatite Deposition
D. Could be anything…

Calcific Tendonitis

Self limiting (but painful) deposition of calcium hydroxyapatite within a tendon.

Essential Trivia:

- The most common location is the rotator cuff, usually the supraspinatous tendon. The "critical zone" of the tendon, just before the foot print, is the most susceptible - as it has the least oxygen tension.

- Even though the rotator cuff is classic, the deposition can occur in any tendon in the body.

- Pain occurs when the mineralization extravasates into adjacent soft tissues (for example the subacromial bursa)

- Hydroxyapatite deposition does not occur in joint cartilage, if you see that - you are most likely dealing with CPPD.

- Classic Imaging Features:
  • *Plain Film:* "Globular" or "Amorphous" with poor margins.
  • *Ultrasound:* It will shadow - just like a stone anywhere else.
  • *MRI:* Dark on T1 and T2, with blooming on gradient.

Case 41 - Pain

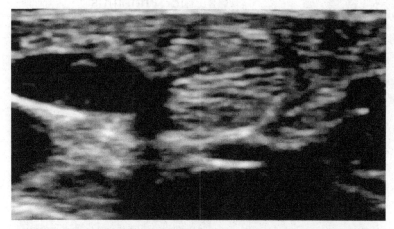

Same Tendon Time Point 1

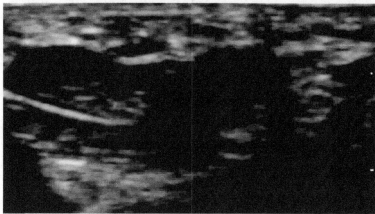

Same Tendon 5 seconds later in exam

1. What is the explanation?
A. The tendon spontaneously tore
B. The tech turned the probe

2. Does this artifact have a name?
A. Magic Angle
B. Anisotropy
C. Chemical Shift
D. Truncation

3. The tendon becomes dark when ?
A. It's seen perpendicular to the sound beam
B. It's NOT perpendicular to the sound beam

Aunt Minnie 91

Case 41 - Anisotropy

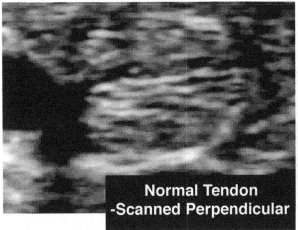

Normal Tendon -Scanned Perpendicular

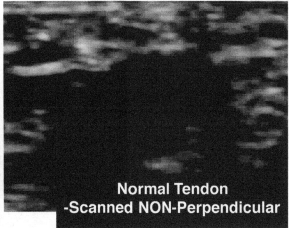

Normal Tendon -Scanned NON-Perpendicular

1. What is the explanation?
A. The tendon spontaneously tore
B. The tech turned the probe

2. Does this artifact have a name?
A. Magic Angle
B. Anisotropy
C. Chemical Shift
D. Truncation

3. The tendon becomes dark when?
A. It's seen perpendicular to the sound beam
B. It's NOT perpendicular to the sound beam

Anisotropy

A common artifact in MSK Ultrasound that can mimic a tendon tear

Essential Trivia:

- The echogenicity of a tendon depends on the orientation of the beam relative to the tendon structure. If the tendon is perpendicular it is bright, and you can see the fibers. If it's not perpendicular then it looks dark.

- This can be used to your advantage when distinguishing a hyper echoic tendon from a hyper echoic blob of fat.

- The artifact is the biggest pain in the ass at the supraspinatous (as it curves along the contours of the humeral head), and the long head of the biceps in the bicipital groove

Case 42 - Pain

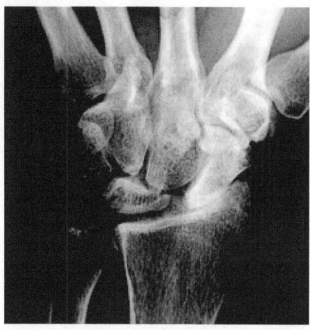
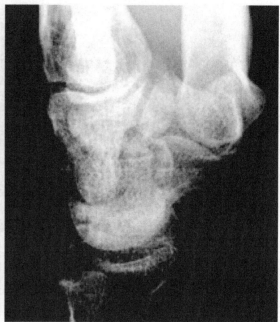

1. What is the diagnosis?
A. SNAC
B. SLAC
C. Ulnar Styloid Impaction Syndrome
D. Lunotriquetral Ligament Injury (VISI)

2. This injury is associated with ?
A. VISI
B. DISI

3. With this diagnosis, arthritis classically occurs FIRST in what location?
A. Between scaphoid and radius
B. Between capitate and lunate
C. Between lunate and radius
D. Between the triquetrum and ulna

Case 42 - SLAC Wrist with DISI

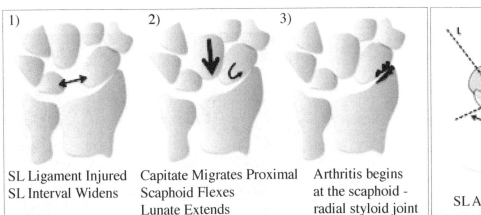

1) SL Ligament Injured
SL Interval Widens

2) Capitate Migrates Proximal
Scaphoid Flexes
Lunate Extends

3) Arthritis begins at the scaphoid - radial styloid joint

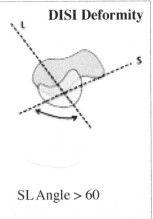

DISI Deformity

SL Angle > 60

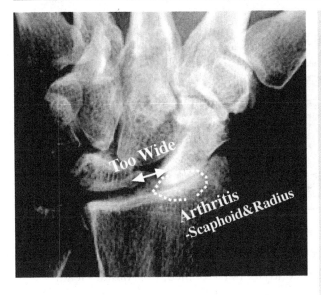

Too Wide

Arthritis -Scaphoid & Radius

SLAC Wrist
"Scapholunate Advanced Collapse."

Progressive instability in the scapho-lunate ligaments lead to progressive instability, and eventual advanced arthritis.

Essential Trivia:

- The general idea is that the scaphoid always wants to flex (tilt volar), and the lunate always wants to extend (tilt dorsal). Normally these opposite ideas hold each other neutral, but if the S-L ligament breaks they rotate towards their natural inclination. This rotary subluxation leads to abnormal articulation, which leads to instability and advanced arthritis (first at the radial-scaphoid joint).

- For multiple choice just remember it's always DISI (never VISI), and that CPPD can be a cause of weakened ligaments.

1. What is the diagnosis?
A. SNAC
B. SLAC
C. Ulnar Styloid Impaction Syndrome
D. Lunotriquetral Ligament Injury (VISI)

2. This injury is associated with ?
A. VISI
B. DISI

3. With this diagnosis, arthritis classically occurs FIRST in what location?
A. Between scaphoid and radius
B. Between capitate and lunate
C. Between lunate and radius
D. Between the triquetrum and ulna

Case 43 - Pain

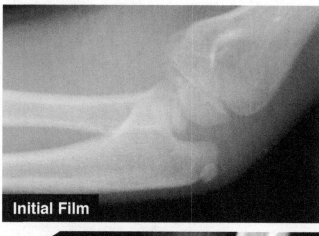

Initial Film

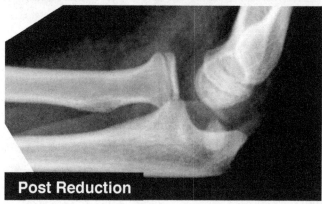

Post Reduction

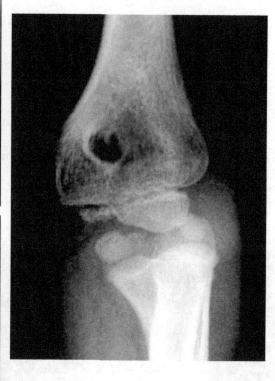

1. What is the usual order of elbow ossification?
A. (1) Capitellum, (2) Olecranon, (3) Medial Epicondyle, (4) Trochlea, (5) Radial Head, (6) Lateral Epicondyle
B. (1) Capitellum, (2) Radial Head, (3) Lateral Epicondyle, (4) Trochlea, (5) Olecranon, (6) Medial Epicondyle
C. (1) Capitellum, (2) Radial Head, (3) Lateral Epicondyle, (4) Olecranon (5) Trochlea, (6) Medial Epicondyle
D. (1) Capitellum, (2) Radial Head, (3) Medial Epicondyle, (4) Trochlea, (5) Olecranon, (6) Lateral Epicondyle

2. What is the pathology in this case?
A. Displaced medial epicondyle
B. Displaced lateral epicondyle
C. Bro, this case is normal

3. Which fractures are more common?
A. Medial epicondyle more common than medial condyle
B. Lateral epicondyle more common than lateral condyle
C. Medial condyle more common than medial epicondyle
D. All statements are false

Aunt Minnie 95

Case 43 - Displaced Medial Epicondylar FX

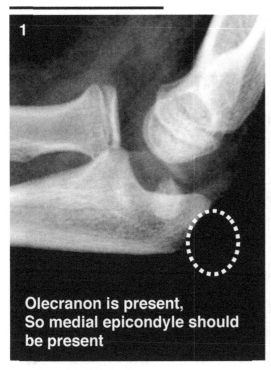

Olecranon is present, So medial epicondyle should be present

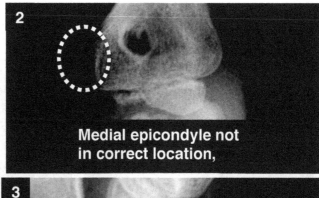

Medial epicondyle not in correct location,

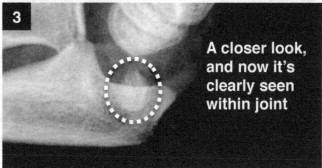

A closer look, and now it's clearly seen within joint

1. What is the usual order of elbow ossification?
A. (1) Capitellum, (2) Olecranon, (3) Medial Epicondyle, (4) Trochlea, (5) Radial Head, (6) Lateral Epicondyle
B. (1) Capitellum, (2) Radial Head, (3) Lateral Epicondyle, (4) Trochlea, (5) Olecranon, (6) Medial Epicondyle
C. (1) Capitellum, (2) Radial Head, (3) Lateral Epicondyle, (4) Olecranon (5) Trochlea, (6) Medial Epicondyle
D. **(1) Capitellum, (2) Radial Head, (3) Medial Epicondyle, (4) Trochlea, (5) Olecranon, (6) Lateral Epicondyle**

2. What is the pathology in this case?
A. **Displaced medial epicondyle**
B. Displaced lateral epicondyle
C. Bro, this case is normal

3. Which fractures are more common?
A. **Medial epicondyle more common than medial condyle**
B. Lateral epicondyle more common than lateral condyle
C. Medial condyle more common than medial epicondyle
D. All statements are false

The Dreaded Peds Elbow

So many little bones… damn these peds elbows

There are two major tricks with this one. (1) Because the medial epicondyle is an extra articular structure, its avulsion **will not necessarily result in a joint effusion**. (2) It **can get interposed** between the articular surface of the humerus and olecranon. Avulsed fragments can get stuck in the joint, even when there is no dislocation.

Anytime you see a dislocation – ask yourself - Is the patient 5 years old? And if so where is the medial epicondyle.

Remember CRITOE, you should never see the **TOE** before the **I**.

Lateral Condyle and Medial Epicondyle Fxs are common, the other ones aren't.

Case 44 - Chest Pain

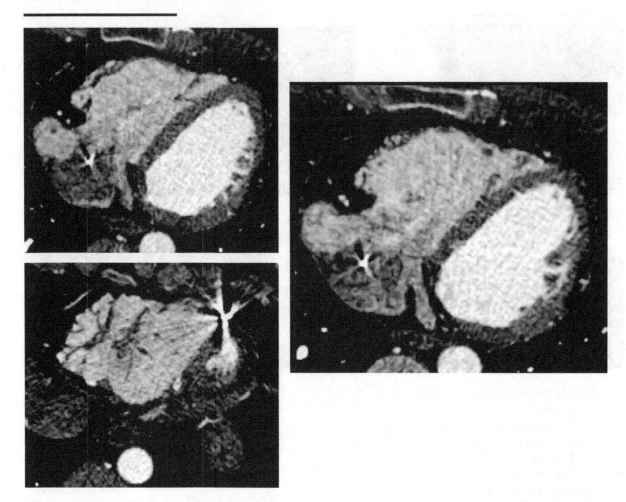

1. What is the diagnosis?
A. Hypertrophic Cardiomyopathy
B. Non-Compaction
C. Arrhythmogenic Right Ventricular Cardiomyopathy (ARVC)
D. TB

2. How do you get this?
A. Too much Burger King
B. Not enough Burger King
C. Smoking
D. Bad Luck (It's inherited).

3. What causes death (usually) ?
A. Ventricular Arrhythmia with Left Bundle Branch Blocks
B. A-Fib -> Stroke

Case 44 - ARVC

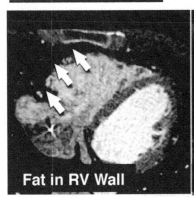
Fat in RV Wall

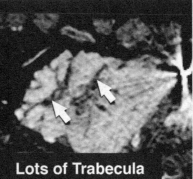
Lots of Trabecula

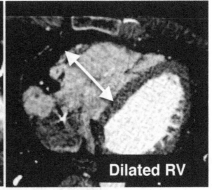
Dilated RV

1. What is the diagnosis?
A. Hypertrophic Cardiomyopathy
B. Non-Compaction
C. Arrhythmogenic Right Ventricular Cardiomyopathy (ARVC)
D. TB

2. How do you get this?
A. Too much Burger King
B. Not enough Burger King
C. Smoking
D. Bad Luck (It's inherited).

3. What causes death (usually) ?
A. Ventricular Arrhythmia with Left Bundle Branch Blocks
B. A-Fib -> Stroke

Arrhythmogenic Right Ventricular Cardiomyopathy (ARVC)

Inherited cardiomyopathy that causes sudden death in young men

Essential Trivia:

- Characterized by fibrofatty degeneration of the RV leading to arrhythmia and sudden death.

- Features include: dilated RV with reduced function, fibrofatty replacement of the myocardium, and normal LV.

- Cardiac MRI can do a lot of sneaky things. In particular, (1) High T1 signal in the RV wall — from all the fat, and (2) fat sat showing signal drop out in the RV.

- People use this major/minor criteria system that includes a bunch of EKG changes that no radiologist could possibly understand (if they are stupid enough to ask just say left bundle branch block).

Case 45 - History Withheld

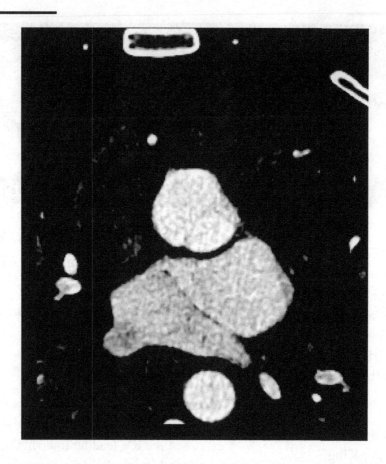

1. What is the diagnosis?
A. Hypoplastic Left Heart
B. Truncus Arteriosus
C. Cor Triatriatum Sinistrum
D. Tetrology of Fallot (TOF)

2. This structural abnormality mimics what valular disorder?
A. Aortic Stenosis
B. Mitral Stenosis
C. Tricuspid Regurgitation
D. Tricuspid Stenosis

3. The classic history is?
A. Pulmonary Hypertension in a newborn (unexplained)
B. Fainting spells in a teenager
C. Chest Pain in a 10 year old
D. It's totally asymptomatic - seen on autopsy incidentally

Case 45 - Cor Triatriatum Sinistrum

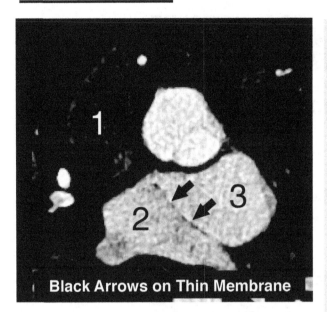

Black Arrows on Thin Membrane

Cor Triatriatum Sinistrum

Congenital heart defect where the left atrium is subdivided by a thin membrane - creating a 3 chamber look.

Essential Trivia:

- This is a very rare situation where you have an abnormal pulmonary vein draining into the left atrium (sinistrum meaning left) with an unnecessary fibromuscular membrane that causes a sub division of the left atrium.

- This creates the appearance of a tri-atrium heart.

- It can occur on the right side - and is called "dextrum" instead of "sinistrum", but this is extremely rare and is very unlikely to be tested (mainly because no one can find a case of it to show).

- This can be a cause of <u>unexplained pulmonary hypertension</u> in the peds setting.

- Basically it <u>acts like mitral stenosis</u>, and can cause pulmonary edema.

- The outcomes are often bad (fa b tal within two years), depending on surgical intervention and associated badness.

1. What is the diagnosis?
A. Hypoplastic Left Heart
B. Truncus Arteriosus
C. Cor Triatriatum Sinistrum
D. Tetrology of Fallot (TOF)

2. This structural abnormality mimics what valular disorder?
A. Aortic Stenosis
B. Mitral Stenosis
C. Tricuspid Regurgitation
D. Tricuspid Stenosis

3. The classic history is?
A. Pulmonary Hypertension in a newborn (unexplained)
B. Fainting spells in a teenager
C. Chest Pain in a 10 year old
D. It's totally asymptomatic - seen on autopsy incidentally

Case 46 - Chest Pain

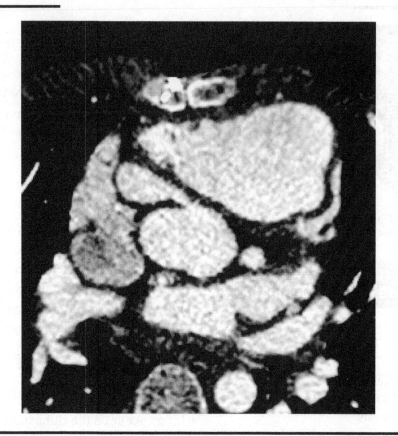

1. What is the diagnosis?
A. Anomalous Left Coronary Artery from the Pulmonary Artery (ALCPA)
B. Aberrant Course of the Left Coronary Artery
C. Coronary Artery Aneurysm
D. Endocarditis

2. In the United States what is the most common cause for this diagnosis?
A. Post Viral
B. Autoimmune
C. Too much Burger King (Atherosclerosis)
D. Not enough Burger King (Bacon Deficiency)

3. In children, this "?" is an important cause
A. Myocardial Bridging
B. Takayasu Arteritis
C. Kawasaki Arteritis
D. Atherosclerosis

Case 46 - Coronary Artery Aneurysm

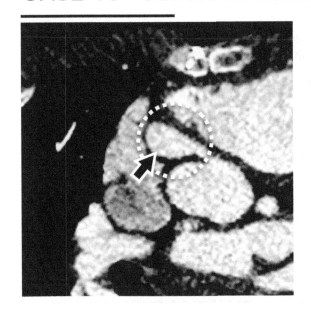

Coronary Artery Aneurysm

Dilated coronary 1.5 x the diameter of normal vessel.

Essential Trivia:

- If the coronary vessel has a fusiform dilation morphology think about a high flow state - i.e. coronary fistula

- In an adult think about atherosclerosis

- In a child think about Kawasaki

- Kawasaki can progress to coronary aneurysm about 25% of the time (if they don't get aspirin and gamma-globulin).

- A large percentage (like 50%) of the kawasaki aneurysms will regress.

- Cardiac cath is an important cause of these things as well. The testable pearl regarding that is that **caths cause pseudo aneurysms**, not the regular three wall dilations.

1. What is the diagnosis?
A. Anomalous Left Coronary Artery from the Pulmonary Artery (ALCPA)
B. Aberrant Course of the Left Coronary Artery
C. Coronary Artery Aneurysm
D. Endocarditis

2. In the United States what is the most common cause for this diagnosis?
A. Post Viral
B. Autoimmune
C. Too much Burger King (Atherosclerosis)
D. Not enough Burger King (Bacon Deficiency)

3. In children, this "?" is an important cause
A. Myocardial Bridging
B. Takayasu Arteritis
C. Kawasaki Arteritis
D. Atherosclerosis

Case 47 - Chest Pain

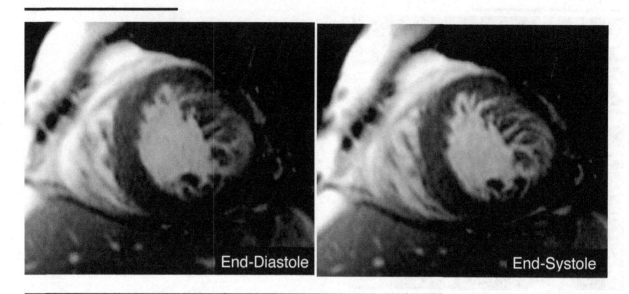

1. What is the diagnosis?
A. Hypertrophic Cardiomyopathy
B. Non-Compaction
C. Arrhythmogenic Right Ventricular Cardiomyopathy (ARVC)
D. TB

2. What is the "buzzword" for this condition?
A. Hypertrabeculated
B. Hypotrabeculated
C. Cylinder Heart
D. Vase Shaped Heart

3. On MRI the measurement made to make this diagnosis is performed during?
A. End Systole
B. End Diastole

Case 47 - Non-Compaction

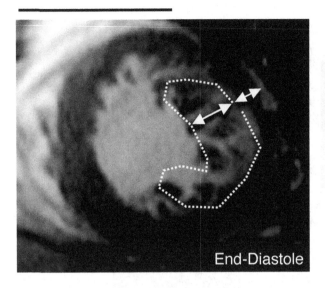

- Dilated LV with **very prominent trabeculation,**
- The trabeculated portion of the wall measures greater than 2.3 times the thickness of the compacted myocardial wall.

End-Diastole

1. What is the diagnosis?
A. Hypertrophic Cardiomyopathy
B. Non-Compaction
C. Arrhythmogenic Right Ventricular Cardiomyopathy (ARVC)
D. TB

2. What is the "buzzword" for this condition?
A. Hypertrabeculated
B. Hypotrabeculated
C. Cylinder Heart
D. Vase Shaped Heart

3. On MRI the measurement made to make this diagnosis is performed during?
A. End Systole
B. End Diastole

Non-Compaction

Uncommon congenital cardiomyopathy that is the result of loosely packed myocardium.

Essential Trivia:

- The left ventricle has a spongy appearance with increased trabeculations and deep intertrabecular recesses.

- The buzzword used is "Hyper-Trabeculated"

- Not only is the trabecula malformed, but the underlying capillary beds are screwed up too. This sets them up for ischemia, infarct, and fibrosis.

- As you might expect these guys get heart failure at a young age.

- With MRI, the diagnosis is made from a ratio of non-compacted **end-diastolic** myocardium to compacted **end-diastolic** myocardium of more than 2.3:1. *With ECHO this ratio is measured on end-systole.*

Case 48 - Chest Pain

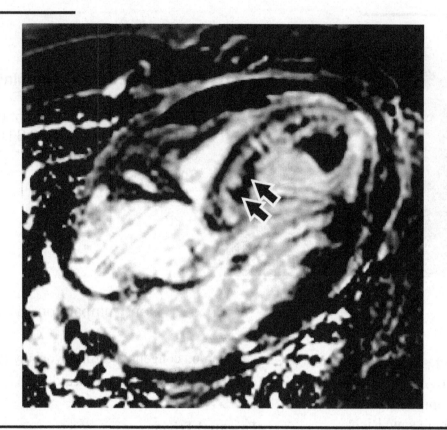

1. What is the diagnosis?
A. Hypertrophic Cardiomyopathy
B. Amyloidosis
C. Chronic Infarct
D. Acute Infarct

2. With regard to the finding near the arrow, is this a good thing?
A. Yes - it's associated with rapid recovery
B. Nope - it's associated with a lack of functional recovery

3. Which of the following is true?
A. Microvascular obstruction can be seen in both acute and chronic infarct
B. Chronic Infarct will have thickened myocardium, from hypertrophic scarring
C. In the setting of ischemia T2 bright tissue may represent salvageable tissue
D. Chronic Infarct will have delayed enhancement, Acute infarct will NOT

4. What vascular distribution is this in?
A. RCA
B. LAD
C. LCx (Circumflex)

Case 48 - Acute Infarct

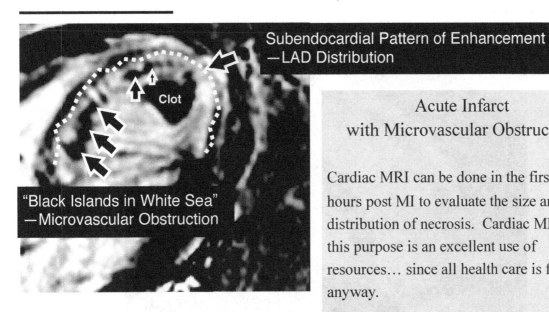

1. What is the diagnosis?
A. Hypertrophic Cardiomyopathy
B. Amyloidosis
C. Chronic Infarct
D. Acute Infarct

2. With regard to the finding near the arrow, is this a good thing?
A. Yes - it's associated with rapid recovery
B. Nope - it's associated with a lack of functional recovery

3. Which of the following is true?
A. Microvascular obstruction can be seen in both acute and chronic infarct
B. Chronic Infarct will have thickened myocardium, from hypertrophic scarring
C. In the setting of ischemia T2 bright tissue may represent salvageable tissue
D. Chronic Infarct will have delayed enhancement, Acute infarct will NOT

4. What vascular distribution is this in?
A. RCA
B. LAD
C. LCx (Circumflex)

Acute Infarct with Microvascular Obstruction

Cardiac MRI can be done in the first 24 hours post MI to evaluate the size and distribution of necrosis. Cardiac MRI for this purpose is an excellent use of resources... since all health care is free anyway.

Essential Trivia:

- Classic Look: zone of enhancement that extends from the subendocardium toward the epicardium in a vascular distribution

- *Microvascular obstruction* will present as islands of dark signal in the enhanced tissue and this represents an acute and subacute finding (**NOT Chronic**).

- Microvascular Obstruction is a poor prognostic finding, associated with lack of functional recovery

- In the acute setting (1 week) injured myocardium will have increased T2 signal, which can be used to estimate the area at risk.

- Both Acute and Chronic MI will have delayed enhancement.

- Acute MI can have normal thickness, Chronic tends to thin up.

Case 49 - Chest Pain

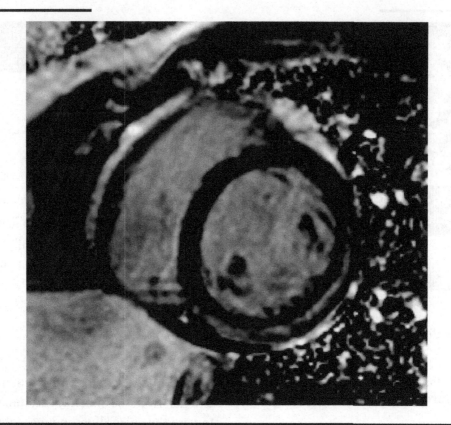

1. What is the diagnosis?
A. Constrictive Pericarditis
B. Myocarditis
C. Chronic Infarct
D. Acute Infarct

2. What vascular territory does this diagnosis favor?
A. LAD
B. RCA
C. LCX
D. Classically has a non-coronary distribution

3. The most common cause of this entity is?
A. Viral (Coxsackie virus B)
B. Bacterial (Strep)
C. Fungal (Candida)
D. Inherited (genetic)

Case 49 - Myocarditis

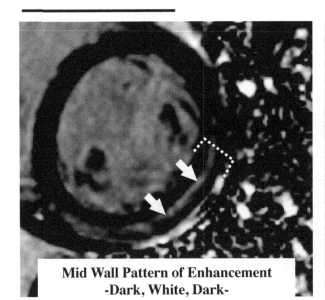

**Mid Wall Pattern of Enhancement
-Dark, White, Dark-**

1. What is the diagnosis?
A. Constrictive Pericarditis
B. Myocarditis
C. Chronic Infarct
D. Acute Infarct

2. What vascular territory does this diagnosis favor?
A. LAD
B. RCA
C. LCX
D. Classically has a non-coronary distribution

3. The most common cause of this entity is?
A. Viral (Coxsackie virus B)
B. Bacterial (Strep)
C. Fungal (Candida)
D. Inherited (genetic)

Myocarditis

Inflammation of the myocardium, from any number of random causes (drugs, viral, Lupus, parasites i.e. Trypanosome Cruzi / Chagas).

Essential Trivia:

- Inflammation of the heart can come from lots of causes (often viral i.e. Coxsackie virus).

- The late Gd enhancement follows a **non-vascular distribution** preferring the lateral free wall.

- The pattern will be epicardial or mid wall (**NOT subendocardial**).

- The main predictor of death (or transplant) is bi-ventricular wall motion abnormality

Cardiac MRI - Essential Trivia

Physics / Basic Technique

There are 3 main sequences you should be able to recognize, and understand.

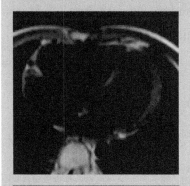 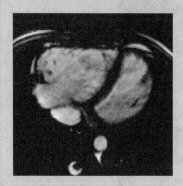 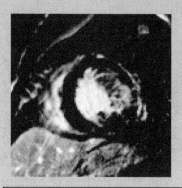

Dark Blood
-This is created with a *spin echo sequence*.
-More specifically a **"double inversion"** is used to null signal from flowing blood.
-The sequences take longer, but are better for anatomy, and more resistant to metal artifact.

Bright Blood
-This is created with a **gradient sequence**.
-The sequences are shorter and are considered the "work-horse" of the modality.
-This is used for ventricular function, blood velocity, & flow measurements.
-Just remember *"SSFP" steady state free precision*

Inversion Recovery
- The *"PSIR"* or Phase Sensitive Inversion Recovery
-Myocardium is nulled by selecting the correct T.I. - usually around 330 msec but this varies.
-The <u>T.I. is chosen when the myocardium is the darkest</u> (lets you see the white delayed enhancement the best).

Coronary Distributions

You should be able to recognize and distinguish the 3 territories on all axises. The "what vessel is involved?" questions, are just too easy to give up.

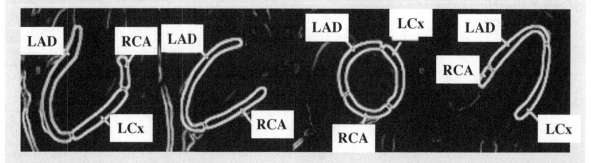

Aunt Minnie 109

Late Gad Enhancement Patterns

The last general topic to have cold for cardiac MRI is to have the distributions of late GD enhancement.

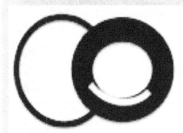
Subendocardial: Infarct

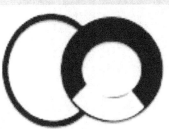
Transmural: Infarct

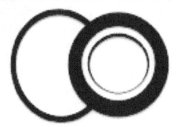
Subendocardial Circumferential Amyloidosis

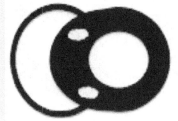
Mid-Wall "Cloudy" HOCM

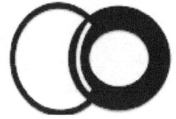
Mid-Wall - Crescent-Septal
Myocarditis, Idiopathic Dilated CM

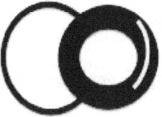
Mid-Wall Crescent -Lateral
Myocarditis, Sarcoidosis

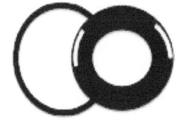
Epicardial:
Myocarditis, Sarcoidosis

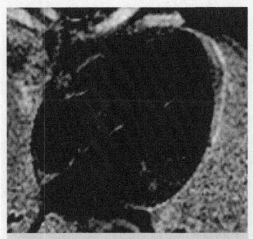
Blood Darker Than Myocardium on Inversion Recovery Sequence

Amyloid

Deposits in the myocardium causes abnormal diastolic function.

Classic Findings:
- Late Gd enhancement over the entire subendocardial circumference.
- The **myocardium is often difficult to suppress** (T.I. like 350 milliseconds). TI will be so long that the blood pool may be darker than the myocardium.

Case 50 - Chest Pain

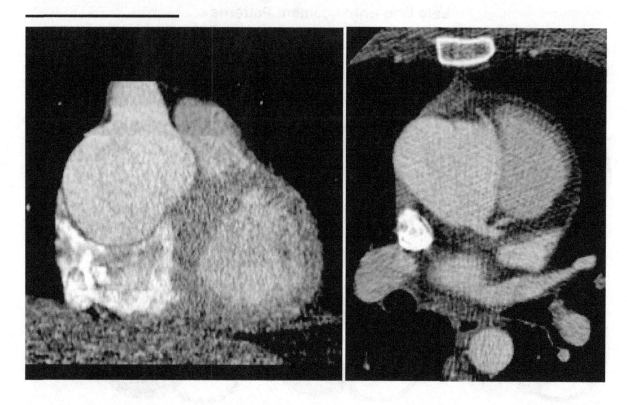

1. What is the diagnosis?
A. Ascending (tubular) Aortic Aneurysm
B. Coronary Artery Aneurysm
C. Coronary Sinus Aneurysm
D. Sinus of Valsalva Aneurysm

2. What part is most commonly involved?
A. Right
B. Left
C. Non coronary

3. What procedure is done to fix this?
A. Bentall
B. Glenn
C. Fontan
D. Jatene

Case 50 - Sinus of Valsalva Aneurysm

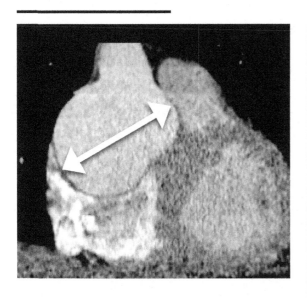

1. What is the diagnosis?
A. Ascending (tubular) Aortic Aneurysm
B. Coronary Artery Aneurysm
C. Coronary Sinus Aneurysm
D. Sinus of Valsalva Aneurysm

2. What part is most commonly involved?
A. Right
B. Left
C. Non coronary

3. What procedure is done to fix this?
A. Bentall
B. Glenn
C. Fontan
D. Jatene

Sinus of Valsalva Aneurysm

Aneurysm of of the Sinus of Valsalva (or the aortic sinus) are rare but do occur.

Essential Trivia:

- Valsalva sinus aneurysm occurs above the aortic valve annulus ("prolapsing aortic cusp" occurs below the annulus).

- These are seen in Marfans and Ehlers Danlos patients, but can also be acquired from infection.

- Most commonly involves the right coronary sinus

- VSD is the most common associated cardiac anomaly.

- Rupture can lead to cardiac tamponade.

- Surgical repair with Bentall procedure (graft replacement of the aortic root, ascending aorta, re-implantation of the coronaries, and replacement of the valve).

Case 51 - Tachyarrhythmia

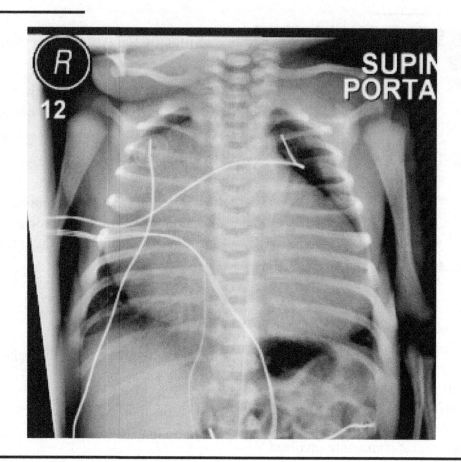

1. What is the diagnosis?
A. VSD
B. PDA
C. Tetralogy of Fallot
D. Ebsteins

2. What valve is abnormal?
A. Mitral
B. Tricuspid
C. Aortic

3. What teratogenic medication is often the culprit?
A. Coumadin
B. Valproic Acid
C. Lithium
D. ACE Inhibitors

CASE 51 - EBSTEIN'S ANOMALY

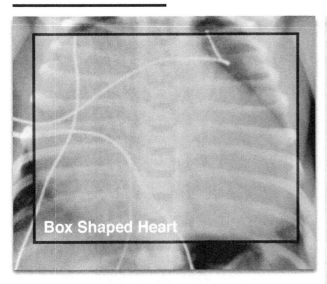

1. What is the diagnosis?
A. VSD
B. PDA
C. Tetralogy of Fallot
D. Ebsteins

2. What valve is abnormal?
A. Mitral
B. Tricuspid
C. Aortic

3. What teratogenic medication is often the culprit?
A. Coumadin
B. Valproic Acid
C. Lithium
D. ACE Inhibitors

Ebsteins Anomaly

Congenital Heart disease secondary to a malformed tricuspid valve. It produces a classic "box shaped" heart of CXR, and therefore is highly testable.

Essential Trivia:

- Seen in children whose moms used Lithium (most cases are actually sporadic).

- The **tricuspid valve is hypoplastic and the posterior leaf is displaced apically** (downward).

- The result is enlarged RA, decreased RV ("atrialized"), and tricuspid regurgitation.

- Often presents with fetal tachy-arrhythmia.

- Cyanosis depends on the degree of atrial shunting.

- The ASD is commonly associated.

- *Imaging Findings:*

  - CXR: They have the massive "**box shaped" heart**.

  - CT / MRI — if the tricuspid septal attachment lies more than 2 cm "beneath" (towards the apex) the mitral septal attachment, this is Ebstein anomaly.

Case 51 - Cyanosis

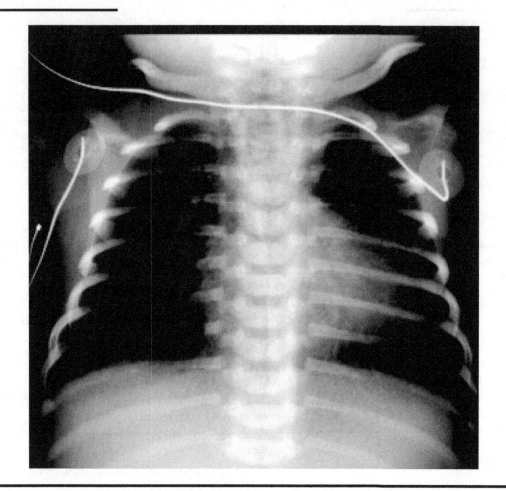

1. What is the diagnosis?
A. VSD
B. ASD
C. Tetralogy of Fallot
D. Truncus Arteriosus

2. In this disorder, the degree of symptoms is related to ?
A. How big the VSD is
B. How big the ASD is
C. The presence or absence of an aortic coarctation
D. How severe the RVOT obstruction is

3. The *"Blalock Taussig Shunt"* is a communication between?
A. Pulmonary Artery and Subclavian Vein
B. Pulmonary Artery and Subclavian Artery
C. Pulmonary Artery and SVC
D. Pulmonary Artery and Aorta

Case 51 - Tetralogy of Fallot (TOF)

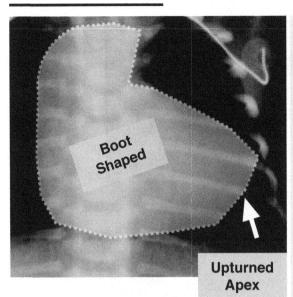

1. What is the diagnosis?
A. VSD **not cyanotic*
B. ASD **not cyanotic*
C. **Tetralogy of Fallot**
D. Truncus Arteriosus ** *would have increased pulmonary vasculature*

2. In this disorder, the degree of symptoms is related to ?
A. How big the VSD is
B. How big the ASD is
C. The presence or absence of an aortic coarctation
D. **How severe the RVOT obstruction is**

3. The *"Blalock Taussig Shunt"* is a communication between?
A. Pulmonary Artery and Subclavian Vein
B. **Pulmonary Artery and Subclavian Artery**
C. Pulmonary Artery and SVC
D. Pulmonary Artery and Aorta

Tetralogy of Fallot (TOF)

The "most common cyanotic heart disease."

Essential Trivia:

- Describes 4 major findings:
    (1) VSD,
    (2) RVOT Obstruction – often from valvular obstruction,
    (3) Overriding Aorta,
    (4) RV hypertrophy (develops after birth).

- The "boot shape" - with the upturned apex will not be present at birth, because the RV hypertrophy hasn't kicked it.

- The degree of severity in symptoms is related to how bad the RVOT obstruction is.

- Pentaology of Fallot if there is an ASD.

- Surgically it's usually fixed with primary repair. The various shunt procedures (Blalock-Taussig being the most famous) is only done if the kid is inoperable or to bridge until primary repair.

- Blalock-Taussig is a shunt between the PA and the Subclavian Artery

CXR Findings:

- Right Arch (I look for this first), TOF and Truncus are the Cyanotics that classically have it).

- Decreased/Normal Pulmonary Vasculature

- "Boot Shaped Heart" with upturned apex.

Case 52 - Cyanosis

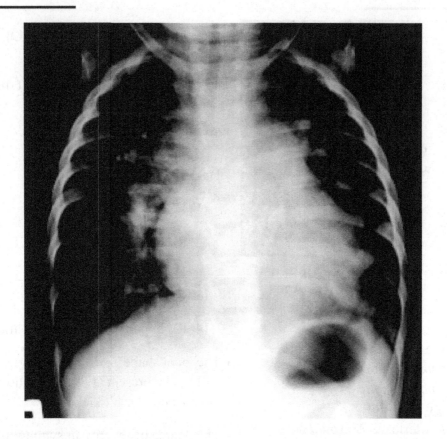

1. What is the diagnosis?
A. PDA
B. VSD
C. Supra-cardiac Total anomalous pulmonary venous return
D. Infra-cardiac Total anomalous pulmonary venous return

2. Which of the follow is commonly seen with this form of heart disease?
A. Polysplenia
B. Asplenia
C. Malrotation
D. Hirschsprung disease

3. What is required to survive with this form of heart disease
A. Aortic Stenosis
B. Left Ventricular Hypertrophy
C. Large PFO
D. Courage

Case 52 - Supra-Cardiac TAPVR

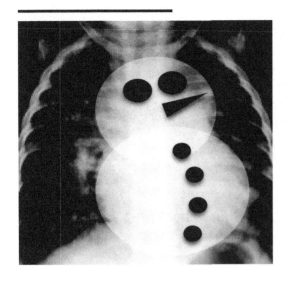

1. What is the diagnosis?
A. PDA ** *this is not cyanotic*
B. VSD ** *this is not cyanotic*
C. **Supra-cardiac Total anomalous pulmonary venous return**
D. Infra-cardiac Total anomalous pulmonary venous return ** *this tends to cause massive pulmonary edema in newborn, and not snowman*

2. Which of the follow is commonly seen with this form of heart disease?
A. Polysplenia
B. **Asplenia * seen with lots of cyanotic heart disease, but especially this one.**
C. Malrotation
D. Hirschsprung disease

3. What is required to survive with this form of heart disease
A. Aortic Stenosis
B. Left Ventricular Hypertrophy
C. **Large PFO**
D. Courage ** *although admirable sometimes that's just not enough, be your adversary cyanotic heart disease or a badly written multiple choice test.*

Tetralogy of Fallot (TOF)

A cyanotic heart disease characterized by all of the pulmonary venous system draining to the right side of the heart

Essential Trivia:

- There are 3 types, but only two are likely to be tested (cardiac type II just doesn't have good testable features).

  - Type I - Supra-Cardiac, the most common type. Veins drain ABOVE the heart giving you a **snowman** look to the heart

  - Type III - Infra-Cardiac. Veins drain BELOW the diaphragm (either into the IVC or hepatic veins), and classically get obstructed on the way back through the diaphragm - causing **full on pulmonary edema**

- Large PFO (or ASD) needed to survive

- **Asplenia** – 50% of asplenia patients have congenital heart issues, of those nearly 100% include TAPVR, (85% have additional endocardial cushion defects).

Congenital Heart - Essential Trivia

Cyanotic or NOT

I talk about this in greater depth in my book "Crack the CORE Exam," but you need to have a few lists memorized to help you eliminate distractors on multiple choice tests. The *first one and most important one is "Cyanotic or Not,"* this information is often found in the header of the question.

Cyanotic: Things that start with "T" ; TOF, TAPVR, Transposition, Truncus, Tricuspid Atresia.

NOT Cyanotic: ASD, VSD, PDA, PAPVR, and Aortic Coarctation (post ductal-adult type).

Congenital Heart Buzzwords

- I say "pulmonary edema is a newborn", you say TAPVR Type III (infracardiac)
- I say "small heart", you say Adrenal Insufficiency (Addison's) - "the Grinch who stole Christmas" would also be correct.
- I say "most common congenital heart disease - in child," you say VSD
- I say "most common congenital heart disease - in adult" you say Bicuspid AV
- I say "most common cyanotic heart disease," you say TOF
- I say "box shaped heart," you say Ebsteins
- I say "boot shaped heart," you say TOF
- I say "snow man shaped heart," you say TAPVR Type I (Supracardiac)
- I say "egg on a string shaped heart," you say Transposition
- I say "Right Arch," you say TOF or Truncus
- I say "Splaying the carina," you say left atrial hypertrophy
- I say "Right Sided PAPVR," you say Sinus Venosus ASD
- I say "Rib Notching," you say Aortic Coarctation
- I say "Aortic Coarctation," you say Bicuspid Valve
- I say "L-Type Transposition," you say "Lucky Type"
- I say "D-Type Transposition," you say "Doomed Type"
- I say "Asplenia," you say cyanotic heart disease (usually TAPVR)
- I say "Anterior indentation on esophagus," you say Pulmonary Sling
- I say "Supra-valvular aortic stenosis," you say Williams Syndrome
- I say "Right upper lobe pulmonary edema," you say mitral regurgitation

Congenital Heart Surgeries

Glenn:

This is a communication made between the SVC to the pulmonary artery (usually the right one).

It's done for tricuspid atresia and part of the staged hypo plastic heart repair.

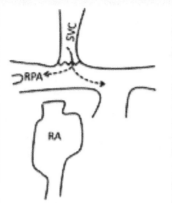

Glenn =
Vein to Artery
SVC to R-PA

Blalock Taussig Shunt:

Originally developed for use with TOF. Shunt is created between the Subclavian artery and the pulmonary artery.

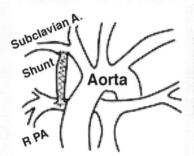

BT Shunt =
Artery to Artery
Subclavian A to PA

Ross Procedure:

Performed for Diseased Aortic Valves in Children. Replaces the aortic valve with the patient's pulmonary valve and replaces the pulmonary valve with a cryopreserved pulmonary valve homograft.

Ross =
-Aortic Valve Fix Using Pulmonic Valve
-Pulmonic Valve Gets a Homograft

Aortic Switch Procedures:

Used for transposition of the great vessels.

- **Senning** - Baffle (shunt thingy) - created from the right atrial wall and atrial septal tissue WITHOUT use of extrinsic material. *RV still systemic pump.*

- **Mustard** - Involves the resection of the atrial septum and creation of a baffle using pericardium (or synthetic material). *RV still systemic pump.*

- **Rastelli** - Baffle placed within the right ventricle diverting flow from the VSD to the aorta, essentially using the VSD as part of the LVOT. ***Pro - LV is systemic pump***, Con - kid will need multiple surgeries as he/she grows.

- **Jatene** - No baffle. Instead a direct resection of aorta and pulmonary artery, and direct switch. Requires coronary re-implantation. ***Pro - LV is systemic pump***, Con - very technically difficult surgery.

Case 53 - Chart Says "SOB," but He seems like a nice Guy to Me.

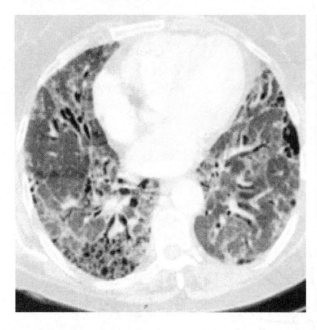
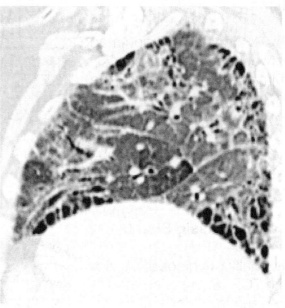

1. What is the diagnosis?
A. NSIP
B. DIP
C. UIP
D. COP

2. What is the trademark feature of this process?
A. Ground Glass
B. Nodules (Centrilobular)
C. Nodules (Perilymphatic)
D. Honeycombing

3. Where is the disease classically worse?
A. Apex
B. Base
C. There is typically no gradient

4. Could this be end stage sacroid?
A. Sure
B. Nope

Case 53 - UIP (Usual Interstitial Pneumonia)

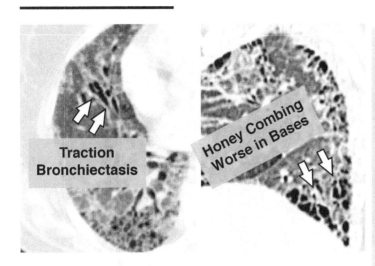

1. What is the diagnosis?
A. NSIP
B. DIP
C. UIP
D. COP

2. What is the trademark feature of this process?
A. Ground Glass
B. Nodules (Centrilobular)
C. Nodules (Perilymphatic)
D. Honeycombing

3. Where is the disease classically worse?
A. Apex
B. Base
C. There is typically no gradient

4. Could this be end stage sacroid?
A. Sure
B. **Nope** * *honeycombing is uncommon in end stage sarcoid. Also, that typically has an apical predominant pattern.*

UIP

This is the most common Interstitial Lung Disease. When the cause is idiopathic it is called IPF.

Essential Trivia:

- UIP describes a set of morphologic changes. You can get these changes from idiopathic disease (IPF) or from known end stage disease (RA, Scleroderma, etc…).

- The prognosis sucks (similar to lung CA)

- *CT Findings:*
  - Apical to basal gradient (worse in bases)
  - Traction bronchiectasis
  - Honeycombing is found 70% of the time, and people expect you to knee jerk UIP when that term is uttered.

- *CXR Findings:*
  - Low Lung Volumes (Fibrosis)
  - Reticular pattern in the posterior costophrenic angle is supposedly the first finding on CXR.

Case 54 - The ED is convinced he has a PE

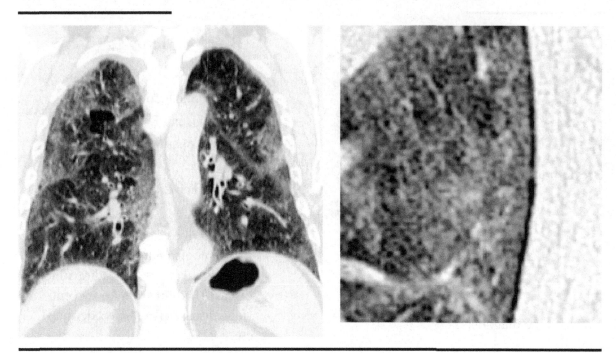

1. What interstitial lung disease does this dude have?
A. NSIP
B. DIP
C. UIP
D. COP

2. What is the trademark feature of this lung process?
A. Ground Glass
B. Nodules (Centrilobular)
C. Nodules (Perilymphatic)
D. Honeycombing

3 What is the "buzzword" for this disease?
A. Honey combing
B. Reticulation
C. Sub pleural sparing

Case 54 - NSIP (Nonspecific Interstitial Pneumonia)

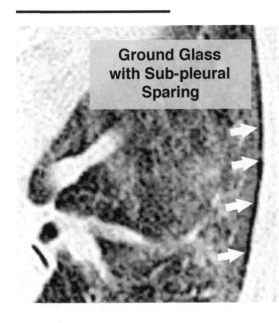

1. What interstitial lung disease does this dude have?
A. **NSIP**
B. DIP
C. UIP
D. COP

2. What is the trademark feature of this lung process?
A. **Ground Glass**
B. Nodules (Centrilobular)
C. Nodules (Perilymphatic)
D. Honeycombing

3. What is the "buzzword" for this disease?
A. Honey combing
B. Reticulation
C. **Sub pleural sparing**

NSIP

Less Common than UIP. Even though the name infers that its non-specific, it's actually a specific entity.

Essential Trivia:

- Histologically it is homogeneous inflammation or fibrosis (UIP was heterogeneous).

- It is a common pattern in collagen vascular disease, and drug reactions.

- It is the **most common interstitial lung disease seen with scleroderma**

- There are two flavors: cellular (the good one - with mostly ground glass), and fibrotic (the bad one with bronchiectasis)

- *CT Findings:*

  - Distribution is lower lobe, posterior, and peripheral predominant

  - Sparing of the immediate sub pleural lung from the ground glass is seen in 50% of cases, and is "classic"

  - Honeycombing (when present, and lower lobe predominant) is *"the most useful HRCT feature"* to differentiate histologic UIP from either fibrotic or cellular NSIP. In other words, **lower lobe honeycombing = UIP.**

Case 55 - Chest Pain

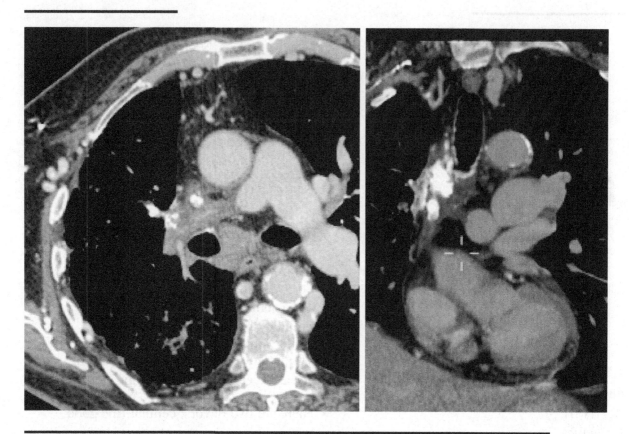

1. What is the diagnosis?
A. Lymphoma (not treated)
B. RA
C. Fibrosing Mediastinitis
D. Mediastinal Lipomatosis

2. What is the "classic cause" (not necessarily the most common) ?
A. Histoplasmosis
B. EBV
C. AIDS
D. Varicella

3. What is the dreaded complication when present in this location?
A. Metastasis to the myocardium
B. Metastasis to the lung parenchyma
C. Superior Vena Cava Syndrome
D. MI

Case 55 - Fibrosing Mediastinitis

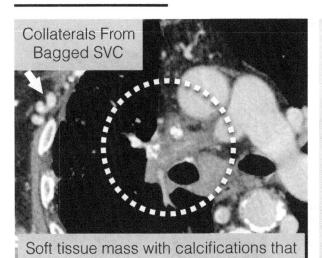

Soft tissue mass with calcifications that infiltrates the normal fat planes.

1. What is the diagnosis?
A. Lymphoma (not treated)
B. RA
C. Fibrosing Mediastinitis
D. Mediastinal Lipomatosis

2. What is the "classic cause" (not necessarily the most common) ?
A. Histoplasmosis
B. EBV
C. AIDS
D. Varicella

3. What is the dreaded complication when present in this location?
A. Metastasis to the myocardium
B. Metastasis to the lung parenchyma
C. Superior Vena Cava Syndrome
D. MI

Fibrosing Mediastinitis

Non malignant fibrous tissue proliferative condition occurring within the mediastinum.

Essential Trivia:

- It's classically caused by histoplasmosis (but the most common cause is actually idiopathic).

- Other causes include TB, radiation, and Sarcoid.

- It's a soft tissue mass with calcifications that infiltrates the normal fat planes.

- It has been known to cause superior vena cava syndrome.

- It's associated with retroperitoneal fibrosis when idiopathic - in the "IgG4" spectrum / associated disorders.

- IgG4s that go together *(if you see one think of the others... the test writers will)*:

  - Fibrosing Mediastinitis
  - Retroperitoneal Fibrosis
  - Autoimmune Pancreatitis
  - Tubulointerstitial nephritis
  - Orbital Pseudotumor

  - *Basically all the weird fibrosing shit*

Case 56 - Cough

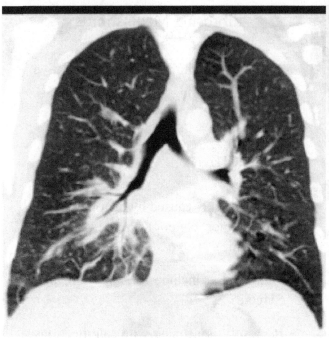
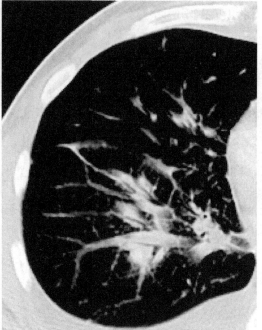

1. What is the diagnosis (*did I mention he enjoys unprotected sex with multiple anonymous partners while at the same time experimenting with mind altering IV drugs*) ?
A. PCP
B. CMV
C. Kaposi Sarcoma
D. AIDS related pulmonary lymphoma

2. Your attending thinks it's either Kaposi Sarcoma or Lymphoma- how can you tell the difference (other than the classic CT findings seen in this case) ?
A. Kaposi is Thallium Positive, Gallium Negative, Lymphoma is Thallium Positive
B. Kaposi is Thallium Positive, Gallium Positve, Lymphoma is Thallium Negative
C. Kaposi is Thallium Negative, Gallium Negative, Lymphoma is Thallium Positive
D. They are both negative on Thallium and Gallium… *clinical correlation*

3. For this disease to occur, the CD4 count must be less than?
A. 400
B. 200
C. 50

Case 56 - Kaposi Sarcoma:

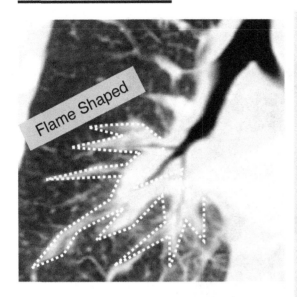

1. What is the diagnosis (*did I mention he enjoys unprotected sex with multiple anonymous partners while at the same time experimenting with mind altering IV drugs*) ?
   A. PCP
   B. CMV
   C. Kaposi Sarcoma
   D. AIDS related pulmonary lymphoma

2. Your attending thinks it's either Kaposi Sarcoma or Lymphoma- how can you tell the difference (other than the classic CT findings seen in this case) ?
   A. Kaposi is Thallium Positive, Gallium Negative, Lymphoma is Thallium Positive
   B. Kaposi is Thallium Positive, Gallium Positve, Lymphoma is Thallium Negative
   C. Kaposi is Thallium Negative, Gallium Negative, Lymphoma is Thallium Positive
   D. They are both negative on Thallium and Gallium... *clinical correlation*

3. For this disease to occur, the CD4 count must be less than?
   A. 400
   B. 200
   C. 50

Kaposi Saarcoma

Tumor caused by Herpes Virus 8, and commonly seen in AIDS patient

Essential Trivia:

- This is the most common lung tumor in AIDS patients (Lymphoma is number two).

- A CD4 count less than 200 is needed

- The tracheobronchial mucosa and perihilar lung are favored.

- The buzzword is **"flame shaped."**

- A bloody pleural effusion is common (50%).

- Hypervascular lymph nodes *(also seen in Castlemans)*

- Slow Growth, with asymptomatic patients (despite lungs looking terrible)

- Nukes correlations:

  - *Kaposi:*
    - **Gallium Negative**
    - Thallium Positive

  - *Lymphoma*
    - Gallium Positive
    - Thallium Postitive

The way to remember this is that Thallium works on the Na/K+ pump mimicking K+, it needs a living cell to work. Gallium just works with inflammation and Kaposi is not that inflammatory (why the lungs look worse than the patient feels).

Case 57 - Cough:

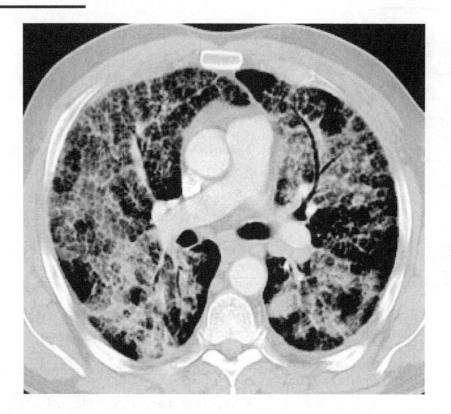

1. What is the diagnosis ?
A. Castlemans
B. PAP
C. Lipoid Pneumonia
D. Hypersensitivity Pneumonia

2. This is *"Strongly Associated with the Disease"* ?
A. EtOH Abuse
B. AIDS
C. Smoking
D. Anti-Rejection Drugs

3. This patient has a brain abscess, what do you think the culture is gonna grow?
A. Strep
B. Staph
C. Nocardia
D. Neurocysticercosis

Case 57 - Pulmonary Alveolar Proteinosis (PAP)

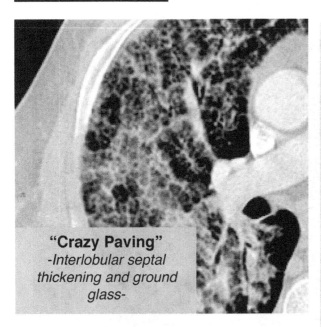

"Crazy Paving"
-Interlobular septal thickening and ground glass-

1. What is the diagnosis ?
A. Castlemans
B. PAP
C. Lipoid Pneumonia
D. Hypersensitivity Pneumonia

2. This is *"Strongly Associated with the Disease"* ?
A. EtOH Abuse
B. AIDS
C. Smoking
D. Anti-Rejection Drugs

3. This patient has a brain abscess, what do you think the culture is gonna grow?
A. Strep
B. Staph
C. Nocardia
D. Neurocysticercosis

PAP

Rare lung disease secondary to abnormal surfactant accumulation.

Essential Trivia:

- This can be primary (90%), or secondary (10%). Secondary causes include cancer or inhalation (silico-proteinosis).

- They are at increased risk of Nocardia infections, and can have nocardia brain abscess.

- Smoking is strongly associated with the disease.

- When seen in children (presenting before age 1) there is a known association with alymphoplasia.

- Can progress to pulmonary fibrosis (30%).

Crazy Paving - The classic imaging finding.

- *Interlobular septal thickening and ground glass.*

- This isn't always PAP, in fact in real life that it is usually NOT PAP. There is a differential that includes common things like edema, hemorrhage, BAC, Acute Interstitial Pneumonia.

- Just know that for the purpose of multiple choice test the answer is almost always PAP.

Case 58 - Wheezy

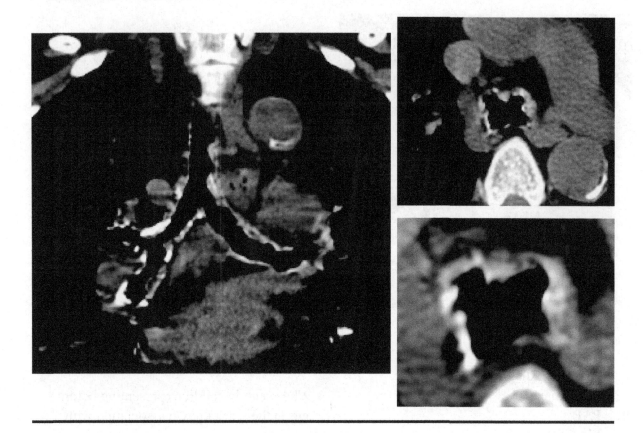

1. What is the diagnosis ?
A. Wegeners
B. Amyloid
C. Tracheobronchopathia Osteochondroplastica (TBO)
D. Saber Sheath Trachea

2. This is finding is critical to narrowing your differential:
A. Involvement of the left main stem
B. Involvement of the right main stem
C. Sparing of the posterior membrane
D. Lung Parenchymal Involvement

3. Relapsing Polychondritis (which has a similar look), differs from this entity by?
A. Sparing of the posterior membrane
B. Involving of the posterior membrane
C. Involvement of the right main stem
D. Smooth Thickening (instead of bumpy nodules)

Case 58 - Tracheobronchopathia Osteochondroplastica (TBO)

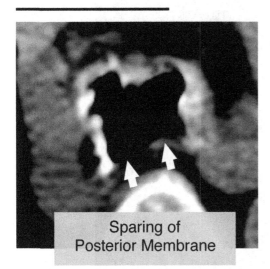

Sparing of Posterior Membrane

1. What is the diagnosis ?
A. Wegeners
B. Amyloid
C. Tracheobronchopathia Osteochondroplastica (TBO)
D. Saber Sheath Trachea

2. This is finding is critical to narrowing your differential:
A. Involvement of the left main stem
B. Involvement of the right main stem
C. Sparing of the posterior membrane
D. Lung Parenchymal Involvement

3. Relapsing Polychondritis(which has a similar look), differs from this entity by?
A. Sparing of the posterior membrane
B. Involving of the posterior membrane
C. Involvement of the right main stem
D. Smooth Thickening (instead of bumpy nodules)

Tracheobronchopathia Osteochondroplastica (TBO)

Rare airway disease characterized by the presence of nodules on the trachea and bronchial walls.

Essential Trivia:

- **Spares the posterior membrane.**

- You have development of cartilaginous and osseous nodules within the submucosa of the tracheal and bronchial walls.

- Classically involves the lower 2/3rds of the trachea and proximal portions of the bronchi.

- *Most patients are asymptomatic*, and it's an incidental findings. (Sometimes they ulcerate & bleed -> hemoptysis in the setting of infection).

- **DDx:**

  - *Relapsing Polychondritis* - Also **spares the posterior membrane.** But, has smooth narrowing (not nodules). These guys have symptoms, and get systemic cartilage issues & recurrent pneumonia.

  - *Amyloid* - Can involve the trachea, but typically **does involve the posterior membrane.**

  - *Wegeners* - The trachea is often involved. *Does involve the posterior membrane.*

Case 59 - History withheld

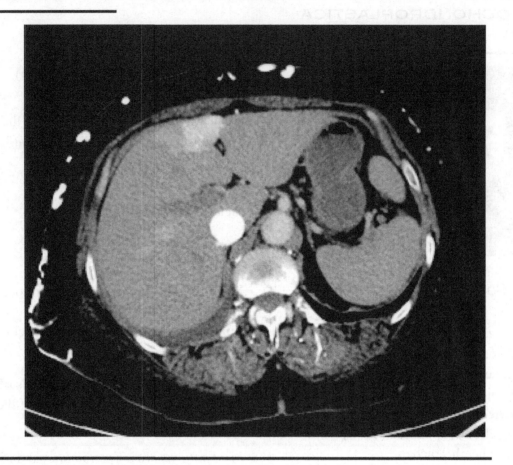

1. Where should you look next?
A. The Brain
B. The Scrotum
C. The Mediastinum
D. The Colon

2. The most common etiology for the underlying cause of this finding is?
A. Malignancy (Lung CA or Lymphoma)
B. Malignancy (Colon CA)
C. Malignancy (HCC)
D. Histoplasmosis

Case 59 - HOT Quadrate Sign - SVC Obstruction

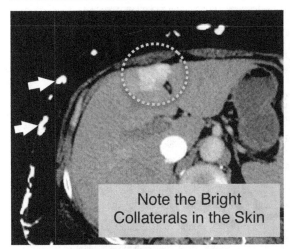

Note the Bright Collaterals in the Skin

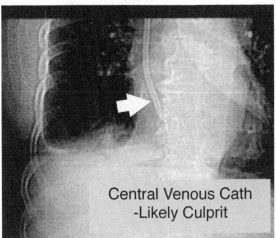

Central Venous Cath - Likely Culprit

1. Where should you look next?
A. The Brain
B. The Scrotum
C. The Mediastinum
D. The Colon

2. The most common etiology for the underlying cause of this finding is?
A. Malignancy (Lung CA or Lymphoma)
B. Malignancy (Colon CA)
C. Malignancy (HCC)
D. Histoplasmosis

HOT Quadrate / SVC Obstruction

A well described finding of SVC Obstruction, which can trick the un-initiated… but we are initiated.

Essential Trivia:

- The mechanism is complicated, and involves disruption of collateral pathways. The gist of it is, extra blood is forced into the umbilical and paraumbilical veins which preferentially drain into the left branch of the portal vein. All this extra flow results in a systemic-portal shunt, causing increased blood flow in the arterial phase of the liver supplied by the left branch of the portal vein - hence the hot quadrate.

- **SVC syndrome** is one of only two reasons a radiation oncologist has to get out of bed at night (the other is cauda equina syndrome).

- Obstruction of the SVC - most commonly from a malignancy (lung or lymphoma) can cause facial swelling, arm swelling, and generalized badness.

- Other causes include scarring from central venous catheters (as in this case), pace maker wires, or fibrosing mediastinitis.

Case 60 - Belly Pain

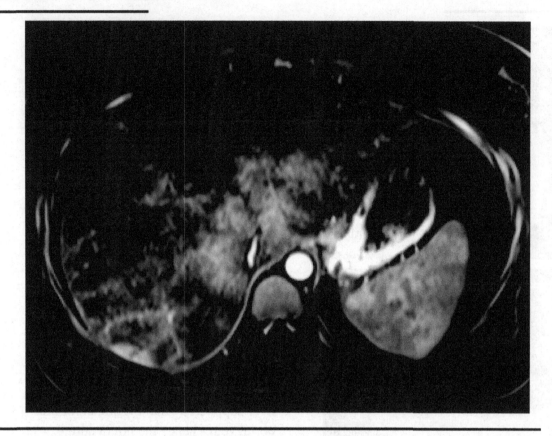

1. What is the diagnosis ?
A. HCC
B. Cholangiocarcinoma
C. Budd Chiari
D. Hemochromatosis

2. The most common etiology for the underlying cause of this finding is?
A. Birth Control
B. Protein C and/or S def
C. Idiopathic
D. Pregnancy

3. Which part of the liver classically enlarges with this entity?
A. Quadrate
B. Caudate
C. Segment 3
D. Segment 5

Case 60 - Budd Chiari Syndrome

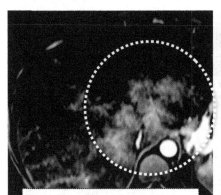

Enhancement Centrally, with Delayed Perfusion Peripherally

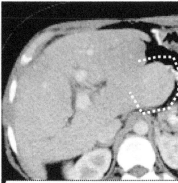

Caudate Lobe Hypertrophy

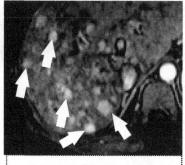

Hyperplastic Nodules - Enhancing vascular Nodules seen in Budd Chiari (they aren't cancer)

1. What is the diagnosis ?
A. HCC
B. Cholangiocarcinoma
C. Budd Chiari
D. Hemochromatosis

2. The most common etiology for the underlying cause of this finding is?
A. Birth Control
B. Protein C and/or S def
C. Idiopathic
D. Pregnancy

3. Which part of the liver classically enlarges with this entity?
A. Quadrate
B. Caudate
C. Segment 3
D. Segment 5

Budd Chiari

Hepatic vein outflow obstruction.

Essential Trivia:

- Presentation can be acute or chronic.

    - Acute from thrombus into the hepatic vein or IVC. These guys will present with rapid onset ascites.

    - Chronic from fibrosis of the intrahepatic veins, presumably from inflammation.

Classic Findings

- Massive **caudate lobe hypertrophy** (spared from separate drainage into the IVC).

- The enhancement pattern will be "flip-flopped" with enhancement of the central liver early, and peripheral portion later.

- The liver has been described as **"nutmeg"** with an inhomogeneous mottled appearance, and delayed enhancement of the periphery of the liver.

- Regenerative (Hyperplastic) Nodules - big and multiple - ** *vascular nodules that simulate HCC.*

Case 62 - Belly Pain After Bicycle Wreck (Age 5)

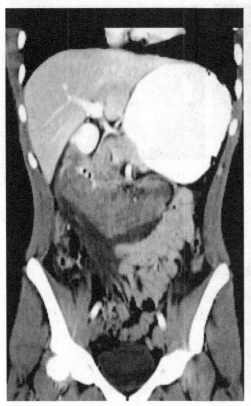
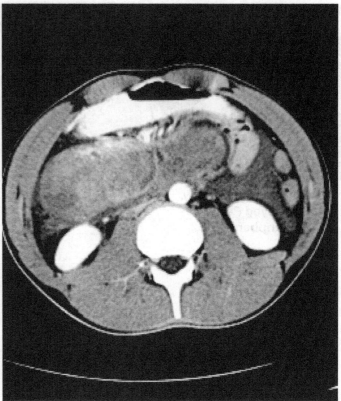

1. What is the diagnosis of exclusion for this same finding in a 6 month old?
A. Adenocarcinoma
B. Intussusception
C. Non-Accidental Trauma
D. Neuroblastoma

2. What finding would make a bad situation worse for this kid?
A. Adjacent fluid collection without contrast
B. Duodenal wall thickening
C. Free Air in the Retroperitoneum
D. Aspiration Pneumonia

3. What is the most common cause of pancreatitis in a child?
A. Gallstones
B. EtOH
C. Medication Induced
D. ERCP
E. Trauma

Case 62 - Duodenal Hematoma

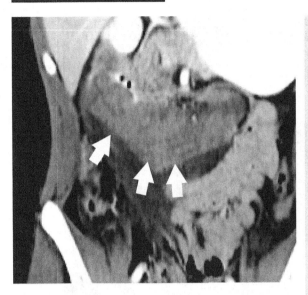

1. What is the diagnosis of exclusion for this finding in a 6 month old?
   A. Adenocarcinoma
   B. Intussusception
   C. Non-Accidental Trauma
   D. Neuroblastoma

2. What finding would make a bad situation worse for this kid?
   A. Adjacent fluid collection without contrast
   B. Duodenal wall thickening
   C. Free Air in the Retroperitoneum
   D. Aspiration Pneumonia

3. What is the most common cause of pancreatitis in a child?
   A. Gallstones
   B. EtOH
   C. Medication Induced
   D. ERCP
   E. Trauma

Duodenal Hematoma

Hepatic vein outflow obstruction.

Essential Trivia:

- If you see these findings (or traumatic pancreatitis) in any kid to young to ride a bike you have to think about non-accidental trauma.

- The case becomes surgical if there is perforation (which is not uncommon). You have to look for gas or contrast in the retroperitoneum

- Fluid collections (without contrast) can be seen without perforation - they aren't that helpful.

- If it's not perforated - they can usually manage it conservatively.

- Back in the stone ages ED Docs / Surgeons did a thing called *"peritoneal lavage"* where they would try and aspirate the peritoneum looking for blood. This would *cause a false positive for rupture on the later CT (air bubbles in the retro-peritoneum)*. Since this practice hasn't been performed since the Cretaceous period it's unlikely that the "test of the future" would ask anything about it. Unless the person writing the questions trained during that period (which is likely).

Case 63 - Belly Pain

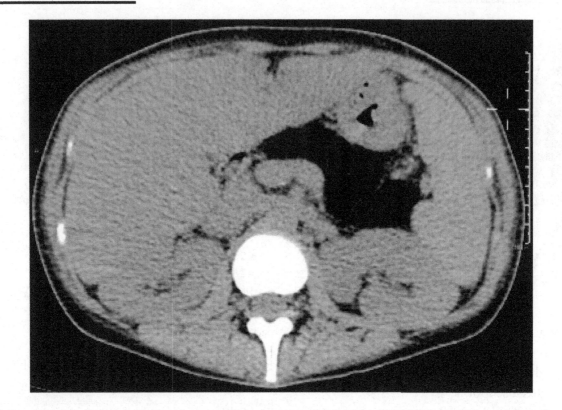

1. What is the diagnosis ?
A. Neuroblastoma
B. Sickle Cell
C. Non-Accidental Trauma
D. Cystic Fibrosis

2. What if I told you this kid is short and has bad eczema (and no friends) ?
A. Dorsal Pancreatic Agenesis
B. Shwachman-Diamond Syndrome
C. Alagille Syndorme
D. Blackfan-Diamond Anemia

3. Where is the pancreas located?
A. Intraperitoneal
B. Retroperitoneal

Case 63 - Cystic Fibrosis

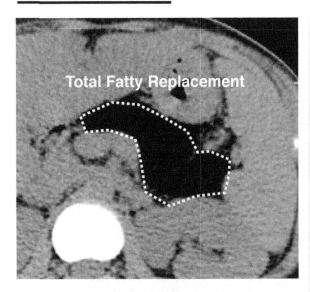

1. What is the diagnosis ?
A. Neuroblastoma
B. Sickle Cell
C. Non-Accidental Trauma
D. Cystic Fibrosis

2. What if I told you this kid is short and has bad eczema (and no friends) ?
A. Dorsal Pancreatic Agenesis
B. Shwachman-Diamond Syndrome
C. Alagille Syndorme
D. Blackfan-Diamond Anemia

3. Where is the pancreas located?
A. Intraperitoneal
B. Retroperitoneal *the tail can be intraperiotneal*

Cystic Fibrosis

"Lipomatous pseudohypertrophy of the pancreas," as seen commonly in CF.

Essential Trivia:

- The pancreas is affected in 85-90% of CF patients.

- Inspissated secretions cause proximal duct obstruction leading to the two main changes in CF:

    - (1) Fibrosis (decreased T1 and T2 signal) and the more common one

    - (2) Fatty replacement (increased T1).

- Patient's with CF, who are diagnosed as adults, tend to have more pancreas problems than those diagnosed as children.

- Those with residual pancreatic exocrine function can have bouts of recurrent acute pancreatitis.

- Small (1-3mm) pancreatic cysts are common.

- **Fibrosing Colonopathy:** Wall thickening of the proximal colon as a complication of enzyme replacement therapy.

- **Shwachman-Diamond Syndrome:** It also causes lipomatous pseudohypertrophy of the pancreas, and is the 2nd most common cause of pancreatic insufficiency in kids (CF #1). Basically, it's a kid with diarrhea, short stature (metaphyseal chondroplasia), and eczema.

Case 64 - Belly Pain

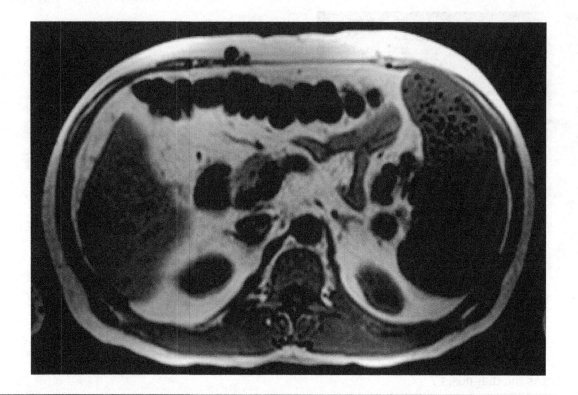

1. What is the diagnosis ?
A. Peliosis
B. Multiple Hemangiomas
C. Sarcoidosis
D. Portal Hypertension

2. What sequence on MRI would be the most sensitive for this finding?
A. Turbo Spin Echo
B. Fast Spin Echo
C. STIR
D. Gradient

3. This finding is the result of?
A. Micro-hemorrhage in the setting of metastatic invasion
B. Micro-hemorrhage seen after a trauma
C. Micro-hemorrhage in the setting of portal hypertension
D. A side effect of endoleak treatment

Case 64 - Gamna Gandy Bodies

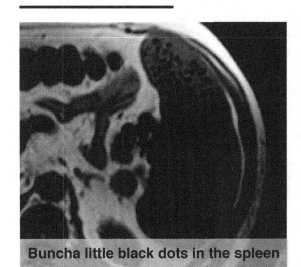

Buncha little black dots in the spleen

1. What is the diagnosis ?
A. Peliosis
B. Multiple Hemangiomas
C. Sarcoidosis
D. Portal Hypertension

2. What sequence on MRI would be the most sensitive for this finding?
A. Turbo Spin Echo
B. Fast Spin Echo
C. STIR
D. Gradient

3. This finding is the result of?
A. Micro-hemorrhage in the setting of metastatic invasion
B. Micro-hemorrhage seen after a trauma
C. Micro-hemorrhage in the setting of portal hypertension
D. A side effect of endoleak treatment

Gamna Gandy Bodies

Also called Siderotic Nodules, they are basically small foci of hemosiderin.

Essential Trivia:

- *Mechanism:* Micro-hemorrhage resulting in hemosiderin and calcium deposition followed by fibroblastic reaction.

- *Who gets them?* Classically **Portal Hypertension**, but they can also be seen in sickle cell (and a whole bunch of other random things).

- They are gonna be dark on T1 and T2 but remember that Gradient is going to be most sensitive because of the local field effects (Spin Echo sequences make a more homogeneous field because of the 180 degree refocusing pulse).

Case 65 - Rectal Bleeding

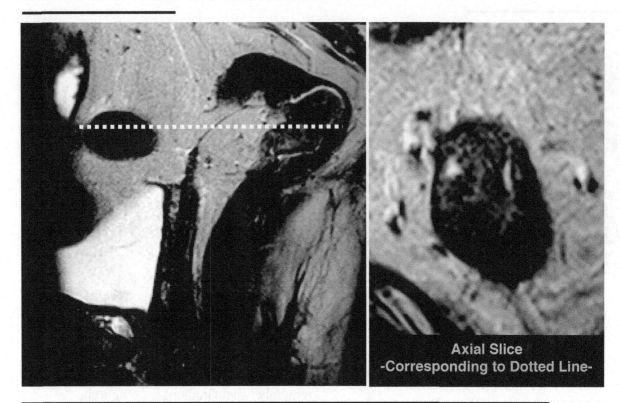

Axial Slice
-Corresponding to Dotted Line-

1. What stage is it ?
A. T1
B. T2
C. T3
D. T4

2. What changes surgically between Stage 2 and Stage 3?
A. Stage 2 gets Chemo, Stage 3 is palliative only
B. Stage 2 gets Surgery, Stage 3 is palliative only
C. Stage 2 gets Surgery, Stage 3 gets chemo/radiation first (then surgery)
D. Stage 2 gets Radiation only, Stage 3 gets chemo and radiation

3. What changes surgically between cancer in the lower 3rd vs middle 3rd?
A. Lower 1/3 gets a Lower Anterior Resection and keeps continence - no diaper :)
B. Lower 1/3 gets a Lower Anterior Resection and loses continence - diaper time :(
C. Lower 1/3 gets a Abdominal Perineal Resection and keeps continence - no diaper :)
D. Lower 1/3 gets a Abdominal Perineal Resection and loses continence - diaper time :(

Case 65 - Rectal Cancer - Stage 3

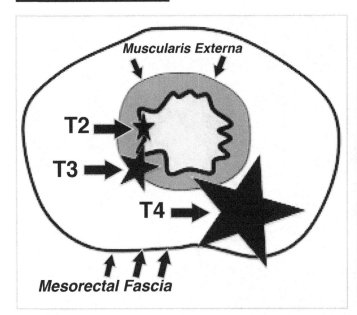

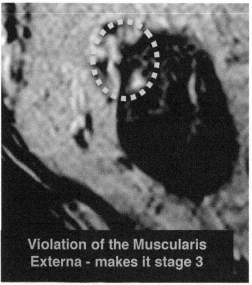

Violation of the Muscularis Externa - makes it stage 3

1. What stage is it ?
A. T1
B. T2
C. T3
D. T4

2. What changes surgically between Stage 2 and Stage 3?
A. Stage 2 gets Chemo, Stage 3 is palliative only
B. Stage 2 gets Surgery, Stage 3 is palliative only
C. Stage 2 gets Surgery, Stage 3 gets chemo/ radiation first (then surgery)
D. Stage 2 gets Radiation only, Stage 3 gets chemo and radiation

3. What changes surgically between cancer in the lower 3rd vs middle 3rd?
A. Lower 1/3 gets a Lower Anterior Resection and keeps continence - no diaper :)
B. Lower 1/3 gets a Lower Anterior Resection and loses continence - diaper time :(
C. Lower 1/3 gets a Abdominal Perineal Resection and keeps continence - no diaper :)
D. Lower 1/3 gets a Abdominal Perineal Resection and loses continence - *Diaper Time :(*

Rectal Cancer

Essential Trivia:

- Nearly always (98%) adenocarcinoma

- If the path says Squamous - the cause was HPV (use your imagination on how it got there).

- Total mesorectal excision is standard surgical method

- Lower rectal cancer (0-5 cm from the anorectal angle), has the highest recurrence rate, and gets the dreaded APR for surgery resulting in the loss of continence. LAR is used for tumors in the upper 2/3 and preserves sphincter function.

- MRI is used to stage (contrast is NOT needed).

- Stage T3 - called when tumor breaks out of the muscularis externa (outer layer of rectum) and into the peri-rectal fat.

- Stage T4 - called when the tumor abuts the mesorectal fascia (this is bad news).

Case 66 - Belly Pain

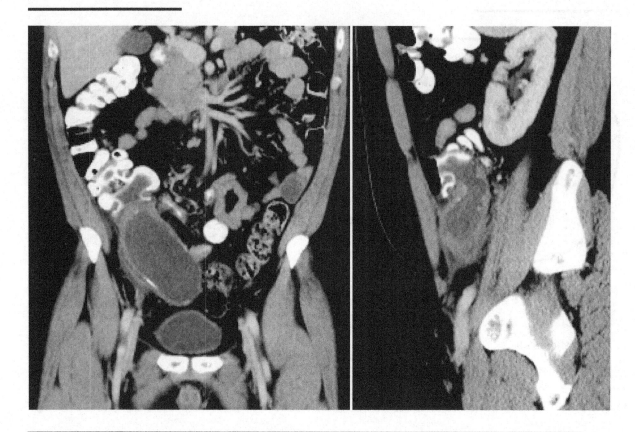

1. What is the diagnosis?
A. Carcinoid
B. Crohns
C. Ulcerative Colitis
D. Appendiceal Mucocele

2. This thing isn't cancer right?
A. Oh no way, that thing is fine. It's just a giant snot booger.
B. That thing is totally cancer - this guy is screwed.
C. It's hard to tell… could be.

3. What is a feared complication of this entity?
A. Paraneoplastic syndrome (SIADH)
B. Bowel Infarct
C. Stricture from chronic inflammation
D. Pseudomyxoma peritonei

Case 66 - Appendiceal Mucocele

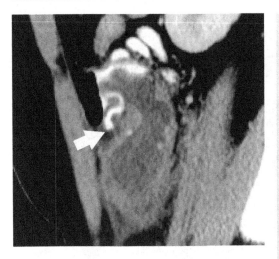

1. What is the diagnosis?
A. Carcinoid
B. Crohns
C. Ulcerative Colitis
D. **Appendiceal Mucocele**

2. This thing isn't cancer right?
A. Oh no way, that thing is fine. It's just a giant snot booger.
B. That thing is totally cancer - this guy is screwed.
C. **It's hard to tell… could be.**

3. What is a feared complication of this entity?
A. Paraneoplastic syndrome (SIADH)
B. Bowel Infarct
C. Stricture from chronic inflammation
D. **Pseudomyxoma peritonei**

Appendiceal Mucocele

Essential Trivia:

- Cystic dilation of the appendix thought to be secondary to proximal luminal obstruction (fecalith, adhesions, a cancer, etc..) leading to accumulation of mucus and dilation of the distal appendix.

- The term mucocele is misleading as it is inclusive of both benign and malignant lesions.

- All mucoceles greater than 2 cm should be excised to remove premalignant lesions

- It's still usually benign, and found incidentally.

- *Complications:*

  - Cancer (underlying primary lesion causing the obstruction)

  - Rupture may lead to pseudomyxoma peritonei

  - Can act as a lead point for ileocolic intussusception

Case 67 - Belly Pain

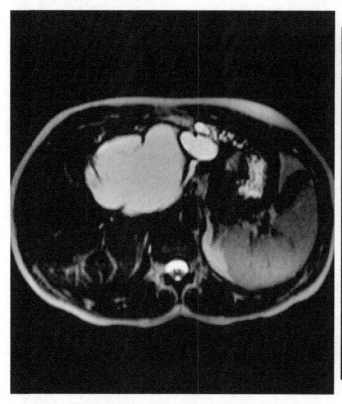
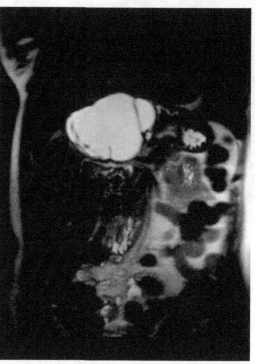

1. What is the diagnosis?
A. Hemangioma
B. Focal Nodular Hyperplasia
C. Biliary Cystadenoma
D. Von Meyenburg Complex

2. This thing isn't cancer right?
A. Oh no way, that thing is fine.
B. That thing is totally cancer - this guy is screwed.
C. It's hard to tell… could be.

3. If you resect it and it grows back that means it's cancer right?
A. Yes, get wider margins next time
B. Not necessarily, some times they just grow back

Case 67 - Biliary Cystadenoma

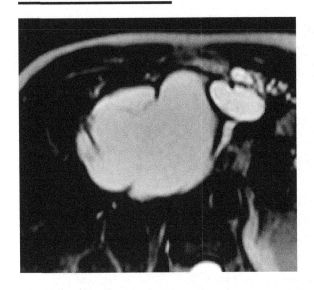

1. What is the diagnosis?
A. Hemangioma
B. Focal Nodular Hyperplasia
C. Biliary Cystadenoma
D. Von Meyenburg Complex

2. This thing isn't cancer right?
A. Oh no way, that thing is fine.
B. That thing is totally cancer - this guy is screwed.
C. It's hard to tell… could be.

3. If you resect it and it grows back that means it's cancer right?
A. Yes, get wider margins next time
B. Not necessarily, some times they just grow back

Biliary Cystadenoma

Benign cystic neoplasm of the liver.

Essential Trivia:

- Intra-hepatic cyst (uni-locular or multi-locular) made of biliary epithelium.

- There are no specific imaging features to differentiate these things from their cancerous cousin the cystadenocarcinoma.

- Some people consider them on a continuum and therefore call them "pre-malignant."

- Even though they are benign they can still reoccur after resection.

- They can exert local mass effect and have been known to cause obstructive jaundice.

Case 68 - Septic ICU Bomb

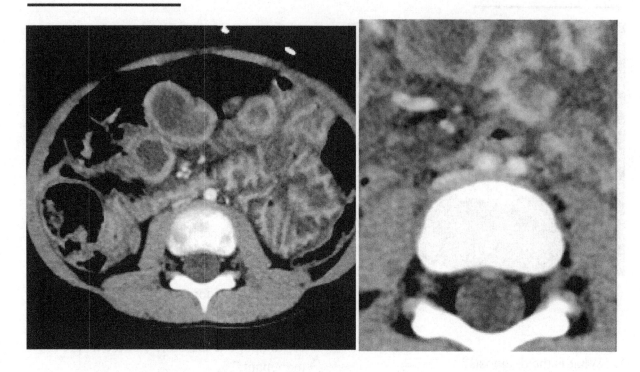

1. What is the diagnosis?
A. Inflammatory Bowel Disease
B. Severe Hypotension
C. Pseudomyxoma Peritonei
D. Portal Hypertension

2. If this was a non-contrasted study, what would you expect the bowel to look like?
A. Denser than the psoas
B. Less Dense than the psoas
C. Equally Dense to the psoas

3. With this diagnosis you expect the Liver to enhance ?
A. More than the spleen
B. Less than the spleen
C. Equal to the spleen

Case 68 - Hypoperfusion Complex

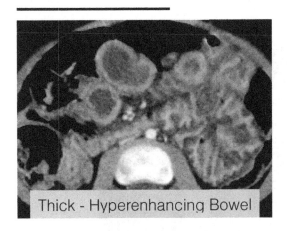
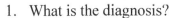
Thick - Hyperenhancing Bowel

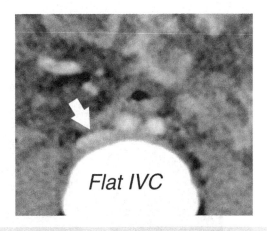
Flat IVC

Shock Bowel

Radiologic features of severe hypotension.

Essential Trivia:

- CT Features include:

  - Thickened Enhancing Bowel Loops (small bowel affected more than larger bowel)

  - On Non-Contrast, bowel loops may appear denser than the psoas

  - Collapsed IVC

  - HYPO-enhancement of solid organs (liver and spleen)

  - HYPER-enhancement of the adrenals

1. What is the diagnosis?
A. Inflammatory Bowel Disease
B. Severe Hypotension
C. Pseudomyxoma Peritonei
D. Portal Hypertension

2. If this was a non-contrasted study, what would you expect the bowel to look like?
A. Denser than the psoas
B. Less Dense than the psoas
C. Equally Dense to the psoas

3. With this diagnosis you expect the Liver to enhance ?
A. More than the spleen
B. **Less than the spleen** * *classic teaching is 25 H.U. less than spleen , although both liver and spleen hypo-perfuse relative to a normal scan.*
C. Equal to the spleen

Case 69 - Belly Pain (this guy has a Transplanted Kidney)

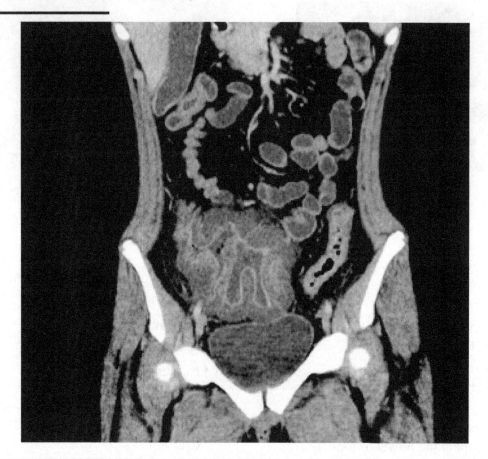

1. What is the diagnosis?
A. Inflammatory Bowel Disease
B. Typhlitis
C. C-Diff
D. Ischemic Colitis

2. What part of the bowel does TB favor?
A. Proximal Small Bowel
B. Terminal Ileum
C. Transverse Colon
D. Rectum

3. Toxic Megacolon classically causes massive dilation of the?
A. Proximal Small Bowel
B. Terminal Ileum
C. Transverse Colon
D. Rectum

Case 69 - Typhlitis

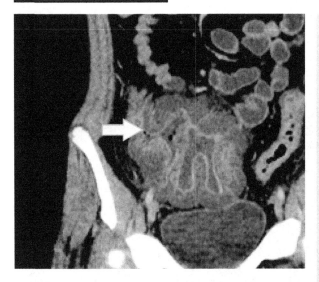

1. What is the diagnosis?
A. Inflammatory Bowel Disease
B. Typhlitis
C. C-Diff
D. Ischemic Colitis

2. What part of the bowel does TB favor?
A. Proximal Small Bowel
B. Terminal Ileum
C. Transverse Colon
D. Rectum

3. Toxic Megacolon classically causes massive dilation of the?
A. Proximal Small Bowel
B. Terminal Ileum
C. Transverse Colon
D. Rectum

Thyphlitis

Also called "Neutropenic Colitis," this is the pattern of colitis in the severely immunosuppressed population.

Essential Trivia:

- *Mechanism:* Intramural bacterial invasion without an inflammatory reaction.

- *Classic Look:* Wall thickening, stranding, and maybe pneumatosis primarily centered around the cecum.

- *Contraindication:* They should NEVER get a barium enema - they will perforate.

Other Random Infectious Bowel Trivia:

- **Entamoeba Histolytica** - Scars the cecum, but spares the terminal ileum (T.I.)

- **TB** - Classically involves the T.I.

- **Yersinia** - Classically involves the T.I.

- **C-Diff / Toxic Megacolon** - Dilates the colon (most notably the transverse colon).

- **Giardia & Strongyloides** - Classically likes the proximal small bowel.

Case 70 - Headache

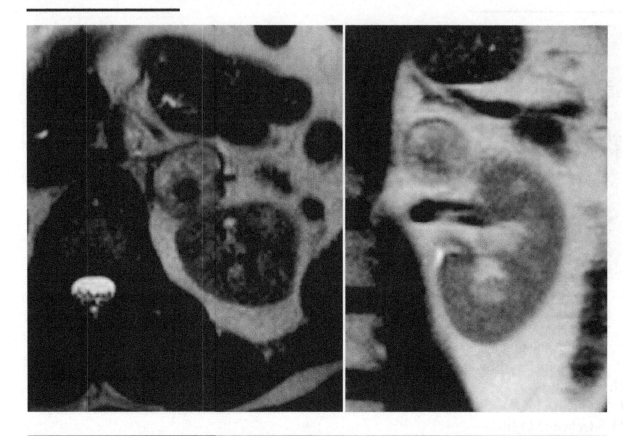

1. What is the diagnosis?
A. Adrenal Adenoma (lipid rich)
B. Adrenal Adenoma (lipid poor)
C. Pheochromocytoma
D. Wollman Syndrome

2. Where is the Organ of Zuckerkandl usually located?
A. SMA
B. IMA
C. Right Iliac
D. Carotid Bifurcation

3. This diagnosis is included in what syndrome?
A. Carney's Complex
B. MEN I
C. MEN IIa
D. Angelman Syndrome

Case 70 - Pheochromocytoma

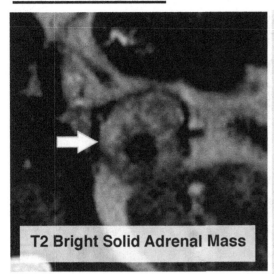

T2 Bright Solid Adrenal Mass

1. What is the diagnosis?
A. Adrenal Adenoma (lipid rich)
B. Adrenal Adenoma (lipid poor)
C. Pheochromocytoma
D. Wollman Syndrome

2. Where is the Organ of Zuckerkandl usually located?
A. SMA
B. IMA *these neuro-crest cells actually extend from the SMA down to the aortic bifurcation, but are MOST concentrated at the IMA*
C. Right Iliac
D. Carotid Bifurcation

3. This diagnosis is included in what syndrome?
A. Carney's Complex ** *Carney's Syndrome has pheos, the "complex" is cardiac stuff*
B. MEN I
C. MEN IIa
D. Angelman Syndrome

Pheochromocytoma

A rare neuro-endocrine tumor of the adrenal or extra-adrenal tissue.

Essential Trivia:

- Uncommon in real life (common on multiple choice tests).

- They are usually large at presentation (larger than 3cm).

- Rule of 10s: 10% are extra adrenal (Organ of Zuckerkandl – usually at the IMA), 10% are bilateral, 10% are in children, 10% are hereditary, 10% are NOT active (no HTN).

- *Imaging Features:*

  - *CT:* Heterogeneous mass on CT.

  - *MRI:* They are **T2 bright.**

  - *Nukes:* Both MIBG and Octreotide could be used (but MIBG is better since Octreotide also uptakes in the kidney).

- Syndromic Associations:

  - *MEN IIa:* Medullary Thyroid Cancer (100%), Parathyroid hyperplasia, Pheochromocytoma (33%)

  - *MEN IIb:* Medullary Thyroid Cancer (80%), Pheochromocytoma (50%), Mucosal Neuroma, Marfanoid Body Habitus

  - *Carney's Syndrome:* Extra-Adrenal Pheo, GIST, and Pulmonary Chondroma (hamartoma).

  - *Von Hippel Lindau:* Bilateral Renal Cell Carcinoma, Pheos, and Hemangioblastomas

Case 71 - Belly Pain

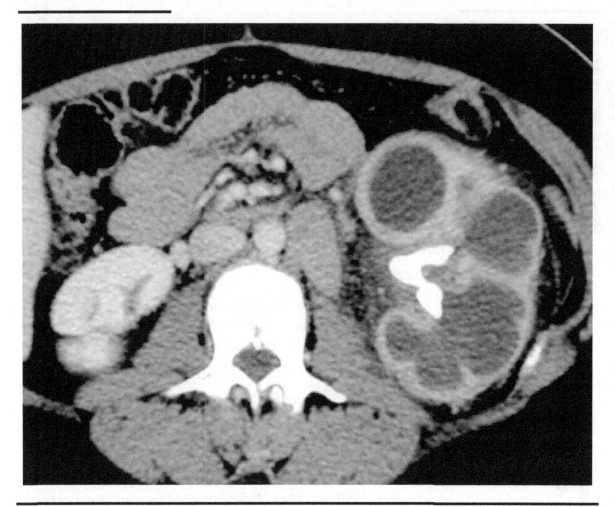

1. What is the diagnosis?
A. Renal Cell Carcinoma
B. Multi-locular Cystic Nephroma
C. Pheochromocytoma
D. Xanthogranulomatous Pyelonephritis

2. What is "always" associated?
A. A big stag-horn stone
B. Diabetes
C. History of lithotripsy
D. Bladder cancer

3. What is the treatment?
A. Lots of antibiotics
B. Needs a tube, gotta drain that beast. Then it will get better.
C. Nephrectomy - that thing is toast.

Case 71 - Xanthogranulomatous Pyelonephritis (XGP)

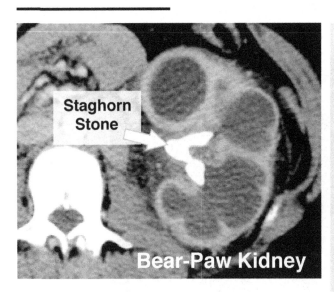

1. What is the diagnosis?
A. Renal Cell Carcinoma
B. Multi-locular Cystic Nephroma
C. Pheochromocytoma
D. Xanthogranulomatous Pyelonephritis

2. What is "always" associated?
A. A big stag-horn stone
B. Diabetes
C. History of lithotripsy
D. Bladder cancer

3. What is the treatment?
A. Lots of antibiotics
B. Needs a tube, gotta drain that beast. Then it will get better.
C. Nephrectomy - that thing is toast.

Xanthogranulomatous Pyelonephritis (XGP)

Uncommon form of chronic pyelonephritis resulting in a non-functioning kidney.

Essential Trivia:

- Chronic destructive granulomatous process that is basically **always seen with a staghorn stone** acting as a nidus for recurrent infection.

- You can have an associated psoas abscess with minimal peri-renal infection.

- It's an Aunt Minnie, with a very characteristic "Bear Paw" appearance on CT.

- The kidney is not functional, and often nephrectomy is done to treat it.

Case 72- Belly Pain (Patient's Age is 40)

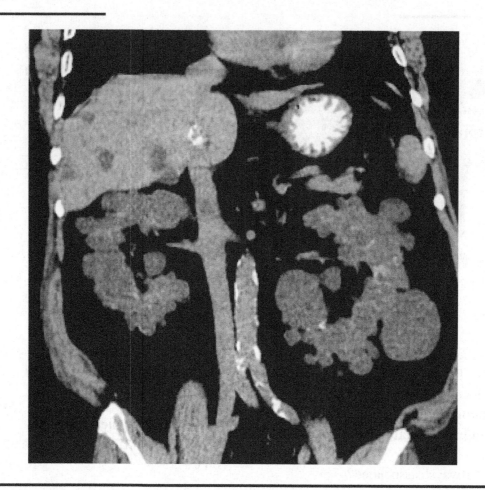

1. What is the diagnosis?
A. AD Polycystic Kidney Disease
B. AR Polycystic Kidney Disease
C. Von Hippel Lindau
D. Tuberous Sclerosis

2. This patient is NOT on dialysis. Are they are increased risk for RCC?
A. Yes
B. No

3. With regard to **AR** Polycystic Kidney Disease, if the disease in the kidneys is bad…?
A. The liver fibrosis is bad too
B. The liver fibrosis is better
C. The cysts in the liver are bad too
D. The cysts in the liver are better

Case 72 - AD - Polycystic Kidney Disease

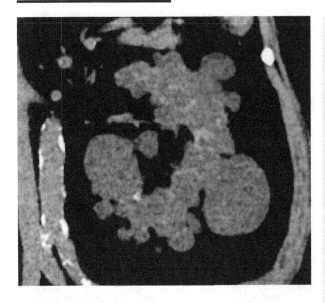

1. What is the diagnosis?
A. AD Polycystic Kidney Disease
B. AR Polycystic Kidney Disease
C. Von Hippel Lindau
D. Tuberous Sclerosis

2. This patient is NOT on dialysis. Are they are increased risk for RCC?
A. Yes
B. No

3. With regard to AR Polycystic Kidney Disease, if the disease in the kidney's is bad…?
A. The liver fibrosis is bad too
B. The liver fibrosis is better
C. The cysts in the liver are bad too
D. The cysts in the liver are better

Autosomal Dominant Polycystic Kidney Disease

Hereditary form of adult cystic renal disease

Essential Trivia:

- "AD" is seen in ADults

- Kidneys get progressively larger and lose function (you get dialysis by 5th decade).

- They get cysts in the liver 70% of the time.

- They get Berry Aneurysms (which can rupture and kill).

- They don't have an intrinsic risk of cancer, but do get cancer once they are on dialysis.

AR-PKD (The Pediatric Form):

- The liver involvement is different than the adult form. Instead of cysts they have abnormal bile ducts and fibrosis. This congenital hepatic fibrosis is ALWAYS present in ARPKD. The ratio of liver and kidney disease is inverse. The worse the liver is the better the kidneys do. The better the liver is the worse the kidneys are.

Case 73 - Belly Pain

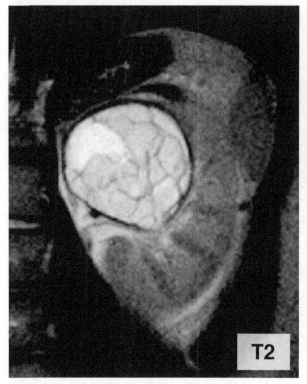
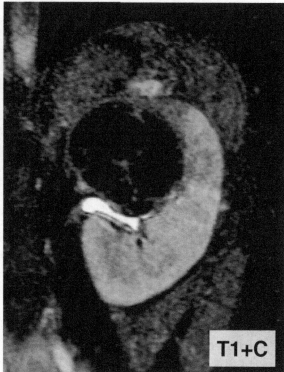

1. What is the diagnosis?
A. AD Polycystic Kidney Disease
B. Multi-locular Cystic Nephroma
C. Multicystic Dysplastic Kidney
D. Oncocytoma

2. What is the classic demographic?
A. Young Boys and Girls
B. Middle Aged Men, and Younger Girls
C. Young Boys, Middle Aged Women
D. Middle Aged Men and Women

3. In an adult you can be 100% sure this is benign right?
A. Oh yeah, there is no way that's cancer
B. Um… can't tell. You can never tell with kidneys.

4. What's the buzzword for these things?
A. "Multiple thin walled cysts"
B. "Protrudes into the renal pelvis"
C. "Bulges the renal contour"

Case 73 - Multi-locular Cystic Nephroma

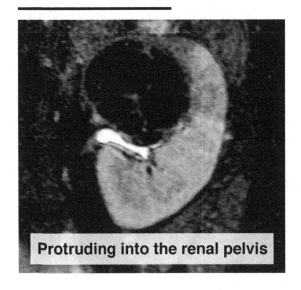

Protruding into the renal pelvis

1. What is the diagnosis?
A. AD Polycystic Kidney Disease
B. Multi-locular Cystic Nephroma
C. Multicystic Dysplastic Kidney
D. Oncocytoma

2. What is the classic demographic?
A. Young Boys and Girls
B. Middle Aged Men, and Younger Girls
C. Young Boys, Middle Aged Women
D. Middle Aged Men and Women

3. In an adult you can be 100% sure this is benign right?
A. Oh yeah, there is no way that's cancer
B. Um… can't tell. You can never tell with kidneys.

4. What's the buzzword for these things?
A. "Multiple thin walled cysts"
B. "Protrudes into the renal pelvis"
C. "Bulges the renal contour"

Multi-locular Cystic Nephroma

Rare benign cystic neoplasm of the kidney.

Essential Trivia:

- "Non-communicating, fluid-filled locules, surrounded by thick fibrous capsule."

- By definition these things are characterized by the absence of a solid component or necrosis.

- Buzzword is "protrude into the renal pelvis."

- The question is likely the bimodal occurrence (4 year old boys, and 40 year old women). I like to think of this as the *Michael Jackson lesion* – it loves young boys and middle aged women.

- It's not a cancer, but you can't tell it from a cystic RCC in an adult, or a cystic Wilms in a kid. So they typically end up with radical (or partial nephrectomy).

Cystic Renal Disease - Essential Trivia

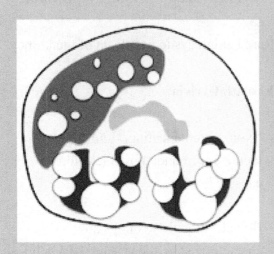

AD Polycystic Kidney Disease

- Cysts in Kidneys
- Kidneys are BIG
- Cysts in Liver

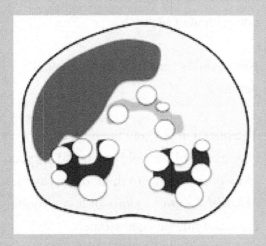

Von Hippel Lindau

- Cysts in Kidneys
- RCCs in the Kidneys
- Cysts in *Pancreas*

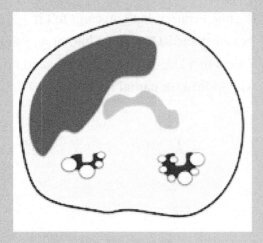

Uremic Cystic Disease

- Cysts in Kidneys
- Kidneys are SMALL

About 40% of patients with end stage renal disease develop cysts. This rises with time of dialysis with about 90% in patients after 5 year of dialysis. The thing to know is: *Increased risk of malignancy with dialysis.*

Multicystic Dsyplastic Kidney

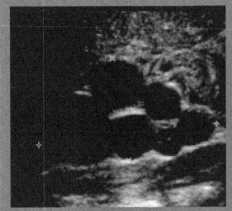

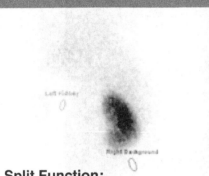

Split Function:
- Right 100%
- Left 0%

This is a peds thing, where you have multiple tiny cysts forming in utereo.

What you need to know is :

(1) There is "no functioning renal tissue," - this is proven with a MAG 3 scan.
(2) Contralateral renal tract abnormalities occur like 50% of the time - think about UPJ Obstruction.

How Can You tell MCDK vs Bad Hydro?

In hydronephrosis the cystic spaces are seen to communicate. "Cystic Spaces that Do NOT communicate" is often a buzzword - for this very reason.

In the real world renal scintigraphy (MAG 3) can be useful. MCDK will show no excretory function.

Lithium Nephropathy *"History of Bi-Polar Disease"*

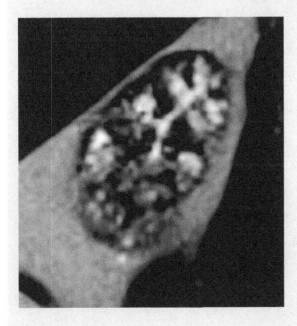

- Occurs in patients who take lithium long term.

- Can lead to diabetes insipidus and renal insufficiency.

- The kidneys are normal to small in volume with multiple (innumerable) tiny cysts, usually 2-5mm in diameters.

- These "microcysts" are distinguishable from the larger cysts associated with acquired cystic disease of uremia.

Case 74 - History Of UnProtected Sex with Multiple Anonymous Partners

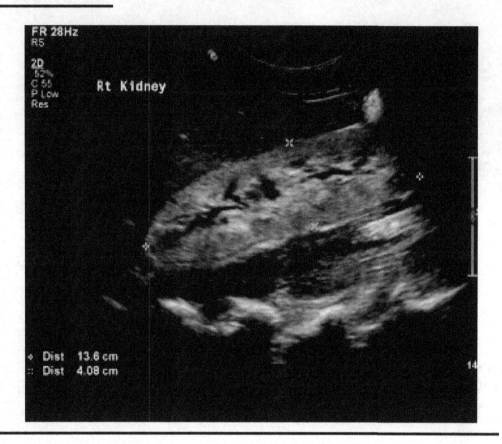

1. What is the diagnosis?
A. Pyelonephritis
B. Pyonephrosis
C. Disseminated PCP
D. HIV Nephropathy

2. What other finding (not well seen on this case) has been classically described with this diagnosis ?
A. Cortical Calcifications
B. Medullary Calcifications
C. Extra fat in the renal sinus
D. Loss of fat in the renal sinus

3. In the same patient population (same demographic risk factors) what would *punctate cortical calcifications* make you think of?
A. Xanthogranulomatous Pyelonephritis
B. CMV Infection
C. PCP Infection

Case 74 - HIV Nephropathy

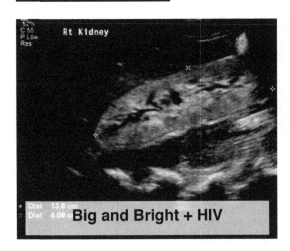

Big and Bright + HIV

1. What is the diagnosis?
A. Pyelonephritis
B. Pyonephrosis
C. Disseminated PCP
D. HIV Nephropathy

2. What other finding (not well seen on this case) has been classically described with this diagnosis?
A. Cortical Calcifications
B. Medullary Calcifications
C. Extra fat in the renal sinus
D. Loss of fat in the renal sinus

3. In the same patient population (same demographic risk factors) what would *punctate cortical calcifications* make you think of?
A. Xanthogranulomatous Pyelonephritis
B. CMV Infection
C. PCP Infection

HIV Nephropathy

Common cause of chronic renal failure in HIV positive patients.

Essential Trivia:

- If you see **BIG BRIGHT Kidneys in a patient with HIV,** then this is the answer.

- Loss of the renal sinus fat appearance has also been described (it's edema in the fat, rather than loss of the actual fat).

- There will / may be a history of proteinuria (they typically present in nephrotic syndrome).

- The biopsy results will show "focal segmental glomerulosclerosis"

- The prognosis typically sucks

Other AIDS Related Renal Trivia:

- **Disseminated PCP** in HIV patients can result in *punctate (primarily cortical) calcifications.*

-**TB:** The most common extrapulmonary site of infection is the urinary tract. The features are papillary necrosis and parenchymal destruction. You can have extensive calcifications. Basically you end up with a *shrunken calcified kidney "putty kidney."* This end stage appearance is essentially an auto nephrectomy.

Case 75 - Pelvic Pain

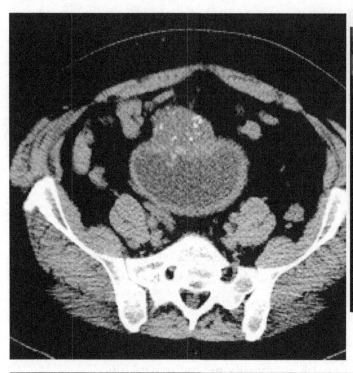
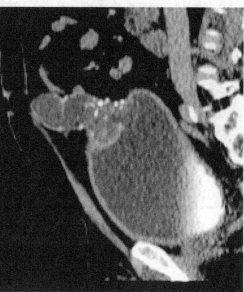

1. What is the diagnosis?
A. Hutch Diverticulum
B. Bladder Ears
C. Cloacal Malformation
D. Bladder cancer

2. What cell type ?
A. Transitional Cell
B. Adenocarcinoma
C. Squamous Cell
D. Rhabdomyosarcoma

3. Schistosomiasis is a common cause of bladder cancer world wide. What is the cell line for those bladder cancers?
A. Transitional Cell
B. Adenocarcinoma
C. Squamous Cell
D. Rhabdomyosarcoma

Case 75 - Urachal Adenocarcinoma

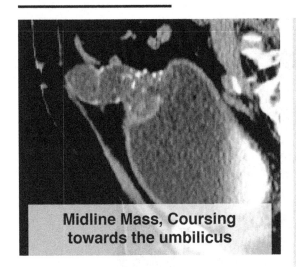

Midline Mass, Coursing towards the umbilicus

1. What is the diagnosis?
   A. Hutch Diverticulum
   B. Bladder Ears
   C. Cloacal Malformation
   D. Bladder cancer

2. What cell type?
   A. Transitional Cell
   B. Adenocarcinoma
   C. Squamous Cell
   D. Rhabdomyosarcoma

3. Schistosomiasis is a common cause of bladder cancer world wide. What is the cell line for those bladder cancers?
   A. Transitional Cell
   B. Adenocarcinoma
   C. Squamous Cell
   D. Rhabdomyosarcoma

Urachal Adenocarcinoma

The urachus is the umbilical attachment of the bladder (initially the allantois then urachus).

Essential Trivia:

- It usually atrophies and becomes the umbilical ligament (as the bladder descends into the pelvis).

- A persistent patent urachus can result in urine flow from the bladder to the umbilicus (and then likely someone's unsuspecting face).

- There is a spectrum of these things from: patent -> sinus -> diverticulum --> Cyst.

- They can get infected.

- Really the main thing to know is that <u>they get adenocarcinoma.</u>

- It's midline and they get adenocarcinoma

- ***Bladder Cancer Key Trivia:***

    - Typical = Transitional Cell
    - Schistosomiasis = Squamous
    - Urachus = Adenocarcinoma
    - Kids = Rhabdomyosarcoma

Case 76 - Pelvic Pain (History of Breast CA)

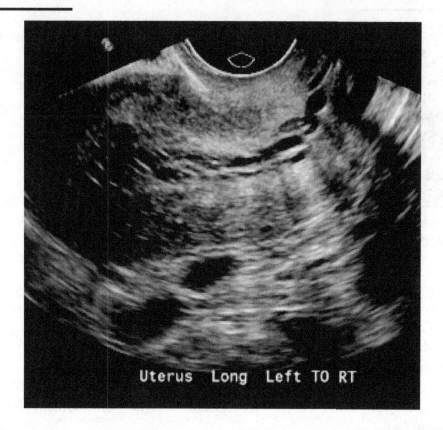

1. What is the diagnosis?
A. Normal Proliferative Phase Uterus
B. Normal Secretory Phase Uterus
C. Adenomyosis
D. Tamoxifen Related Changes
E. Nabothian Cysts

2. The GYN resident is very concerned for an underlying polyp, what would be the best way to tell if one is hiding in there?
A. Intra-operative D&C
B. Repeat Ultrasound with patient in prone position
C. Repeat Ultrasound with provocative maneuvers (have her bare down)
D. Repeat Ultrasound as a sonohysterogram

3. A post menopausal patient, presents with a history of bleeding. Her Endometrial thickness is measured at 4mm. What is the likely cause for her bleeding?
A. Cancer
B. Endometrial Polyp
C. Atrophy
D. Endometrial Hyperplasia

4. Endometrial Hyperplasia seen in the setting of an ovarian mass is the classic multiple choice trick for?

A. Granulosa Cell Tumor
B. Brenner Tumor
C. Ovarian Fibrothecoma
D. Ovarian Fibroma

Case 76 - Tamoxifen Related Changes

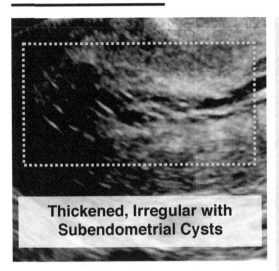

Thickened, Irregular with Subendometrial Cysts

1. What is the diagnosis?
A. Normal Proliferative Phase Uterus
B. Normal Secretory Phase Uterus
C. Adenomyosis
D. Tamoxifen Related Changes
E. Nabothian Cysts

2. The GYN resident is very concerned for an underlying polyp, what would be the best way to tell if one is hiding in there?
A. Intra-operative D&C
B. Repeat Ultrasound with patient in prone position
C. Repeat Ultrasound with provocative maneuvers (have her bare down)
D. Repeat Ultrasound as a sonohysterogram

3. A post menopausal patient, presents with a history of bleeding. Her Endometrial thickness is measured at 4mm. What is the likely cause for her bleeding?
A. Cancer
B. Endometrial Polyp
C. Atrophy
D. Endometrial Hyperplasia

4. Endometrial Hyperplasia seen in the setting of an ovarian mass is the classic multiple choice trick for?

A. Granulosa Cell Tumor *tumor makes estrogen which thickens endometrium*
B. Brenner Tumor
C. Ovarian Fibrothecoma
D. Ovarian Fibroma

Tamoxifen

This is what the uterus of Tamoxifen patient looks like.

Essential Trivia:

- Tamoxifen is a SERM (acts like estrogen in the pelvis, blocks the estrogen effects on the breast).

- It's used to treat hormonally responsive breast cancer, but increases the risk of endometrial cancer.

- Normally post menopausal endometrial tissue shouldn't be thicker than 4mm, but on Tamoxifen the endometrium gets a pass up to 8mm, although the exact number at which you should recommend a biopsy is allusive.

- It seems that most people agree that endometrial cancer typically presents with bleeding, and therefore bleeding patients with thickened endometrium should probably undergo a biopsy.

- If you are wondering if a polyp is hiding you can get a sonohysterogram (ultrasound after instillation of saline).

Classic Imaging Findings:
- Thickened Irregular Appearance of the Endometrium
- Subendometrial cysts,
- Development of endometrial polyps (30%).

Case 77 - Pelvic Pain

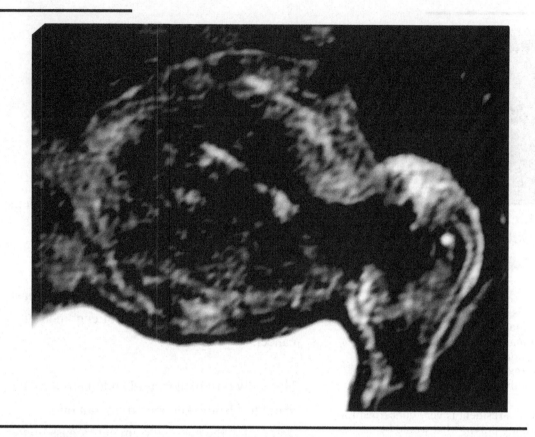

1. What is the diagnosis?
A. Adenomyosis
B. Adenomyomatosis
C. Endometrial hyperplasia
D. Endometrial cancer

2. What measurement is used to define this pathology on MRI?
A. Thickness of the lower uterine segment
B. Number of ovarian follicles
C. Thickness of the junctional zone
D. Thickness of the posterior uterine wall

3. What part of the uterus tends to be most heavily afflicted, what part tends to be spared?
A. Posterior Wall is Favored, Anterior Wall is Spared
B. Cervix is favored, Posterior Wall is spared
C. Inferior wall is favored, Cervix is spared
D. Posterior Wall is Favored, Cervix is spared.

Case 77 - Adenomyosis

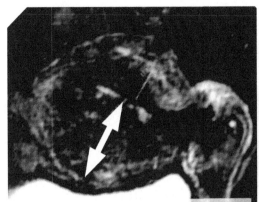

Thickened, Junctional Zone

1. What is the diagnosis?
A. Adenomyosis
B. Adenomyomatosis
C. Endometrial hyperplasia
D. Endometrial cancer

2. What measurement is used to define this pathology on MRI?
A. Thickness of the lower uterine segment
B. Number of ovarian follicles
C. Thickness of the junctional zone
D. Thickness of the posterior uterine wall

3. What part of the uterus tends to be most heavily afflicted, what part tends to be spared?
A. Posterior Wall is favored, Anterior Wall is spared
B. Cervix is favored, Posterior Wall is spared
C. Inferior wall is favored, Cervix is spared
D. Posterior Wall is favored, Cervix is spared.

Adenomyosis

Endometrial tissue that has migrated into the myometrium

Essential Trivia:

- Most commonly in multiparous women of reproductive age, especially if they've had a history of uterine procedures (Caesarian section, dilatation and curettage).

- First Line therapy is typically GnRH agonists – to mess with the normal cyclical hormone induced proliferation.

- Does (probably) respond to uterine artery embolization, although hysterectomy is considered the definitive treatment for severe cases.

Classic Imaging Findings:

Ultrasound:
- Heterogeneous uterus (hyperechoic adenomyosis, with hypoechoic muscular hypertrophy
- Enlargement of the posterior wall, spares cervix.

MRI
- **Thickening of the junctional zone of the uterus to more than 12 mm** (normal is < 5mm). The thickening can be either focal or diffuse.
- Small high T2 signal regions corresponding to regions of cystic change

Case 78 - History Withheld

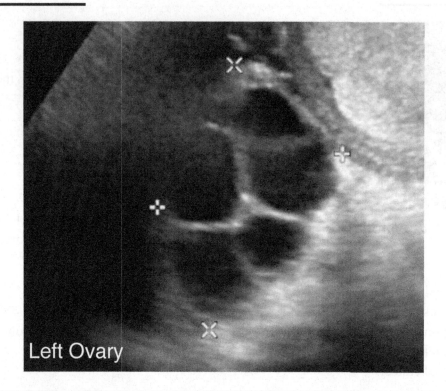

1. What is the diagnosis?
A. Ovarian Torsion
B. Polycystic Ovarian Syndrome *(betcha this chick has a mustache)*
C. Theca Lutein Cysts
D. Hemorrhagic Cyst

2. What measurement is used to define this pathology on MRI?
A. On birth control
B. On fertility meds (clomid)
C. Has some bizarro encephalopathy (anti NMDA)
D. Has gastric cancer

3. Let's say she is pregnant… what's probably true about this pregnancy?
A. Totally normal single gestation
B. Oh it's doomed for sure, probably trisomy 13
C. Multiple Gestations – possible reality tv show in her future

Case 78 - Theca Lutein Cysts

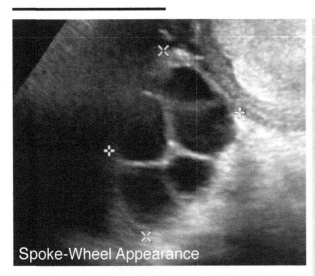
Spoke-Wheel Appearance

1. What is the diagnosis?
A. Ovarian Torsion
B. Polycystic Ovarian Syndrome *(betcha this chick has a mustache)*
C. Theca Lutein Cysts
D. Hemorrhagic Cyst

2. What measurement is used to define this pathology on MRI?
A. On birth control
B. On fertility meds (clomid)
C. Has some bizarro encephalopathy (anti NMDA)
D. Has gastric cancer

3. Let's say she is pregnant… what's probably true about this pregnancy?
A. Totally normal single gestation
B. Oh it's doomed for sure, probably trisomy 13
C. Multiple Gestations – possible reality tv show in her future (followed by a divorce)

Theca Lutein Cysts

This is a type of functional cyst related to overstimulation from b-HCG.

Essential Trivia:

- What you see are large cysts (~ 2-3 cm) and the ovary has a typical multilocular cystic "spoke-wheel" appearance.

- Clinical history might be hyperemesis gravidarum – all that b-HCG causes nausea.

Think about 3 things:
- Multifetal pregnancy,
- Gestational trophoblastic disease (moles), and
- Ovarian Hyperstimulation syndrome.

Ovarian Hyperstimulation syndrome.
- This is a complication associated with fertility therapy (occurs in like 5%). They will show you the ovaries with theca lutein cysts, then ascites, and pleural effusions. They may also have pericardial effusions. Complications include increased risk for ovarian torsion (big ovaries), and hypovolemic shock.

Aunt Minnie 172

Case 79 - Pelvic Pain

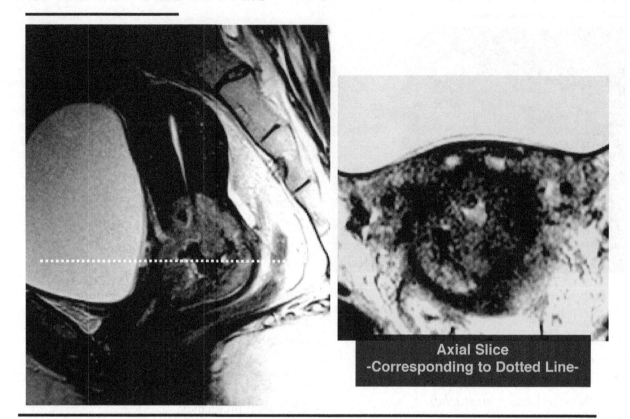

1. What is the diagnosis?
A. Cervical Cancer
B. Nabothian Cyst(s)
C. Vaginal Leiomyoma
D. Skene Gland Cyst

2. What's the stage?
A. Stage 1
B. Stage 2a
C. Stage 2b

3. What is the typical cell type?
A. Transitional Cell
B. Adenocarcinoma
C. Squamous Cell
D. Rhabdomyosarcoma

Case 79 - Cervical Cancer

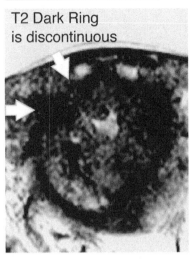
T2 Dark Ring is discontinuous

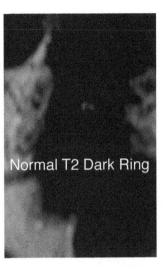
Normal T2 Dark Ring

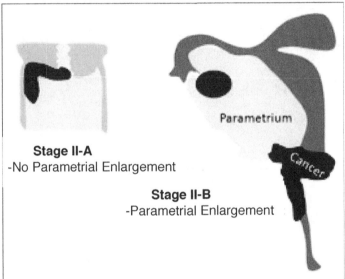
Stage II-A
-No Parametrial Enlargement

Stage II-B
-Parametrial Enlargement

1. What is the diagnosis?
A. Cervical Cancer
B. Nabothian Cyst(s)
C. Vaginal Leiomyoma
D. Skene Gland Cyst

2. What's the stage?
A. Stage 1
B. Stage 2a
C. Stage 2b

3. What is the typical cell type?
A. Transitional Cell
B. Adenocarcinoma
C. Squamous Cell
D. Rhabdomyosarcoma

Cervical Cancer

Essential Trivia:

- It's usually squamous cell, related to HPV (like 90%).

- The big thing to know is parametrial invasion (stage IIb).

- Violation of the normal T2 dark line around the cervix = parametrial invasion

- Stage IIa or below is treated with surgery. Once you have parametrial invasion (stage IIb), or involvement of the lower 1/3 of the vagina it's gonna get chemo/ radiation

- *What is this Parametrium?* The parametrium is a fibrous band that separates the supravaginal cervix from the bladder. It extends between the layers of the broad ligament. The uterine artery runs inside the parametrium, hence the need for chemo – once invaded.

Case 80 - Chest Pain

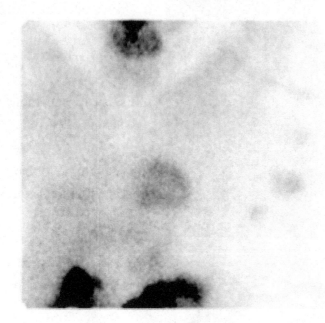

RT ANTERIOR LT

1. What is the tracer (his kidneys are hot)?
A. Gallium
B. MIBG
C. Iodine
D. MIBI

2. What makes uptake of this tracer intense?
A. Blood Flow, and Mitochondria
B. Blood Flow, and Glucose Metabolism
C. Blood Flow and Functionality of the Na/K Pump

3. Bony Uptake of this tracer is considered bad (cancer) ?
A. Iodine
B. MIBG
C. Octreotide
D. All of the above

Case 80 - The Incidental Cancer

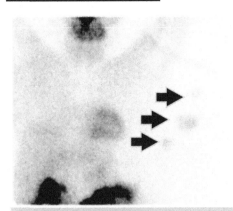

Axillary Nodes Like this are NOT normal!

1. What is the tracer (his kidneys are hot)?
A. Gallium *won't have spleen uptake
B. MIBG *won't have kidney uptake
C. Iodine *won't have heart uptake
D. MIBI

2. What makes uptake of this tracer intense?
A. Blood Flow, and Mitochondria
B. Blood Flow, and Glucose Metabolism
C. Blood Flow and Functionality of the Na/K Pump

3. Bony Uptake of this tracer is considered bad (cancer)?
A. Iodine
B. MIBG
C. Octreotide
D. All of the above

Incidental Cancer

Watch your back... the tiger is in the tall grass.

Essential Trivia:

- Sestamibi - This tracer is used for parathyroid imaging, cardiac imaging, and breast specific gamma imaging.

- It works by having affinity for high blood flow and mitochondria.

- Lymph Nodes - Any lymph nodes seen on BSGI (Breast Specific Gamma Imaging), Cardiac Studies using MIBI, or Parathyroid studies should be considered cancer till proven otherwise. You'll need to recommend something else - ultrasound first (probably) then eventual biopsy.

- As a resident I had an elderly attending who would always give the same answer, when I would ask what I should do with an incidental finding. He would look at me through his thick orange cataracts and say "Biopsy the Mother Fucker!"... He also gave good advice on women.

- *Bad Bones* - You should NEVER see bone uptake on MIBG, I-131, or Octreotide scans. If you see this, you are dealing with bone mets till proven otherwise.

Case 81 - Cough - CD4 Count 30

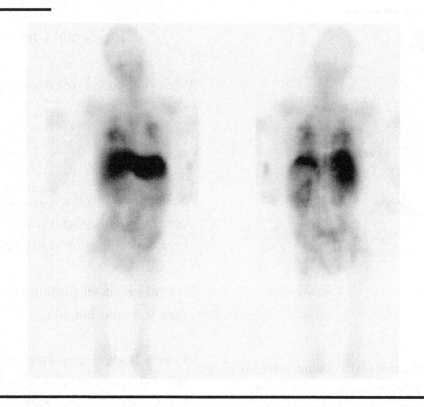

1. What is the tracer ?
A. Gallium
B. MIBG
C. Iodine
D. MIBI

2. What is the mechanism of this tracer?
A. Mimics Iron
B. Mimics Bilirubin
C. Mimics Potassium
D. Mimics Calcium

3. For PCP pneumonia, uptake is classically ?
A. More intense than the liver
B. Less intense than the liver
C. More intense than the kidneys
D. Less intense than the kidneys

4. What is the "critical organ" for this tracer?
A. Bladder
B. Stomach
C. Kidney
D. Colon

Case 81 - Gallium Scan - PCP

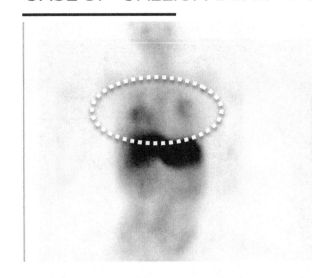

1. What is the tracer ?
A. **Gallium**
B. MIBG
C. Iodine
D. MIBI

2. What is the mechanism of this tracer?
A. **Mimics Iron**
B. Mimics Bilirubin
C. Mimics Potassium
D. Mimics Calcium

3. For PCP pneumonia, uptake is classically ?
A. **More intense than the liver**
B. Less intense than the liver
C. More intense than the kidneys
D. Less intense than the kidneys

4. What is the "critical organ" for this tracer?
A. Bladder
B. Stomach
C. Kidney
D. **Colon**

PCP (Pneumocystis)

Most common opportunistic pulmonary infection found in HIV patients (in the United States).

Essential Trivia:

- An elevated serum lactate dehydrogenase level is very sensitive for PCP (and very non-specific, so family medicine docs probably love it).

- The sensitivity of Gallium scanning for the evaluation of PCP in HIV patients has been reported to be as high as 90-95%.

- *Classic Findings:* **Diffuse heterogeneous pulmonary activity which is more intense than the liver**

- Gallium Mechanism: The body handles Ga+3 the same way it would Fe+3 - which as you may remember from step 1 gets bound (via lactoferrin) and concentrated in areas of inflammation, infection, and rapid cell division. Therefore it's a very non-specific way to look for infection or tumor.

- *"Critical Organ"* - The organ that would first be subjected to radiation in excess of the maximum permissible amount. For Gallium this is the colon.

Case 82 - Confusion

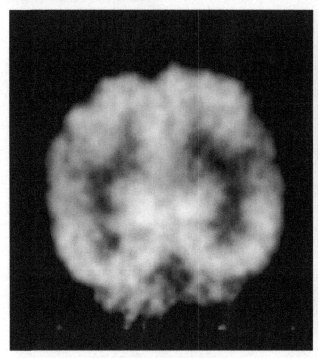
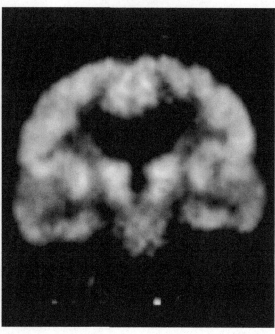

1. What is the energy of the tracer?
A. 140
B. 511
C. 173 & 247
D. 365

2. What is the diagnosis?
A. Alzheimers
B. Vascular Dementia
C. Picks Disease
D. Dementia with Lewy Bodies

3. What part of the brain atrophies first with this diagnosis?
A. Cingulate Gyrus
B. Motor Strip
C. Rectus Gyrus
D. Hippocampus

4. What part of the brain is classically preserved with neurodegenerative disorders?
A. Cingulate Gyrus
B. Motor Strip
C. Rectus Gyrus
D. Hippocampus

Case 82 - Alzheimers

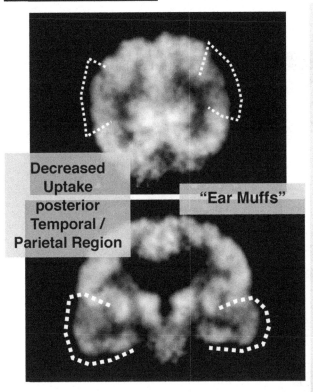

1. What is the energy of the tracer?
A. 140
B. 511 - ** positron emission from FDG*
C. 173 & 247
D. 365

2. What is the diagnosis?
A. Alzheimers
B. Vascular Dementia
C. Picks Disease
D. Dementia with Lewy Bodies

3. What part of the brain atrophies first with this diagnosis?
A. Cingulate Gyrus
B. Motor Strip
C. Rectus Gyrus
D. Hippocampus

4. What part of the brain is classically preserved with neurodegenerative disorders?
A. Cingulate Gyrus
B. Motor Strip
C. Rectus Gyrus
D. Hippocampus

Alzheimer Disease (AD)

The most common cause of dementia in the elderly

Essential Trivia:

- The characteristic progressive atrophy pattern begins in the medial temporal lobes (bilateral hippocampi).

- *PET-FDG as a tracer* - Progressive decrease in glucose metabolism has been shown to correspond to underlying neuronal degeneration in specific patterns - this is exploited for dementia imaging.

- Decreased FDG for AD is in an "ear muffs" appearance - involving the inferior frontal lobe, and posterior temporal / parietal region. The cingulate gyrus is NOT spared.

- The motor cortex is classically spared with neurodegenerative disorders (not necessarily with multi-intact dementia).

- There are kinds of new tracers for AD imaging (none of which will be paid for by insurance) that tag the amyloid and tau proteins. The most famous is the Amyloid plaque sensitive agent "Pittsburgh compound B" or C^{11}-PiB.

Dementia Imaging - Essential Trivia

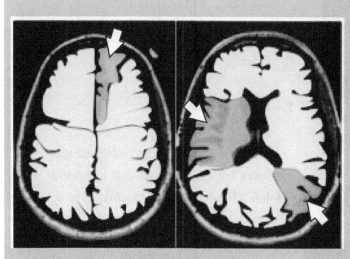

Decreased Uptake in Multiple Vascular Territories

Multi-Infarct Dementia

- This is the second most common cause of dementia.

- Cortical infarcts and lacunar infarcts are seen on MRI.

- PET-FDG will demonstrate multiple scattered areas of decreased activity

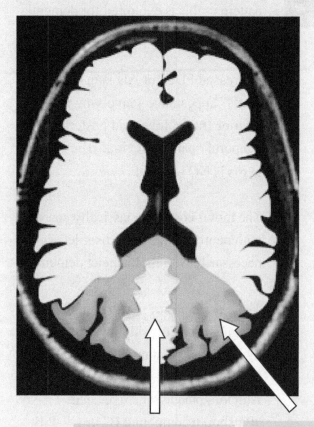

Preservation of the Cingulate Gyrus **Decreased Uptake in the Lateral Occipital Cortex**

Dementia with Lewy Bodies

- This is the third most common cause of dementia (second most common neurodegenerative).

- Very similar clinical picture to the dementia seen with Parkinsons, with the major difference being that in DLB, the dementia comes first.

- The hippocampi remain normal in size (unlike AD).

- PET-FDG will show **decreased uptake in the lateral occipital cortex**, with **sparing of the mid posterior cingulate gyrus (Cingulate Island)**

Picks / Frontotemporal Dementia

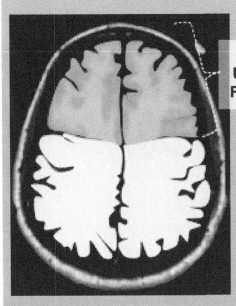

Decreased Uptake in the Frontal Lobes

- The 3rd most common neurodegenerative disorder.

- Atrophy and Decreased FDG patterns vary on the subtype but typically involve the frontal lobe and anterior temporal lobes.

- **Depression can be a mimic** - for the same decreased FDG pattern.

Huntingtons

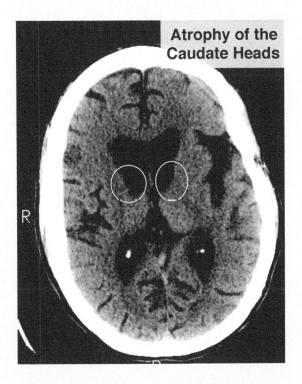

Atrophy of the Caudate Heads

- Inherited (Autosomal Dominant - Triplet Repeat) - neurodegenerative disorder caused by the loss of neurons in the basal ganglia (especially the caudate nucleus)

- Characteristic pattern of **atrophy in the caudate head** - results in a *"box like" configuration of the frontal horns*; which people try and quantify with measurements.

- There is also atrophy and increased T2 signal in the putamen.

- Not surprisingly, FDG-PET will show low activity in caudate nucleus and putamen

Case 83 - Headache

CISTERNOGRAM

ANTERIOR RLAT

1. What is the tracer (most likely)?
A. Gallium
B. MIBG
C. Indium - DTPA
D. MIBI

2. What is the diagnosis?
A. Normal Pressure Hydrocephalus
B. Meningitis
C. Pseudotumor Cerebri

3. Can this study distinguish between communicating and obstructive (non-communicating) hydrocephalus ?
A. Yup
B. Nope

Case 83 - Normal Pressure Hydrocephalus (NPH)

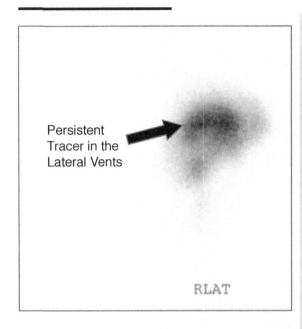

Persistent Tracer in the Lateral Vents

RLAT

1. What is the tracer (most likely)?
A. Gallium
B. MIBG
C. Indium - DTPA
D. MIBI

2. What is the diagnosis?
A. Normal Pressure Hydrocephalus
B. Meningitis
C. Pseudotumor Cerebri

3. Can this study distinguish between communicating and obstructive (non-communicating) hydrocephalus ?
A. Yup
B. Nope

Normal Pressure Hydrocephalus

NPH is an idiopathic decrease in the absorption of CSF. Secondary causes can occur - the main ones being meningitis and subarachnoid hemorrhage.

Essential Trivia:

- NPH is clinically Wet, Wacky, and Wobbly (incontinent, confused, and ataxic) clinically.

- The classic CT findings is "ventricular enlargement out of proportion to atrophy" on CT.

CSF Imaging:

- Tracer (most commonly In-DTPA) is injected intrathecal. You then watch to see if it flows normally.

- The major rule to remember that **at 24 hours it should clear from the basilar cisterns and be over the cerebral convexities**

- Another finding sometimes described is the **early detection of tracer into the lateral ventricles - causing a heart shape** (instead of the normal trident).

- The cisternogram cannot distinguish communicating vs noncommunicating types of hydrocephalus (unless you want to inject tracer directly into the lateral ventricles).

Case 84 - Pre-Natal Check Up

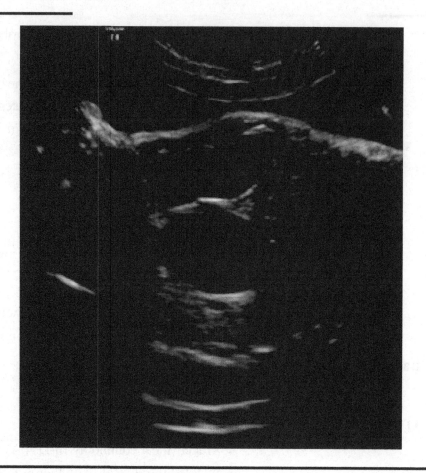

1. What is the diagnosis?
A. Gastric Outlet obstruction
B. Colonic Atresia
C. Duodenal Atresia
D. Malrotation

2. What is a common associated finding on pre-natal ultrasound?
A. Polyhydramnios
B. Oligohydramnios
C. Renal Atresia
D. Limb abnormalities

3. Is this diagnosis typically ?
A. Solitary Atresia
B. One of multiple Atresias

Case 84 - Duodenal Atresia

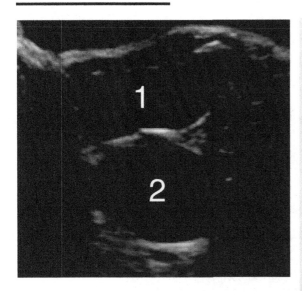

1. What is the diagnosis?
A. Gastric Outlet obstruction
B. Colonic Atresia
C. Duodenal Atresia
D. Malrotation

2. What is a common associated finding on pre-natal ultrasound?
A. Polyhydramnios
B. Oligohydramnios
C. Renal Atresia
D. Limb abnormalities

3. Is this diagnosis typically ?
A. Solitary Atresia
B. One of multiple Atresias

Duodenal Atresia

One of the most common causes of neonatal bowel obstruction.

Essential Trivia:

- *"Double Bubble"* – Because the atretic portion is usually just distal to the ampulla of Vater, you do still have the first portion of the duodenum. The double bubble appearance represents a dilation of the stomach, and this proximal duodenum.

- The double bubble appearance can be seen with annular pancreas but this takes time to develop, and is typically not seen immediately after birth.

- The degree of distention will be more pronounced than with midgut volvulus (which is a more acute process – associated with malrotation).

- Just like a plain film of the belly, this can be seen on pre-natal US (or MRI). On prenatal Ultrasound, the double bubble will not be present till late 2nd or 3rd trimester.

- Polyhydramnios is an associated pre-natal finding.

- Thought to be secondary to failure to canalize during development (often an isolated atresia).

Case 85 - Pre-Natal Check Up

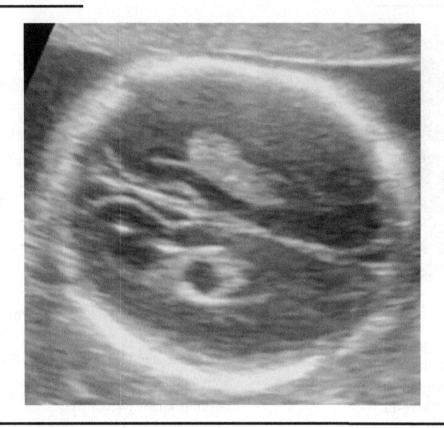

1. What is the diagnosis?
A. Aqueductal stenosis
B. Neonatal Brain Tumor – probably ATRT
C. Choroid Plexus Cyst
D. Holoprosencephaly

2. When this finding is made in isolation, what is it's significance?
A. The kid is screwed – very specific congenital malformation
B. The kid is screwed – very specific for fetal alcohol syndrome
C. The kid will probably be fine – this is very common in the general population

3. What is the **main** syndrome / pathology this is associated with?
A. Trisomy 21
B. Trisomy 18
C. Trisomy 13
D. Turner's Syndrome

Case 85 - Choroid Plexus Cyst

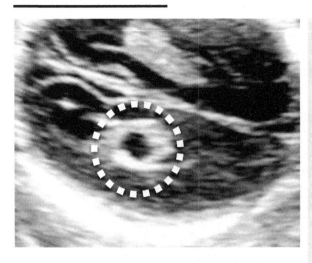

1. What is the diagnosis?
A. Aqueductal stenosis
B. Neonatal Brain Tumor – probably ATRT
C. Choroid Plexus Cyst
D. Holoprosencephaly

2. When this finding is made in isolation, what is it's significance?
A. The kid is screwed – very specific congenital malformation
B. The kid is screwed – very specific for fetal alcohol syndrome
C. The kid will probably be fine – this is very common in the general population

3. What is the **main** syndrome / pathology this is associated with?
A. Trisomy 21
B. Trisomy 18
C. Trisomy 13
D. Turner's Syndrome

Choroid Plexus Cyst

"Soft sign" of chromosome abnormalities.

Essential Trivia:

- Benign and often transient finding seen in about 1% of pregnancies.

- This is one of those incidental findings that in isolation means nothing. It's supposed to make you look closer for other findings.

- **Trisomy 18 is the primary testable association.** Here are the high yield points:

  • CP Cyst by itself gives you about a 1% risk of Trisomy 18
  • CP Cyst with other anomalous gives you about a 4% risk of Trisomy 18
  • The risk for Trisomy 18 is the same regardless of whether you have one cyst or multiple.
  • About 50% of Trisomy 18 babies have/had choroid plexus cysts.

- Other association: trisomy 21, Turner's Syndrome, and Klinefelter's

Case 86 - Pre-Natal Check Up (9 weeks)

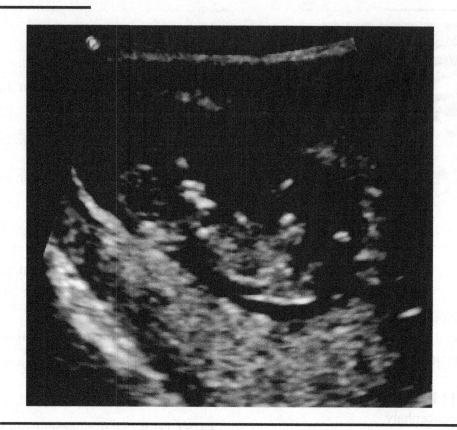

1. What is the diagnosis?
A. Gastroschisis
B. Omphalocele
C. Totally normal at this gestational age

2. Gastroschisis ALWAYS occurs on?
A. The right side
B. The left side

3. Which has more associated syndromes ?
A. Omphalocele
B. Gastroschisis

4. Maternal serum AFP will be elevated with?
A. Omphalocele
B. Gastroschisis
C. Both

Case 86 – Normal Midgut Herniation

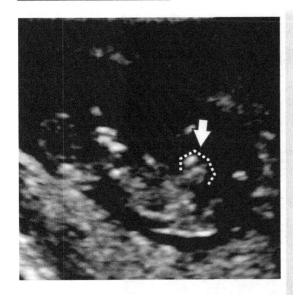

1. What is the diagnosis?
A. Gastroschisis
B. Omphalocele
C. **Totally normal at this gestational age**

2. Gastroschisis ALWAYS occurs on?
A. **The right side**
B. The left side

3. Which has more associated syndromes?
A. **Omphalocele**
B. Gastroschisis

4. Maternal serum AFP will be elevated with?
A. Omphalocele
B. **Gastroschisis**
C. Both

Normal Midgut Herniation

A normal thing, that looks like an omphalocele to the un-initiated.

Essential Trivia:

- *Normal Embryology:*
  - At week 6: The midgut forms a "U shaped loop" which herniates through the umbilical ring.
  - At week 11: The midgut normally rotates 270 degrees counterclockwise around the superior mesenteric artery and returns to the abdominal cavity.
- ****Normal from week 6 - week 11*

- This mimics the appearance of an omphalocele.

Omphalocele – This is a congenital midline defect, with herniation of gut at the base of the umbilical cord.

Trivia to know:
- It DOES have a surrounding membrane (gastroschisis does not), so AFP not elevated.
- Associated anomalies are common (unlike gastroschisis)
- Trisomy 18 is the most common associated chromosomal anomaly
- Other associations: Cardiac (50%), Other GI, CNS, GU, Turners, Klinefelters, Beckwith-Wiedemann.
- Outcomes are not that good, because of associated syndromes.
- Umbilical Cord Cysts (Allantoic Cysts) are associated.

Case 87 - Pre-Natal Check Up (7 weeks)

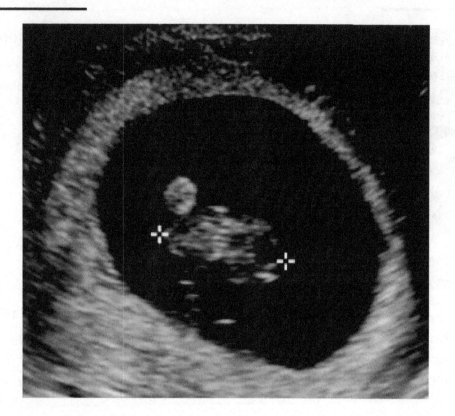

1. What is the diagnosis?
A. Dandy Walker Malformation
B. Hydrocephalus (aqueductal stenosis)
C. Total normal at this gestational age

2. The Rhombencephalon forms what?
A. The Thalamus
B. The Midbrain
C. The Hindbrain (cerebellum, Pons, & medulla)
D. The cerebral hemispheres

3. In a Dandy Walker malformation, what is the relationship between the Torcula and the Lambdoid suture?
A. The Torcula is elevated above it
B. The Torcula is depressed below it
C. They line up perfectly

Case 87 - Normal Cystic Rhombencephalon

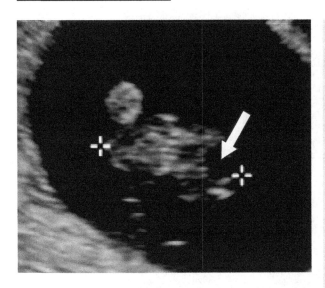

1. What is the diagnosis?
A. Dandy Walker Malformation
B. Hydrocephalus (aqueductal stenosis)
C. **Total normal at this gestational age**

2. The Rhombencephalon forms what?
A. The Thalamus
B. The Midbrain
C. **The Hindbrain (cerebellum, Pons, & medulla)**
D. The cerebral hemispheres

3. In a Dandy Walker malformation, what is the relationship between the Torcula and the Lambdoid suture?
A. **The Torcula is elevated above it**
B. The Torcula is depressed below it
C. They line up perfectly

Normal Cystic Rhombencephalon

A normal thing, that looks like a scary CNS problem.

Essential Trivia:

- *Normal Embryology:*
  - The rhombencephalon is a primary brain "vesicle" that will go on to form the hindbrain (Cerebellum, pons, medulla)
  - Between week 6 and 8 this has a normal cystic appearance, with the cavity forming a normally proportioned 4th ventricle by week 11.
  - ****Normal from week 6 - week 8**

- This is sometimes confused (by the un-initiated) as a Dandy Walker Malformation.

Dandy Walker

The results of a mal-developed roof to the 4th ventricle.

Classically there are 3 findings to know:
(1) Hypoplasia of the vermis
(2) Cystic dilation of the 4th Ventricle
(3) **Torcular-Lambdoid Inversion** *(torcula above the lambdoid suture because of elevation of the tentorium).*

WTF is the Torcula? - It's a fancy word for the confluence of the venous sinuses

Case 88 - Pre-Natal Screen

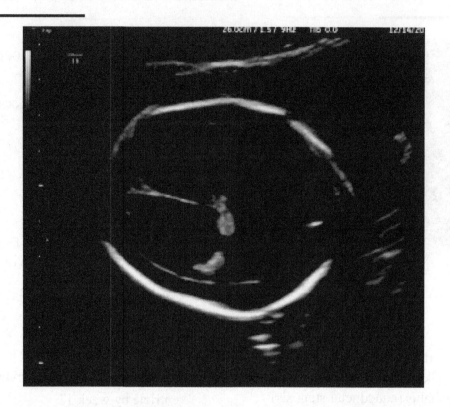

1. What is the diagnosis?
A. Hydrocephalus
B. Hydranencephaly
C. Holoprosencephaly

2. What is the most common congenital cause of this?
A. Stroke
B. Sickle Cell
C. Fetal EtOH Syndrome
D. Aqueductal Stenosis

3. The absence of a cortical mantle (not seen in this case) would suggest?
A. Hydrocephalus
B. Hydranencephaly
C. Holoprosencephaly

Case 88 - Hydrocephalus (Aqueductal Stenosis)

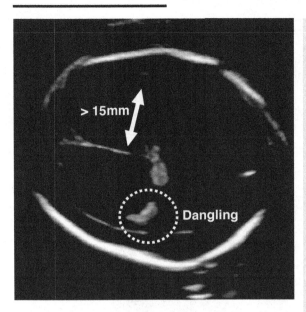

Aqueductal Stenosis

One of the most common causes of congenital obstructive hydrocephalus.

Essential Trivia:

Aqueductal Stenosis:

- Causes can be congenital (from webs or scarring), acquired (from tumors), or intrinsic (from infection or blood).

Fetal Hydrocephalus

- Typically defined as **lateral ventricle size greater than 15mm**

- *"Dangling Choroid Sign"* - this is when you have choroid separated more than 3mm from the margin of the ventricle

- Up to 80% have associated anomalies.

1. What is the diagnosis?
A. Hydrocephalus
B. Hydranencephaly
C. Holoprosencephaly

2. What is the most common congenital cause of this?
A. Stroke
B. Sickle Cell
C. Fetal EtOH Syndrome
D. Aqueductal Stenosis

3. The absence of a cortical mantle (not seen in this case) would suggest?
A. Hydrocephalus
B. Hydranencephaly
C. Holoprosencephaly

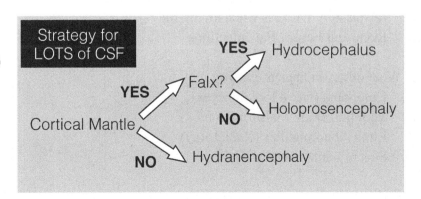

Case 89 - Trouble Breathing

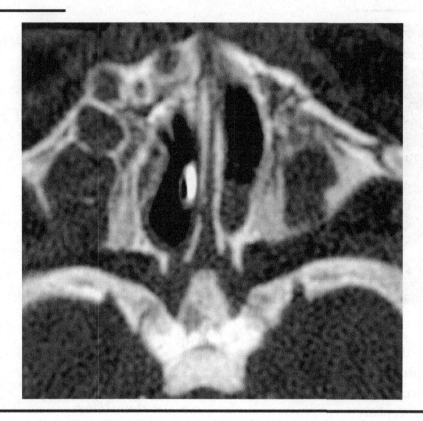

1. What is the diagnosis?
A. Sinonasal Polyposis
B. Choanal Atresia
C. Allergic Sinusitis
D. Holoprosencephaly.

2. What is the most "classic" clinical history?
A. Respiratory Distress when running
B. Respiratory Distress when Feeding
C. Respiratory Distress when laying flat
D. Recurrent Fever / Ear Infections

3. What other findings might you look for?
A. Coloboma (weird looking eyes)
B. Vertebral Body Malformations
C. Limb Abnormalities (Radial Ray)
D. Severe white matter disease

Case 89 - Choanal Atresia

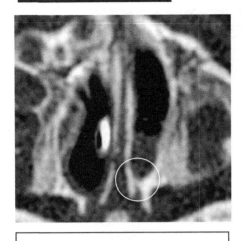
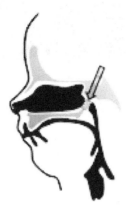
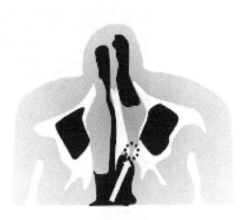

Bony Obstruction of the choanal opening

Air Fluid Level above obstruction point

Medial Bowing of the posterior medial sinus

1. What is the diagnosis?
A. Sinonasal Polyposis
B. Choanal Atresia
C. Allergic Sinusitis
D. Holoprosencephaly.

2. What is the most "classic" clinical history?
A. Respiratory Distress when running
B. Respiratory Distress when Feeding
C. Respiratory Distress when laying flat
D. Recurrent Fever / Ear Infections

3. What other findings might you look for?
A. Coloboma (weird looking eyes)
B. Vertebral Body Malformations
C. Limb Abnormalities (Radial Ray)
D. Severe white matter disease

Choanal Atresia

Congenital lack of formation of the choanal openings.

Essential Trivia:

-Two types: Bony (90%) and Membraneous (10%)

-It's usually unilateral (65%)

-The classic history is either (a) failure to pass the NG tube, or (b) respiratory distress while feeding – can't breathe through nose and you have a bottle / nipple in your mouth.

-Don't forget that infants are obligate nose breathers

-There is a known association with early pregnancy use of antithyroid drugs

-There are multiple syndromes associated with this – the big one to know is **CHARGE** (**C**oloboma, **H**eart Defects, **A**tresia - Choanal, **R**etardation, **G**enital Issues, **E**ar Problems)

Case 90 - Belly Looks Big

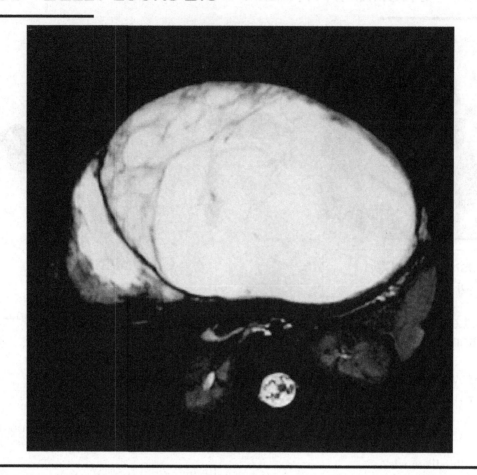

1. What is the diagnosis?
A. Hepatoblastoma
B. Infantile Hemangioendothelioma
C. Mesenchymal Hamartoma
D. HCC (Fibrolamellar)

2. Which is true regarding the age group this tumor is found in?
A. Never seen before 6 months
B. Most commonly seen between age 0-2
C. Most commonly seen between age 5-10
D. Most commonly seen in teenagers

3. What lab would you expect to be elevated?
A. AFP
B. Endothelial Growth Factor
C. Neither

Case 90 - Mesenchymal Hamartoma

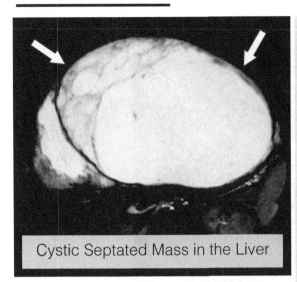

Cystic Septated Mass in the Liver

1. What is the diagnosis?
A. Hepatoblastoma
B. Infantile Hemangioendothelioma
C. Mesenchymal Hamartoma
D. HCC (Fibrolamellar)

2. Which is true regarding the age group this tumor is found in?
A. Never seen before 6 months
B. Most commonly seen between age 0-2
C. Most commonly seen between age 5-10
D. Most commonly seen in teenagers

3. What lab would you expect to be elevated?
A. AFP
B. Endothelial Growth Factor
C. Neither

Mesenchymal Hamartoma

Cystic tumor seen in the liver of neonates

Essential Trivia:

- It's one of the 3 tumors you think about in the liver of a 1 year old (the other two are hepatoblastoma, and infantile hemangioendothelioma).

- This tumor can be distinguished from those 2, because its very cyst like.

- Some people don't even consider this a tumor, but more of a developmental anomaly.

- Symptoms (and possible death) occur from the mass effect this thing delivers.

- AFP is usually negative (classically elevated with hepatoblastoma)

Classic Look:
- Large, mostly cystic, septated mass in the liver of a kid (2 or younger).

DDx:
- *Hepatoblastoma* – Same Age Group, But more solid, and has elevated AFP

- *Infantile Hemangioendothelioma* – Same Age Group, but looks like a vascular lesion (not a cyst). Also has elevated endothelial growth factor.

Case 91 - Infertility Workup

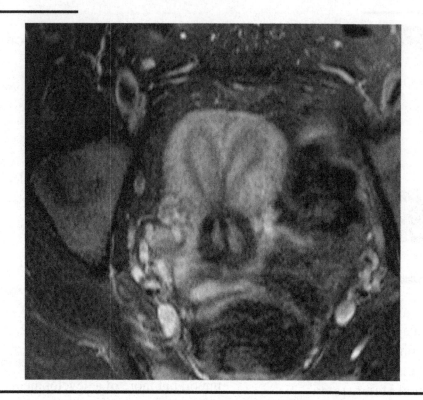

1. What is the diagnosis?
A. Arcuate Uterus
B. T Shaped Uterus
C. Septate Uterus
D. Bicornuate Uterus

2. Is there an increased risk of infertility/fetal loss?
A. Yes
B. Not Usually

3. Which of the following statements is TRUE?
A. DES use was associated with a Bicornuate Uterus
B. Arcuate Uterus has an increased risk of fetal loss
C. Septate Uterus has a NORMAL fundal contour
D. Bicornuate Uterus has a NORMAL fundal contour

Case 91 - Septate Uterus

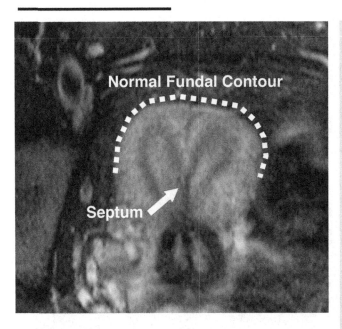

1. What is the diagnosis?
A. Arcuate Uterus
B. T Shaped Uterus
C. Septate Uterus
D. Bicornuate Uterus

2. Is there an increased risk of infertility/fetal loss?
A. Yes
B. Not Usually

3. Which of the following statements is TRUE?
A. DES use was associated with a Bicornuate Uterus ** *"T-Shaped"*
B. Arcuate Uterus has an increased risk of fetal loss ** *Nope it's a normal variant*
C. Septate Uterus has a NORMAL fundal contour
D. Bicornuate Uterus has a NORMAL fundal contour **Nope*

Septate Uterus

Uterine Malformation characterized by a residual septum.

Essential Trivia:

- This one has two endometrial canals separated by a fibrous (or muscular) septum.

- Fibrous vs Muscular can be determined with MRI and this distinction changes surgical management (different approaches).

- Septum is a normal developmental structure that is suppose to resorb (usually resorbing from inferior to superior).

- **There is an increased risk of infertility and recurrent spontaneous abortion** (felt to be secondary to implantation on the septum).

Classic Description:
- **Normal Fundal Contour + Septum**
- 1 Uterus, 1 Cervix, 2 Ovaries --- otherwise normal.

Case 92 - Infertility Workup

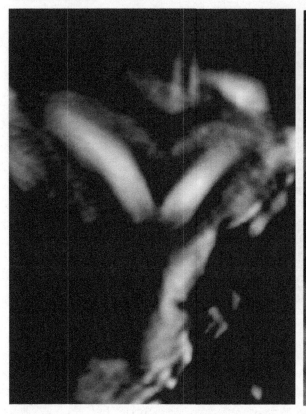 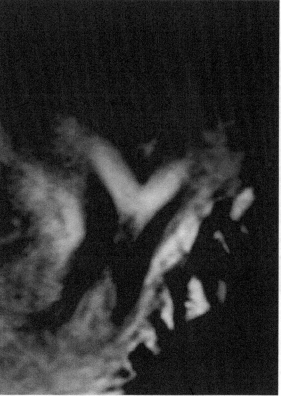

1. What is the diagnosis?
A. Arcuate Uterus
B. T Shaped Uterus
C. Septate Uterus
D. Bicornuate Uterus

2. Is there an increased risk of infertility/fetal loss?
A. Yes
B. Not Usually

3. When you have a mullerian duct anomaly, you should also remember to look at?
A. The heart
B. The pancreas
C. The kidneys
D. The liver

Case 92 - Bicornuate Uterus

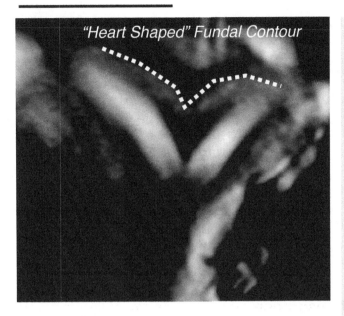

"Heart Shaped" Fundal Contour

1. What is the diagnosis?
A. Arcuate Uterus
B. T Shaped Uterus
C. Septate Uterus
D. Bicornuate Uterus

2. Is there an increased risk of infertility/fetal loss?
A. Yes
B. Not Usually

3. When you have a mullerian duct anomaly, you should also remember to look at?
A. The heart
B. The pancreas
C. The kidneys
D. The liver

Bicornuate Uterus

Uterine Malformation characterized by a **"heart shape"**, with two horns to the uterus.

Essential Trivia:

- This comes in two flavors (one cervix unicollis, two cervix bicollis). There will be separation of the uterus by a deep myometrial cleft.

Bicornuate vs Septate
- This requires some kind of cross sectional imaging (you can't tell by HSG). You distinguish the two by the apex of the fundal contour:
    - Apex of Fundal Contour > 5mm Above Tubal Ostia = Septate
    - Apex of Fundal Contour < 5mm Above Tubal Ostia = Bicornuate

- The risk of fetal loss is much less than septate, and for the most part not a major issue.

- There is a 25% chance of an associated longitudinal vaginal septum

Classic Description:
- ABnormal Fundal Contour (external fundal indentation >1cm)
- Can have one or two cervixes (uni or bi-collis)

Uterine Malformations - Essential Trivia

Lack of Development

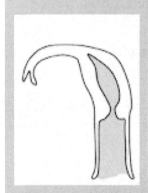
Unicornuate

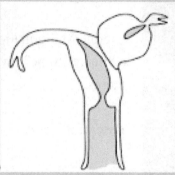
Unicornuate
- with Non-Communicating Rudimentary Horn

Essential Trivia:

- Endometrial tissue in a rudimentary horn (communicating or not – **increases the risk of miscarriage and uterine rupture**

- 40% of these chicks will have renal issues (usually renal agenesis) ipsilateral to the rudimentary horn.

Lack of Resorption

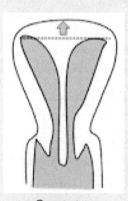
Septate

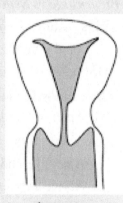
Arcuate

Essential Trivia:

- The Arcuate Uterus is just a concavity to the fundus. **It's a normal variant**, and has no significance clinically.

- Septate Uterus has a normal fundal contour, and a **known increased risk for fetal loss / infertility**.

Lack of Fusion

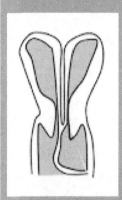
Didelphys

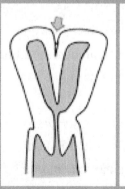
Bicornuate

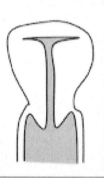
T-Shaped

Essential Trivia:

- Didelphys - if no vaginal septum, it's typically asymptomatic

- T Shaped - This is seen in daughters of patient's who took **DES** (synthetic estrogen) in the 1940s. They **also get vaginal clear cell CA.**

Bicornuate vs Septate

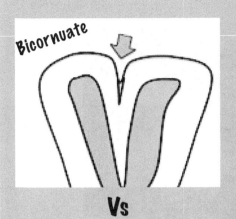

Bicornuate

- **"Heart Shaped"** - Fundal contour is <u>less</u> than 5mm above the tubal ostia

- No significant infertility issues

- Resection of the "septum" results in poor outcomes

Septate

- Fundal contour is **Normal** ; <u>more</u> than 5mm above the tubal ostia

- Legit infertility issues

- Resection of the septum can help

Bicornate vs Didelphus

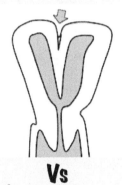

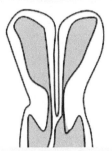

Bicornuate

- *"Partial Fusion"*

- 2 uteri, 1 or partial 2 cervix, 1 vagina

- Vaginal Septum about 25% of the time

- Clinically - between unicornuate / normal

Didelphys

- *NO Fusion*

- 2 uteri, 2 cervix, 2 upper 1/3 vagina

- Vaginal Septum about 75% of the time

- Clinically – like unicornuate

Case 93 - History Withheld

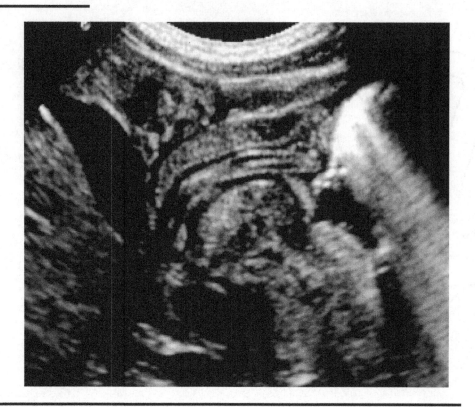

1. What is the diagnosis?
A. Gastric Volvulus
B. Duodenal Web
C. Hypertrophic Pyloric Stenosis
D. Annular Pancreas

2. What is the classic clinical history?
A. Vomiting (Bilious)
B. Vomiting (Non-Bilious)
C. Constipation

3. What age do you see this pathology?
A. You can see it immediately after birth
B. Between 1 week and 3 weeks (rare after 1 month)
C. Between 3 weeks and 3 months
D. Most commonly seen between age 3 and 6

Case 93 - Hypertrophic Pyloric Stenosis

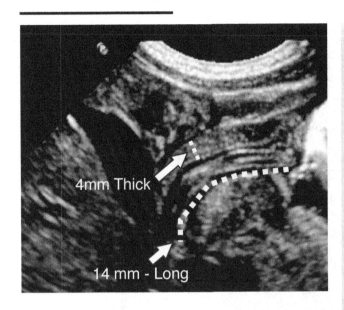

1. What is the diagnosis?
A. Gastric Volvulus
B. Duodenal Web
C. Hypertrophic Pyloric Stenosis
D. Annular Pancreas

2. What is the classic clinical history?
A. Vomiting (Bilious)
B. Vomiting (Non-Bilious)
C. Constipation

3. What age do you see this pathology?
A. You can see it immediately after birth
B. Between 1 week and 3 weeks (rare after 1 month)
C. Between 3 weeks and 3 months
D. Most commonly seen between age 3 and 6

Hypertrophic Pyloric Stenosis

Thickening of the gastric pyloric musculature, which can result in progressive obstruction

Essential Trivia:

- Step 1 buzzword is **"non-bilious vomiting."**

- **Does NOT occur at birth** or after 3 months. There is a specific age range 2-12 weeks (**peak at 3-6 weeks**). ****just think 3wks to 3 months**

- Criteria is 4mm and 14mm (4mm single wall, 14mm length).

- The primary differential is pylorospasm (which will relax during exam).

- The most common pitfall during the exam is gastric over distention, which can lead to displacement of the antrum and pylorus – leading to false negative.

- False positive can result from off axis measurement.

- The phenomenon of "paradoxial aciduria" has been described, and is a common buzzword.

Case 94 - Belly Pain

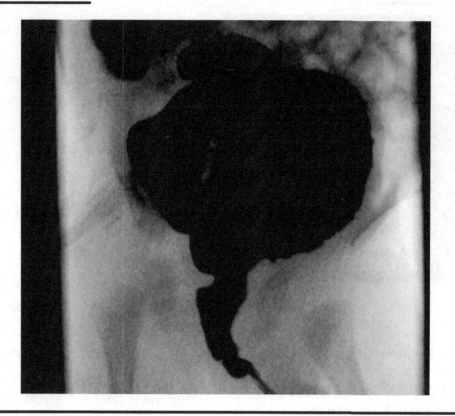

1. What is the diagnosis?
A. Anterior Urethral Valves
B. Posterior Urethral Valves
C. Membranous Urethral Stricture
D. Hutch Diverticulum

2. Who do you see this pathology in?
A. Baby Boys
B. Baby Girls
C. Both Baby Boys and Girls
D. Presents in Boys when they start to toilet train (around age 2)

3. Most cases are ?
A. Sporadic
B. Syndromic

Case 94 - Posterior Urethral Valves

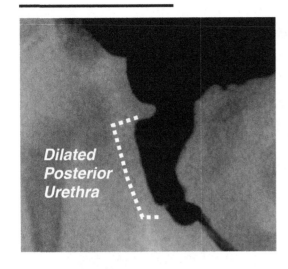

1. What is the diagnosis?
A. Anterior Urethral Valves
B. Posterior Urethral Valves
C. Membranous Urethral Stricture
D. Hutch Diverticulum

2. Who do you see this pathology in?
A. Baby Boys
B. Baby Girls
C. Both Baby Boys and Girls
D. Presents in Boys when they start to toilet train (around age 2)

3. Most cases are ?
A. Sporadic
B. Syndromic

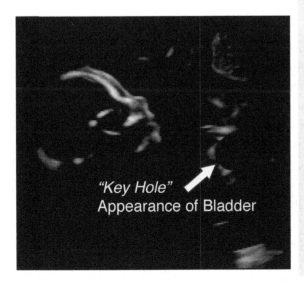

Posterior Urethral Valves

Most common congenital obstructive lesion of the urethra

Essential Trivia:

- A thick valve like membrane, which gets left behind in a failure of regression of the mesonephric duct. It's located at the verumontanum – distal prostatic urethra.

- Only seen in male infants

- Pre-natal US may show oligohydramnios (when severe)

- VCUG (Voiding Cystourethrogram) is the best test. The best phase during this test is the micturition phase. You need a lateral (or oblique view) to actually see the urethra.

Ways this can be shown:
- VCUG demonstrating the Valve (as in this case)
- Neonatal Hydro – prenatal US (3rd trimester)
- Neonatal Hydro – prenatal MRI (3rd trimester)
- *"Keyhole Sign"* – dilation of the posterior urethra can cause a "key hole" like appearance on US.

Case 95 - History Withheld

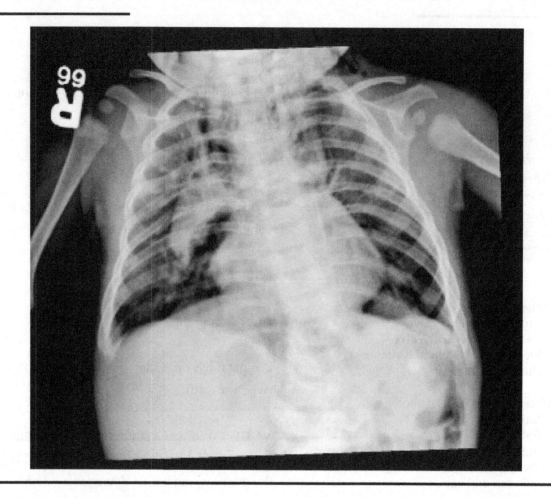

1. What is the diagnosis?
A. Normal Study
B. Thymus is enlarged (possibly rebound)
C. Lymphoma
D. Pneumomediastinum

2. Which of the follow is true ?
A. Thymic hyperplasia is COLD on PET, Lymphoma is HOT on PET
B. Thymic hyperplasia is HOT on PET, Lymphoma is HOT on PET
C. Thymic hyperplasia is COLD on PET, Lymphoma is COLD on PET
D. Thymic hyperplasia is HOT on PET, Lymphoma is COLD on PET

3. Which is true regarding the fat pads of the elbow?
A. The Anterior fat pad should never be visible
B. The Posterior fat pad can sometimes be seen , but the anterior fat pad should never be seen.
C. A false positive posterior fat pad sign can occur from improper positioning

Case 95 - Spinnaker Sail Sign - (Pneumomediastinum)

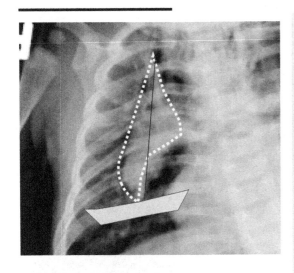

1. What is the diagnosis?
A. Normal Study
B. Thymus is enlarged (possibly rebound)
C. Lymphoma
D. Pneumomediastinum

2. Which of the follow is true?
A. Thymic hyperplasia is COLD on PET, Lymphoma is HOT on PET
B. Thymic hyperplasia is HOT on PET, Lymphoma is HOT on PET
C. Thymic hyperplasia is COLD on PET, Lymphoma is COLD on PET
D. Thymic hyperplasia is HOT on PET, Lymphoma is COLD on PET

3. Which is true regarding the fat pads of the elbow?
A. The Anterior fat pad should never be visible
B. The Posterior fat pad can sometimes be seen, but the anterior fat pad should never be seen.
C. A false positive posterior fat pad sign can occur from improper positioning

Spinnaker Sail Sign

A sign of pneumomediastinum

Essential Trivia:

- This occurs when the thymus is outlined by air and displaced laterally.

Other Sail Signs:
- **Elbow Sail Sign – Joint Effusion**
  - Pearls: Anterior Fat Pad, sometimes seen as a thin sliver. The posterior fat pad should never be seen (if the elbow is correctly positioned, as a true lateral). Joint effusion can float the fat pads out, creating the appearance of a sail – an indicating an occult fracture.

- **Adult Chest Sail Sign (retrocardiac sail)** – Left Lower Lobe Collapse. Collapse of the LLL can create a triangular "sail like" density behind the heart.

Thymic Rebound –
- The thymus shrinks during stress, and then "rebounds" bigger than it was before (usually taking around 9 months). Classic times when this occurs, are post chemo, or after hanging out in the NICU (getting stressed out).

- The trick question is this can be PET Avid, and mimic lymphoma. Supposedly you can tell them apart by morphology (the thymus will still drape over the heart, whereas lymphoma is a ball).

Case 96 - Leg Pain

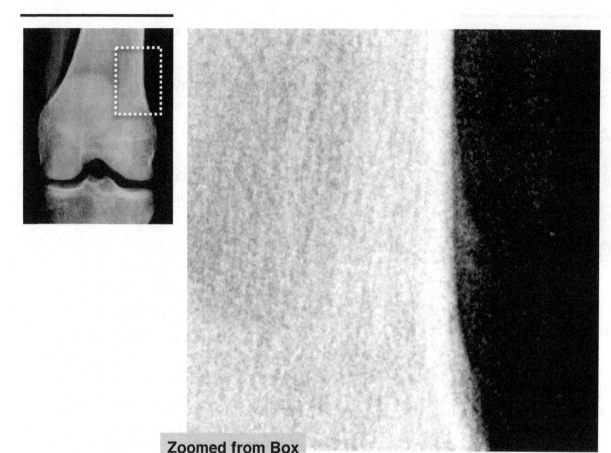

Zoomed from Box

1. What is the diagnosis?
A. Chondrosarcoma
B. Osteosarcoma
C. ABC
D. Myositis Ossificans

2. Which typically has the best prognosis?
A. Conventional (Intramedullary) Type
B. Periosteal
C. Parosteal
D. Telangiectatic

3. Which is true ?
A. The mineralization pattern of osteosarcoma goes from peripheral to central
B. The mineralization pattern of myositis ossificans goes from peripheral to central

4. If this patient had a pneumothorax – what would you say the likely cause was?

A. Family medicine trying to put a central line in on the floor
B. Bleb rupture – (assuming the patient smokes)
C. Metastatic Disease to the lung
D. Chemotherapy induced pneumothorax

Case 96 - Codman's Triangle - Osteosarcoma

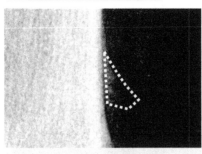

Codman triangle - With aggressive lesions, the periosteum does not have time to ossify completely, so only the edge of the raised periosteum will ossify – creating the appearance of a triangle.

1. What is the diagnosis?
A. Chondrosarcoma
B. Osteosarcoma
C. ABC
D. Myositis Ossificans

2. Which typically has the best prognosis?
A. Conventional (Intramedullary) Type
B. Periosteal
C. Parosteal
D. Telangiectatic

3. Which is true?
A. The mineralization pattern of osteosarcoma goes from peripheral to central
B. The mineralization pattern of myositis ossificans goes from peripheral to central

4. If this patient had a pneumothorax – what would you say the likely cause was?

A. Family medicine trying to put a central line in on the floor
B. Bleb rupture – (assuming the patient smokes)
C. Metastatic Disease to the lung
D. Chemotherapy induced

Essential Trivia:

- There are a bunch of subtypes, but for the purpose of this discussion there are 4. Conventional Intramedullary (85%), Parosteal (4%), Periosteal (1%), Telangiectatic (rare).

- All the subtypes produce bone or osteoid from neoplastic cells, and prefer the femur.

- Most are idiopathic, but the testable causes are: Pagets, Prior Radiation, and Bone Infarct.

Pearls Per Sub-Type:

- **Conventional Intramedullary** – Most Common, typically higher grade than surface types. Occurs between age 10-20.

- **Parosteal** – "BULKY" surface lesion. Typically low grade. Seen in middle aged adults.

- **Periosteal** – Surface lesion, but less bulky. Worse prognosis than parosteal (but better than conventional type). Seen in ages 15-25.

- **Telangiectatic** – Will have fluid-fluid levels on MRI. Kinda looks like an ABC. Prognosis is similar to that of the conventional type. Average age is 20.

High Yield Trivia:

- Osteosarcoma met to the lung is a "classic" (frequently tested) cause of occult pneumothorax.
- "Reverse Zoning Phenomenon" – more dense mature matrix in the center, less peripherally (opposite of myositis ossificans).
- Secondary Osteosarcomas – From Pagets, tend to be very high grade

Case 97 - Daily NICU CXR

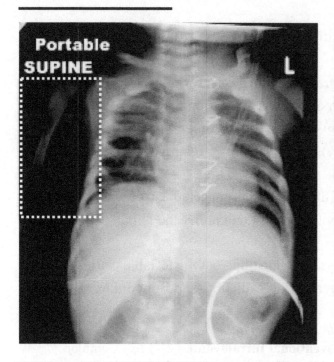
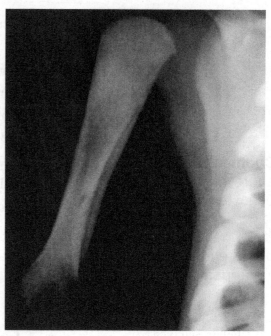

1. What is the most likely cause of the finding?
A. Prostaglandin Therapy
B. Stress from the NICU
C. Chronic Steroid Use
D. Langerhans Cell Histiocytosis

2. Which of the follow is true regarding Physiologic Periostitis of the Newborn ?
A. It occurs in a newborn
B. It occurs in the femur before the tibia
C. It occurs in the metaphysis (never the diaphysis)

3. Where is the classic location for the erosion lesion seen in congenital syphilis?
A. The medial proximal tibia
B. The lateral proximal tibia
C. The lateral distal femur
D. The medial distal femur

Case 97 - Periosteal Reaction (Prostaglandin Therapy)

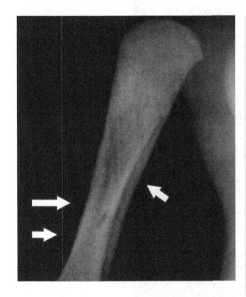

1. What is the most likely cause of the finding?
   A. **Prostaglandin Therapy**
   B. Stress from the NICU
   C. Chronic Steroid Use
   D. Langerhans Cell Histiocytosis

2. Which of the follow is true regarding Physiologic Periostitis of the Newborn ?
   A. It occurs in a newborn
   B. **It occurs in the femur before the tibia** *(proximal before distal)*
   C. It occurs in the metaphysis (never the diaphysis)

3. Where is the classic location for the erosion lesion seen in congenital syphilis?
   A. **The medial proximal tibia**
   B. The lateral proximal tibia
   C. The lateral distal femur
   D. The medial distal femur

Periosteal Reaction

It's a nonspecific finding of periosteal irritation.

Essential Trivia:

- Prostaglandin Therapy – Prostaglandin E1 and E2 (often used to keep a PDA open) can cause a periosteal reaction. The classic trick is to show a chest x-ray with sternotomy wires (or other hints of congenital heart), and then periosteal reaction in the arm bones

Other Causes:

- *"Physiologic Periostitis of the Newborn"* – should never happen in a newborn. You see it around 3 months. There are 3 "Nots" of this Physiologic Periostitis. (1) NOT before 1 month, (2) NOT in the tibia before the femur, (3) NOT Metaphysis (should be diaphysis).

- Periosteal Reaction in the Jaw is **Caffeys disease** (for multiple choice), and bisphosphonate therapy for Osteogenesis Imperfecta in the real world.

- **TORCHS** like Rubella and Syphilis can cause it. Remember "Celery stalk" for rubella, and medial proximal metaphysis of the tibia (Wimberger) for Syphilis

- Never forget that **child abuse** can present as a periosteal reaction (healing fracture)

- **Neuroblastoma mets**

Case 98 - Walking Funny

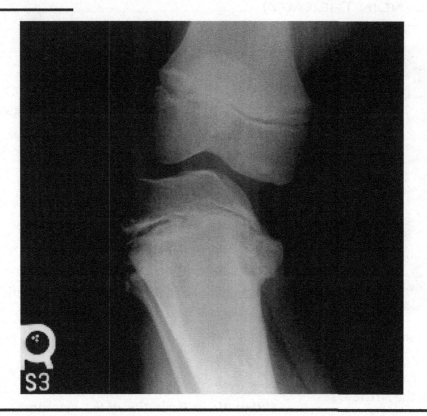

1. What is the diagnosis?
A. Sinding-Larsen Johansson
B. Blounts
C. Congenital Syphilis
D. Congenital Rubella

2. What is the other name for this?
A. Tibia Valga
B. Tibia Vara

3. Which of the follow is true?
A. It's rarely bilateral
B. It's usually seen before age 2
C. When seen in adolescents - it's usually a fat kid
D. It's associated with delayed ambulation ("late walkers")

Case 98 - Blount Disease

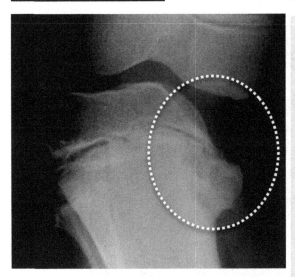

1. What is the diagnosis?
A. Sinding-Larsen Johansson
B. Blounts
C. Congenital Syphilis
D. Congenital Rubella

2. What is the other name for this?
A. Tibia Valga
B. Tibia Vara

3. Which of the follow is true?
A. It's rarely bilateral
B. It's usually seen before age 2
C. When seen in adolescents - it's usually a fat kid
D. It's associated with delayed ambulation ("late walkers")

Blount Disease (Tibia Vara)

Growth disorder of the tibia, which resembles a "bowed leg."

Essential Trivia:

- Varus angulation occurring at the medial aspect of the proximal tibia (varus bowing occurs at the metaphysis not the knee).

- This is often bilateral, and NOT often seen before age 2 *(two sides, not before two)*.

- Later in the disease progression the medial metaphysis will be depressed and an osseous outgrowth classically develops.

- You can see it in two different age groups; (a) early – which is around age 3, and (b) late – which is around age 12.

- The early type is seen in "early walkers"
    - Possible mechanism is stress on a bone that's not ready to bare weight

- The late type is seen in fat kids
    - Possible mechanism is too much Burger King and Taco Bell

Aunt Minnie 216

Case 99 - This Kid Hates To Play Outside

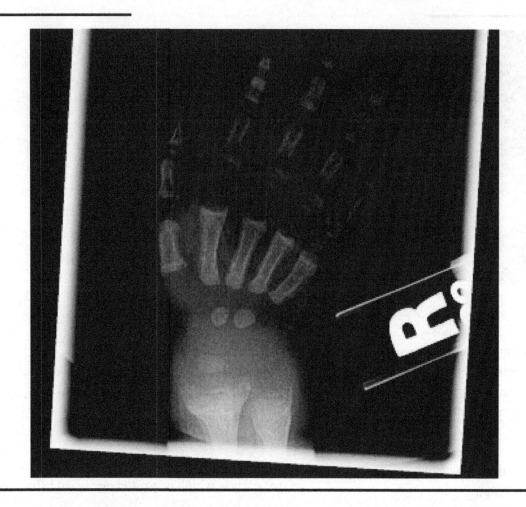

1. What is the diagnosis?
A. Ellis-Van Crevald
B. Rickets
C. Achondroplasia
D. Congenital Rubella

2. Can this disorder occur in a newborn?
A. Yup
B. Nope

3. Which of the following is true?
A. This kid is at increased risk for SCFE
B. The disorder is typically least prominent at the growth plates
C. Leg Bowing classically begins before ambulation
D. The bones are paradoxically increased in strength

Case 99 - Rickets

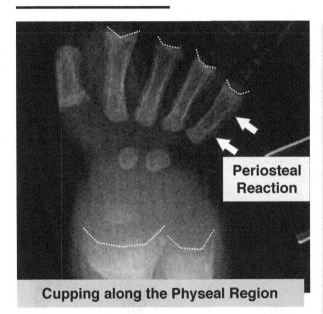

Cupping along the Physeal Region / Periosteal Reaction

Rickets

Metabolic condition that occurs from a lack of Vitamin D (or the inability to use it correctly).

Essential Trivia:

- Targets the most rapidly growing bones (knees and wrists), with features most prominent at the areas of growth (growth plates).

- NOT seen in newborns; the Mother's Vitamin D is still doing it's thing.

- If you see what looks like rickets on x-ray in a newborn the answer is Hypophosphatasia

- These kids are at increased risk for SCFE (and other fractures)

Classic Findings:
- "Cupping / Fraying" of the physeal margins.
- Bowing of the knees - especially once the kid starts walking.
- Involvement of the anterior ribs ends "Rachitic Rosary"

1. What is the diagnosis?
A. Ellis-Van Crevald
B. Rickets
C. Achondroplasia
D. Congenital Rubella

2. Can this disorder occur in a newborn?
A. Yup
B. Nope * when x-ray features are seen on a newborn the answer in Hypophosphatasia

3. Which of the following is true?
A. This kid is at increased risk for SCFE
B. The disorder is typically least prominent at the growth plates
C. Leg Bowing classically begins before ambulation
D. The bones are paradoxically increased in strength

Case 100 - Belly Pain (3 month old)

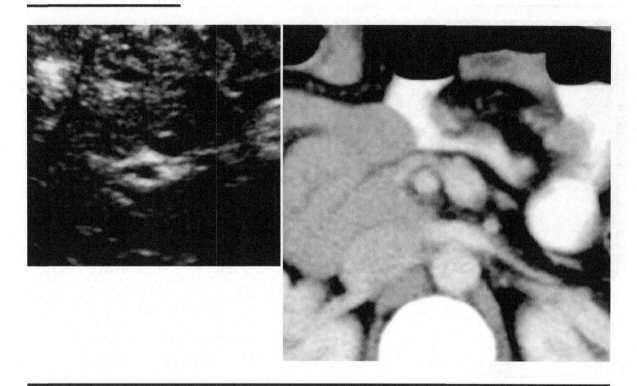

1. What is going on here?
A. Looks normal to me
B. Heterotaxia
C. Malrotation
D. Biliary Atresia

2. What if this kid came in with bilious vomiting ?
A. "Clinical Correlation" , could be viral
B. Could be obstructed needs an Upper GI
C. Could be obstructed needs a water soluble enema
D. Could be obstructed needs a CT

3. What surgical procedure is done on these kids ?
A. Lecompte maneuver
B. Kasai Procedure
C. Ross Procedure
D. Ladds Procedure

Case 100 - Malrotation

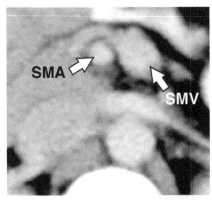

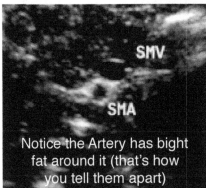

Notice the Artery has bight fat around it (that's how you tell them apart)

1. What is going on here?
A. Looks normal to me
B. Heterotaxia
C. Malrotation
D. Biliary Atresia

2. What if this kid came in with bilious vomiting ?
A. "Clinical Correlation", could be viral
B. Could be obstructed needs an Upper GI
C. Could be obstructed needs a water soluble enema
D. Could be obstructed needs a CT

3. What surgical procedure is done on these kids ?
A. Lecompte maneuver
B. Kasai Procedure
C. Ross Procedure
D. Ladds Procedure

SMA & SMV Reversal - Malrotation

The SMA is normally on the same side as the Aorta (artery with artery). When you seen it reversed - think Malrotation.

Essential Trivia:

- Normally, the developmental rotation of the gut places the ligament of Trietz to the left of the spine (at the level of the duodenal bulb).

- These patients are at increased risk for mid gut volvulus, and internal hernias.

- If you see the appearance of malrotation and the clinical history is bilious vomiting, then you must suspect midgut volvulus.

- In an older chid (or even adults) obstruction + malrotation is from kinking from a "Ladds Band" - which is a stalk of peritoneal tissue.

- The "Ladds Procedure" is done to prevent volvulus. It involves cutting out the Ladds band, and stimulating adhesion formation to tac the bowel down.

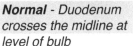

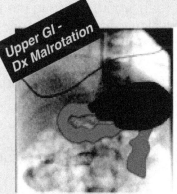
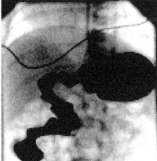

Normal - Duodenum crosses the midline at level of bulb

Malrotation

Random Peds - Essential Trivia

Timed Trivia

Airway/Lungs:
- Croup - Peaks around 1 year
- Epiglottis - Peaks are 3.5 years
- Transient Tachypnea - Should resolve by day 3
- Respiratory Distress Syndrome (Hyaline Membrane) - seen in kids < 32 weeks
- Extralobar Sequestration presents early b/c of heart disease association
- Intralobar Sequestration presents later with recurrent pneumonia

Adrenals/Kidneys/Testicles
- Neuroblastoma - you can be born with
- Wilms tumor - you can NOT be born with (shows up around age 1)
- Kidney Tumors (age < 1) think Nephroblastomatosis - the wilms precursor, and Mesoblastic Nephroma
- Torsion of the Testicular Appendages – most common cause of acute scrotal pain in age 7-14.

GI:
- Hypertrophic pyloric stenosis - NOT in newborn ; think 3 weeks - 3 months
- Intussusception - think 3 months - 3 years
- NEC occurs 90% of the time within the first 10 days of life
- Liver Tumors (age < 1) think Hemangioendothelioma, Hepatoblastoma, and Mesenchymal Hamartoma

Bones:
- Remember the elbow ossifications occur in a set order (CRITOE), Capitellum (Age 1), Radius (Age 3), Internal (medial epicondyle – Age 5), Trochlea (Age 7), Olecranon(Age 9), and External (lateral epicondyle – Age 11).
- Blounts occurs around age 3 (or less commonly in fat adolescents)
- Congenital Syphilis - Bony changes do NOT occur until 6-8 weeks of life
- Congenital Rubella - Bony changes occur in the first week of life
- Caffey's Disease (if it were real) would occur in the first 6 months of life
- Physiologic Periostitis of the Newborn - doesn't occur till around 3 months
- Perthes occurs around age 6
- SCFE occurs around age 12
- Bony changes of Rickets are NOT seen in a newborn, if it looks like Rickets in a newborn the answer is Hypophosphatasia

Neuro:
- Germinal Matrix Hemorrhage is only seen in premature infants - never after 36 weeks

When You See This — You Gotta Look There

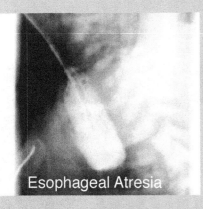
Esophageal Atresia

VACTERL

V – Vertebral Anomalies (37%)
A – Anal (imperforate anus) (63%)
C – Cardiac (77%)
TE – Tracheoesophageal Fistula (40%)
R – Renal (72%)
L – Limb (radial ray) – 58%

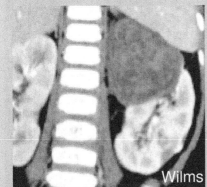
Wilms

Wilms Associations

Beckwith-Weidemann:
-Big Tongue, Omphalocele, Hemihypertrophy

WAGR
-Wilms, Aniridia, Genital, Growth Retardation

Other associations:
- Hepatoblastoma

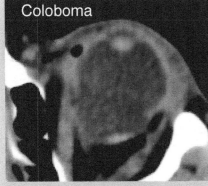
Coloboma

CHARGE Syndrome

- **C**oloboma of the eye,
- **H**eart defects,
- **A**tresia of the choanae,
- **R**etardation of growth and/or development,
- **G**enital and/or urinary abnormalities,
- **E**ar abnormalities/deafness.

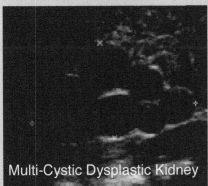
Multi-Cystic Dysplastic Kidney

Multi-Cystic Dysplastic Kidneys

- 50% have a UPJ Obstruction on the other side

- If you see a UPJ Obstruction, Look for "Crossing Vessels," as a possible cause

Case 101 - Palpable Bump

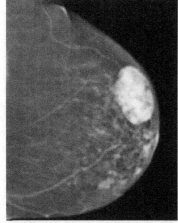
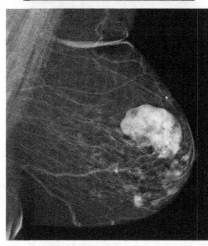
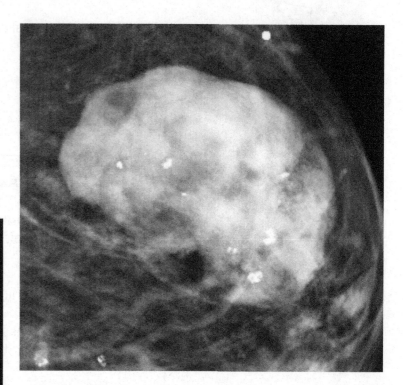

1. What is the diagnosis?
A. Lipoma
B. IDC
C. Island of Normal Breast Tissue
D. Hamartoma

2. Lets say this was biopsied and the path showed Pseudoangiomatous Stromal Hyperplasia, what is the prognosis?
A. Certain Death
B. Might be ok, with Chemo and Radiation - stage the axilla
C. Should be fine , it's a benign entity

3. What subtype of IDC is associated with Radial Scar?
A. Mucinous
B. Medullary
C. Papillary
D. Tubular

Case 101 - Hamartoma

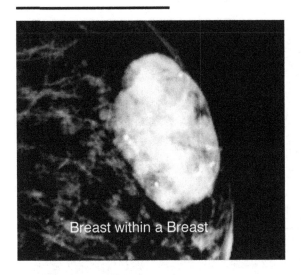

Breast within a Breast

1. What is the diagnosis?
A. Lipoma
B. IDC
C. Island of Normal Breast Tissue
D. **Hamartoma**

2. Lets say this was biopsied and the path showed Pseudoangiomatous Stromal Hyperplasia, what is the prognosis?
A. Certain Death
B. Might be ok, with Chemo and Radiation - stage the axilla
C. **Should be fine, it's a benign entity**

3. What subtype of IDC is associated with Radial Scar?
A. Mucinous
B. Medullary
C. Papillary
D. **Tubular**

Hamartoma

Benign fat containing mass.

Essential Trivia:

- There are five classic fat containing lesions, all of which are benign. The oil cyst / fat necrosis, hamartoma, galactocele, lymph nodes, and lipoma.

- Of these 5, only oil cyst/fat necrosis and lipoma are considered "pure fat containing" masses.

Hamartoma

- The buzzword is "breast within a breast."

- They have an Aunt Minnie appearance on mammography, although they are difficult to see on ultrasound (they blend into the background).

Other Trivia

- *Pseudoangiomatous Stromal Hyperplasia* = Benign thing with a scary sounding name

- *Tubular IDC* - Spiculated cancer, with a good prognosis, and an association with radial scar

Case 102 - "High Risk" Screener

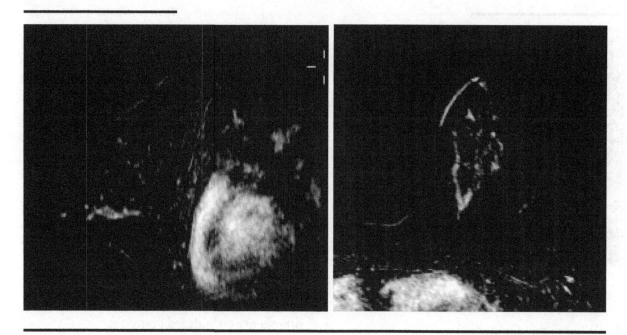

1. What BI-RADS approved vocabulary word would you use for this?
A. Linear / Segmental - Non Mass Like Enhancement (NMLE)
B. Clustered Ring - Non Mass Like Enhancement (NMLE)
C. Irregular Mass
D. Oval Mass

2. What is this "classic" for ?
A. Fibroadenoma
B. ILC
C. IDC
D. DCIS

3. To be considered "high risk" enough to get screening MRI, what must you chance of Breast CA be?
A. Lifetime Risk Greater than 5%
B. Lifetime Risk Greater than 10%
C. Lifetime Risk Greater than 20-25%
D. Lifetime Risk Greater than 50 %

Case 102 - DCIS

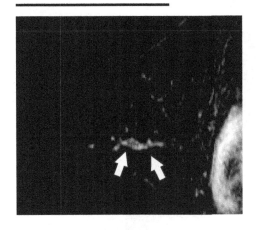

1. What BI-RADS approved vocabulary word would you use for this?
   A. **Linear / Segmental - Non Mass Like Enhancement (NMLE)**
   B. Clustered Ring - Non Mass Like Enhancement (NMLE)
   C. Irregular Mass
   D. Oval Mass

2. What is this "classic" for?
   A. Fibroadenoma
   B. ILC
   C. IDC
   D. **DCIS**

3. To be considered "high risk" enough to get screening MRI, what must you chance of Breast CA be?
   A. Lifetime Risk Greater than 5%
   B. Lifetime Risk Greater than 10%
   C. **Lifetime Risk Greater than 20-25%**
   D. Lifetime Risk Greater than 50%

DCIS

The "earliest form of breast cancer." It can't kill you, but the side-effects from the chemo might.

Essential Trivia:

- "Cancer" is confined to the ducts

DCIS on Mammogram

- Usually a suspicious calcification pattern (fine linear branching or fine pleomorphic)

- 8% of DCIS will present as a mass without calcifications

DCIS On MRI

- Clumped, ductal, linear or segmental non-mass likely enhancement.

- Kinetics are typically NOT helpful for DCIS.

Screening Trivia

- People with a lifetime risk greater than 20-25% qualify for screening MRI.

- Anything that gets you more estrogen increases your risk (obesity, liver damage - leading to less estrogen metabolism).

- 20Gy of Radiation to your chest as a kid buys you a screening MRI – at 25 or 8 years after exposure (*which ever is longer)

Case 103 - Screening Mammogram

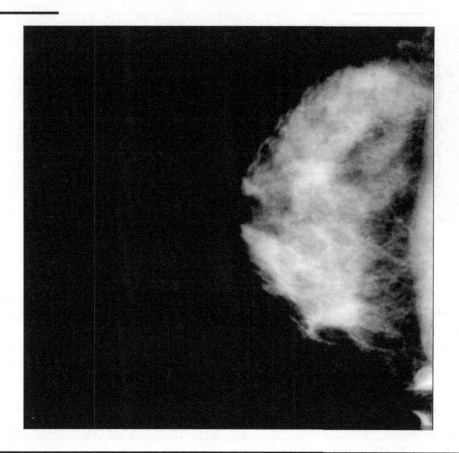

1. What is the "next step" ?
A. Put the patient in ultrasound
B. Get spot compressions
C. Put the patient in the consultation room *("the room of tears")*
D. Look to see if the patient has ever had a chest CT

2. This finding can ONLY be made on ?
A. Screening Mammograms
B. Diagnostic Mammograms
C. A CC View
D. An Ultrasound

3. Which of the following is true
A. It's twice as likely to be bilateral
B. It's twice as likely to be unilateral
C. When present it's unilateral just as often as it is bilateral
D. It's NEVER unilateral

Case 103 - Sternalis Muscle

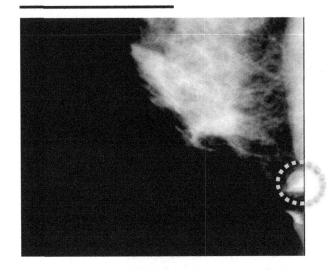
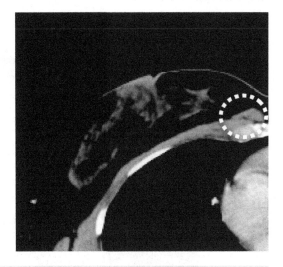

1. What is the "next step"?
A. Put the patient in ultrasound
B. Get spot compressions
C. Put the patient in the consultation room ("the room of tears")
D. Look to see if the patient has ever had a chest CT

2. This finding can ONLY be made on?
A. Screening Mammograms
B. Diagnostic Mammograms
C. A CC View
D. An Ultrasound

3. Which of the following is true
A. It's twice as likely to be bilateral
B. It's twice as likely to be unilateral
C. When present it's unilateral just as often as it is bilateral
D. It's NEVER unilateral

Sternalis

Variant chest wall muscle, that mimics a mass on mammograms.

Essential Trivia:

- It's a non-functional muscle next to the sternum that can simulate a mass.

- It is ONLY SEEN ON THE CC VIEW.

- It's unilateral twice as often as bilateral (when it occurs - which is about 5% of the time).

- Handling this in real life is all about the old gold. Find that thing on the priors (even better is a CT), CC only, never on the MLO.

Case 104 - Chest Pain

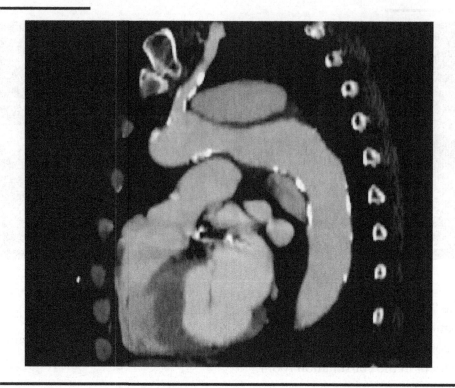

1. What is the major risk for for this?
A. Atherosclerosis
B. Hypertension

2. How would you grade this?
A. Standford A
B. Standford B
C. Standford C

3. What is the difference is management between type A and type B?
A. A is surgical , B is medical
B. A is medical , B is surgical

4. When might this thing get a stent graft?
A. If in involves more than 5cm of the descending thoracic aorta
B. If it persists for longer than 3 months, without thrombosing
C. If the patient has persistent pain despite anti-hypertensive therapy
D. If the flap extends into the SMA or Celiac Trunk

5. Which of the following classically originates from the FALSE lumen ?
A. Right Renal
B. Left Renal
C. SMA
D. Celiac

Case 104 - Aortic Dissection (Type B)

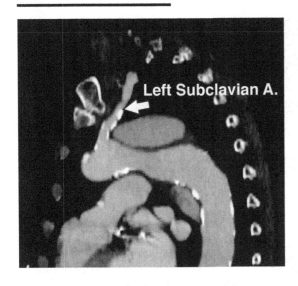

1. What is the major risk for for this?
A. Atherosclerosis
B. Hypertension

2. How would you grade this?
A. Standford A
B. Standford B
C. Standford C

3. What is the difference is management between type A and type B?
A. A is surgical, B is medical
B. A is medical, B is surgical

4. When might this thing get a stent graft?
A. If in involves more than 5cm of the descending thoracic aorta
B. If it persists for longer than 3 months, without thrombosing
C. If the patient has persistent pain despite anti-hypertensive therapy
D. If the flap extends into the SMA or Celiac Trunk

5. Which of the following classically originates from the FALSE lumen?
A. Right Renal
B. Left Renal
C. SMA
D. Celiac

Aortic Dissection

Most common of the acute aortic syndromes, where blood dissects into the potential space between the intima and media

Essential Trivia:

- Caused by Hypertension (70%) - Other causes include cocaine use, marfans, and pregnancy.

- Stanford A: Proximal to the left subclavian artery takeoff
- Stanford B: Distal to the left subclavian artery takeoff

- True Lumen: Typically smaller, surrounded by intimal calcifications

- False Lumen: Typically bigger, and the origin of the left renal artery.

Treatment:
- Type A is surgical, Type B is medical (anti-hypertensives).

- Type B can get an endograft if it's considered "unstable,"
   - Persistent or recurrent pain despite adequate anti-hypertensive therapy
   - Acute expansion of the false lumen
   - Periaortic or mediastinal hematoma (contained rupture)
   - Visceral, renal or limb malperfusion syndrome

Case 105 - Stent Graft Follow-Up

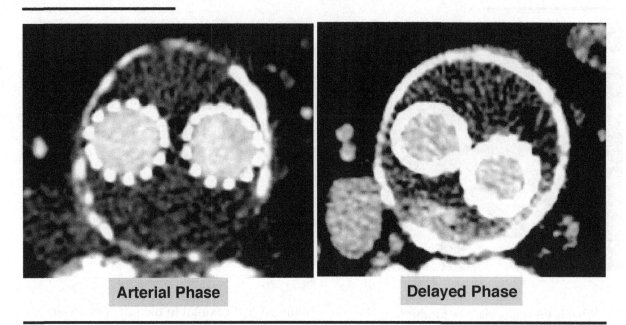

Arterial Phase **Delayed Phase**

1. What is going on here?
A. There is enhancing scar in the graft
B. There is enhancing tumor in the graft
C. The graft is infected
D. The graft is leaking

2. What is the most common type of endo-leak?
A. Type 1A
B. Type 2
C. Type 3
D. Type 4

3. Which endoleak(s) is considered "high pressure" and must be fixed?
A. Type 1A
B. Type 1B
C. Type 2
D. Type 3
E. Type 4
F. Type 2 and Type 3
G. Type 1 and Type 2
H. Type 1 and Type 3

Case 105 - Endoleak

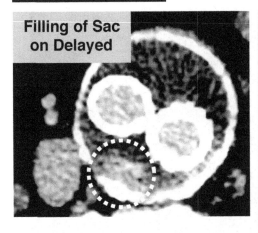

Filling of Sac on Delayed

1. What is going on here?
A. There is enhancing scar in the graft
B. There is enhancing tumor in the graft
C. The graft is infected
D. The graft is leaking

2. What is the most common type of endo-leak?
A. Type 1A
B. Type 2
C. Type 3
D. Type 4

3. Which endoleak(s) is considered "high pressure" and must be fixed?
A. Type 1A
B. Type 1B
C. Type 2
D. Type 3
E. Type 4
F. Type 2 and Type 3
G. Type 1 and Type 2
H. Type 1 and Type 3

Essential Trivia:

- Type 1: Leak at the top (A) or the bottom (B) of the graft. They are typically high pressure and require intervention (or the sac will keep growing).

- Type 2: Filling of the sac via a feeder artery. This is the MOST COMMON type, and is usually seen after repair of an abdominal aneurysm. The most likely culprits are the IMA or a Lumbar artery. They often spontaneously resolve, but may require treatment. Typically, you follow the sac size and if it grows you treat it.

- Type 3: This is a defect/fracture in the graft. It is usually the result of pieces not overlapping.

- Type 4: This is from porosity of the graft. ("4 is from the Pore"). It's of historic significance, and doesn't happen with modern grafts.

- **High Pressure:** Type 1 and Type 3 are considered high pressure, because they communicate directly with systemic blood flow.

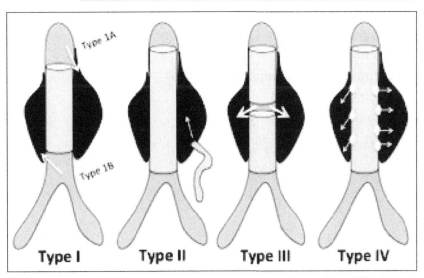

Case 106 - "My Leg Hurts"

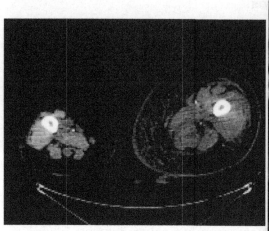
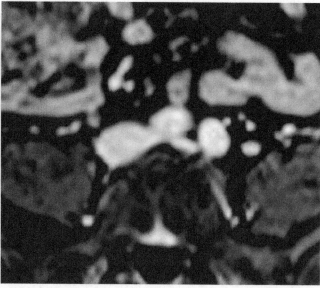

1. What is going on here?
A. The right iliac vein is compressing the left iliac vein
B. The right iliac artery is compressing the right iliac vein
C. The right iliac artery is compressing the left iliac vein
D. The left iliac artery is compressing the left iliac vein

2. Is there an Eponym for this?
A. Dodd-Frank Syndrome
B. Miller-Fisher Syndrome
C. May-Thurner Syndrome
D. Marcus Gunn Phenomenon

3. What is the treatment?
A. Thrombolysis Only
B. Thrombolysis + Angioplasty (no stent)
C. Thrombolysis + Stent
D. Surgical Re-implantation

Case 106 - May-Thurner Syndrome

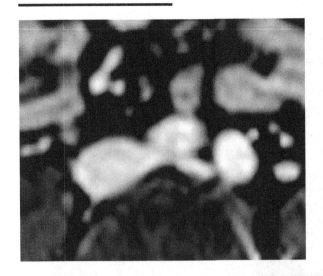
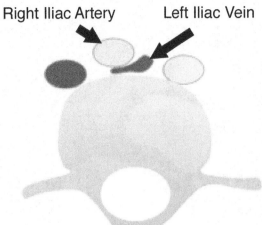

1. What is going on here?
   A. The right iliac vein is compressing the left iliac vein
   B. The right iliac artery is compressing the right iliac vein
   C. The right iliac artery is compressing the left iliac vein
   D. The left iliac artery is compressing the left iliac vein

2. Is there an Eponym for this?
   A. Dodd-Frank Syndrome
   B. Miller-Fisher Syndrome
   C. May-Thurner Syndrome
   D. Marcus Gunn Phenomenon

3. What is the treatment?
   A. Thrombolysis Only
   B. Thrombolysis + Angioplasty (no stent)
   C. Thrombolysis + Stent
   D. Surgical Re-implantation

Essential Trivia:

- A syndrome resulting in DVT of the left common iliac vein.

- The pathology is compression of the left common iliac vein by the right iliac artery.

- *Why the left?* Although both left and right common iliac veins lie deep to the right common iliac artery, the left has a more transverse course and is predisposed to compression (the right has a more vertical course and is therefore not as predisposed).

- *Can you get it on the right?* Yes, but it's rare and unlikely to show up on a multiple choice test.

- Treatment is thrombolysis and stenting.

- If they show you a swollen left leg, this is probably the answer.

Case 107 - "Pretty Sure It's Just A Bakers Cyst"

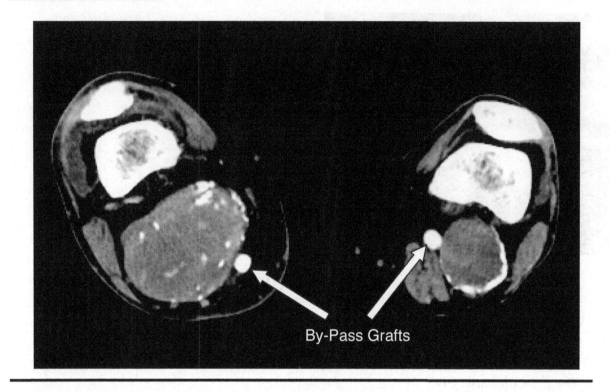

1. Where should you look next ?
A. The brain - for berry aneurysms
B. The liver - for findings or cirrhosis
C. The abdominal aorta - to see if its aneurysmal
D. The kidneys - to check for RCCs

2. What is the most dreaded complication of this finding?
A. An acute limb (foot)
B. Stroke - from DVT
C. PE - from DVT

3. Popliteal Entrapment most commonly occurs secondary to?
A. Compression from the medial head of the gastrocnemius
B. Compression from the lateral head of the gastrocnemius
C. Compression from the semimembranosus
D. Compression from the popliteus

Case 107 - Popliteal Aneurysm

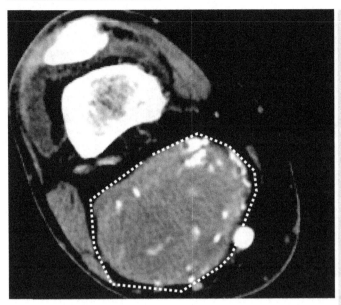

1. Where should you look next ?
A. The brain - for berry aneurysms
B. The liver - for findings or cirrhosis
C. The abdominal aorta - to see if its aneurysmal
D. The kidneys - to check for RCCs

2. What is the most dreaded complication of this finding?
A. An acute limb (foot)
B. Stroke - from DVT
C. PE - from DVT

3. Popliteal Entrapment most commonly occurs secondary to?
A. Compression from the medial head of the gastrocnemius
B. Compression from the lateral head of the gastrocnemius
C. Compression from the semimembranosus
D. Compression from the popliteus

Popliteal Aneurysm

This is the most common peripheral arterial aneurysm (2nd most common overall, to the aorta).

Essential Trivia:

- The main issue with these things is distal thromboembolism, which can be limb threatening.

- There is a strong and frequently tested association with AAA.

- 30-50% of patients with popliteal aneurysms have a AAA

- 10% of patients with AAA have popliteal aneurysms

- 50-70% of popliteal aneurysms are bilateral

- The most dreaded complication of a popliteal artery aneurysm is an acute limb from thrombosis and distal embolization of thrombus pooling in the aneurysm.

Popliteal Entrapment – Symptomatic compression or occlusion of the popliteal artery due to the developmental relationship with the medial head of the gastrocnemius (less commonly the popliteus).

Case 108 - Chest / Arm Pain

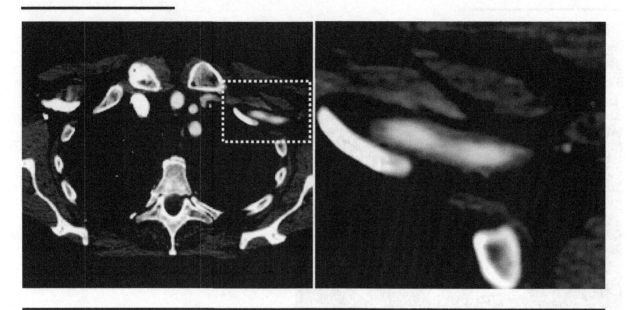

1. What is the diagnosis?
A. Cogan Syndrome
B. PAN (polyarteritis nodosa)
C. Wegeners
D. Giant Cell Arteritis

2. What is the most likely age of the patient ?
A. Less than 30
B. Between 30-50
C. Older than 70

3. Where else in the body does this commonly effect?
A. Renal Arteries
B. Temporal Arteries
C. Infra-renal aorta
D. Iliac Arteries

Case 108 - Giant Cell Arteritis

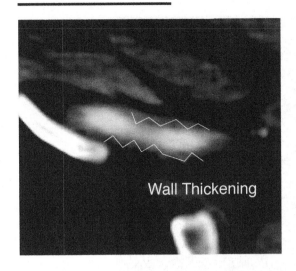

1. What is the diagnosis?
A. Cogan Syndrome
B. PAN (polyarteritis nodosa)
C. Wegeners
D. Giant Cell Arteritis

2. What is the most likely age of the patient?
A. Less than 30
B. Between 30-50
C. Older than 70

3. Where else in the body does this commonly effect?
A. Renal Arteries
B. Temporal Arteries
C. Infra-renal aorta
D. Iliac Arteries

Giant Cell Arteritis

This is the most common primary system vasculitis

Essential Trivia:

- This vasculitis loves old men (usually 70-80).

- This vasculitis involves the aorta and its major branches particularly those of the external carotid (temporal artery).

- This can be shown in two ways: (1) an ultrasound of the temporal artery, demonstrating wall thickening, or (2) CTA / MRA or even angiogram of the arm pit area (Subclavian/ Axillary/ Brachial), demonstrating wall thickening, occlusions, dilations, and aneurysm.

- Think about it as the part of the body that would be compressed by crutches (old men need crutches).

- Trivia worth knowing is that (1) ESR and CRP are markedly elevated, and (2) that the disease responds to steroids.

- "Gold Standard" for diagnosis is temporal artery biopsy (although it's often negative).

Case 109 - MRI Physics (Case 1)

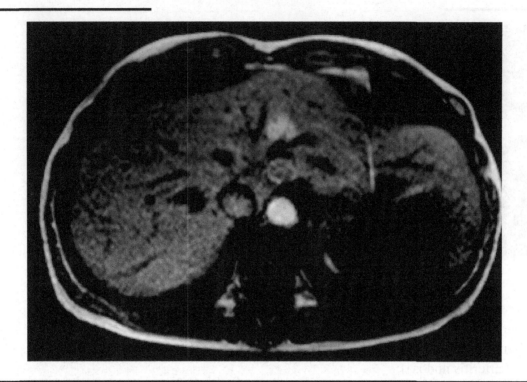

1. What is the artifact?
A. Partial Volume
B. Truncation
C. Motion (Pulsation)
D. Chemical Shift

2. Which direction is this artifact occurring?
A. Phase encoding
B. Frequency encoding

3. If this artifact was obscuring a finding in the liver, what could you do?
A. Increase the matrix
B. Decrease the bandwidth
C. Move the patient from the 3T to a 1.5 T
D. Switch the phase encoding and frequency encoding directions

Case 109 - Pulsation Artifact

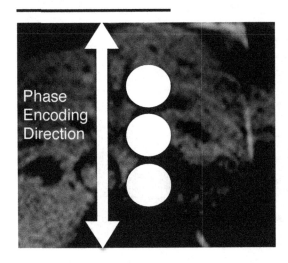

1. What is the artifact?
A. Partial Volume
B. Truncation
C. Motion (Pulsation)
D. Chemical Shift

2. Which direction is this artifact occurring?
A. Phase encoding
B. Frequency encoding

3. If this artifact was obscuring a finding in the liver, what could you do?
A. Increase the matrix
B. Decrease the bandwidth
C. Move the patient from the 3T to a 1.5 T
D. Switch the phase encoding and frequency encoding directions

Pulsation Artifact

A type of motion artifact.

Essential Trivia:

- Motion artifact can be seen with both voluntary and involuntary (cardiac, respiratory) movements.

- Motion creates difference between frequency encoding (which is fast) and phase encoding (which is slow). You will see ghosting or smearing - primarily in the phase encoding direction. You can also see the classic pulsation artifact from the aorta.

- In abdominal imaging the phase encoding step is done in the AP direction (because this is usually the thinner part of the patient, and phase encoding is time intensive). This can be switched to move the artifact off the area of interest.

Case 110 - MRI Physics (Case 2)

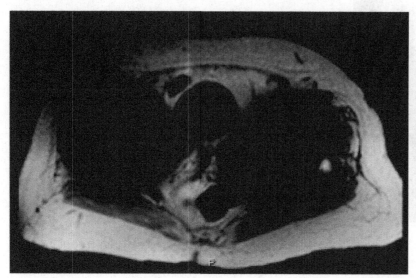 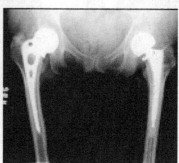

1. What is the artifact?
A. Susceptibility
B. Truncation
C. Zipper
D. Chemical Shift

2. This artifact will be better (less severe) on?
A. Spin Echo Sequences
B. Gradient Echo Sequences

3. Which of the follow is true, regarding this artifact?
A. Better on In-Phase Imaging (relative to out of phase)
B. Better on Out of-Phase Imaging (relative to in phase)
C. Equal on both In-Phase and Out of Phase Imaging

Case 110 - Susceptibility Artifact

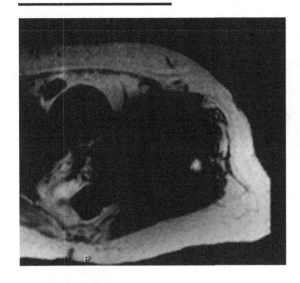

1. What is the artifact?
A. **Susceptibility**
B. Truncation
C. Zipper
D. Chemical Shift

2. This artifact will be better (less severe) on?
A. **Spin Echo Sequences**
B. Gradient Echo Sequences

3. Which of the follow is true, regarding this artifact?
A. Better on In-Phase Imaging (relative to out of phase)
B. **Better on Out of-Phase Imaging (relative to in phase)**
C. Equal on both In-Phase and Out of Phase Imaging

Susceptibility Artifact

Artifact seen in substances that can be magnetized by the external field (metal, & calcium hydroxyapatite are the big ones).

Essential Trivia:

- A less prominent version occurs at tissue interfaces (bone and muscle, or air and bone). The classic location for this is the transition from paranasal sinus to skull base.

- Generally speaking, susceptibility affects all pulse sequences, but is most severe with GRE images and least severe with SE (because of the 180 degree refocusing pulse - to lose those T2* effects).

- Susceptibility artifact worsens on in phase imaging relative to out of phase. This has nothing to do with the phase of water and fat. Instead it has everything to do with in phase being done later. The longer TE, the more susceptibility. Remember, air will do the same thing.

Making it better:
- Using SE and FSE instead of GRE.
- Use a wider receiver bandwidth,
- Align the longitudinal axis of a metal implant with the axis of the main field.
- STIR does way better than frequency selective fat suppression.

Case 111 - MRI Physics (Case 3)

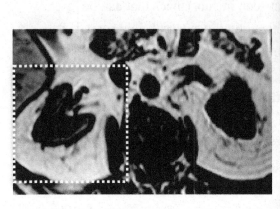
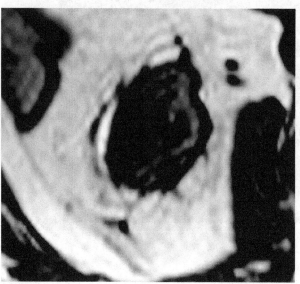

1. What is the artifact?
A. Aliasing
B. Truncation
C. Zipper
D. Chemical Shift (type 1)
E. Chemical Shift (type 2 - india ink)

2. This artifact occurs in the ?
A. Frequency Encoding Direction
B. Phase Encoding Direction

3. This artifact increases with
A. Decreased Field Strength (worse on T 1.5 relative to T3)
B. Increased Gradient Strength
C. Narrower read out bandwidth

Case 111 - Chemical Shift Artifact - Type 1

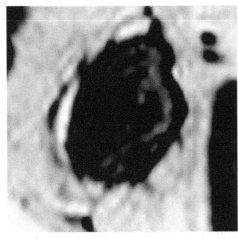

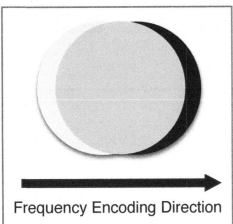

Frequency Encoding Direction

1. What is the artifact?
A. Aliasing
B. Truncation
C. Zipper
D. Chemical Shift (type 1)
E. Chemical Shift (type 2 - india ink)

2. This artifact occurs in the ?
A. Frequency Encoding Direction
B. Phase Encoding Direction

3. This artifact increases with
A. Decreased Field Strength (worse on T 1.5 relative to T3)
B. Increased Gradient Strength
C. Narrower read out bandwidth

Chemical Shift Artifact - Type 1

Artifact seen at fat - water interfaces

Essential Trivia:

- The chemical environments of fat and water are different for protons. This causes these protons to precess at different rates, and results in an error during read out (frequency encoding) direction.

- The type 1 artifact results from a shift in the spatial location of fat voxels. Because of their different environment (and precession speed), voxels containing fat will not have the expected resonance frequency and will be spatially misregistered, causing a shift in the spatial location in the frequency-encode direction. This artifact appears as a white (or dark) band at the interface between fat and water.

Most Testable Facts:
- This "type 1" artifact can occur on gradient or spin echo sequences (Type 2 in only seen on gradient).

- Chemical shift increases with field strength (it's not seen below 1 T)

- Chemical shift decreases with increased gradient strength

- Chemical shift decreases with a wider read out bandwidth

Case 112 - MRI Physics (Case 4)

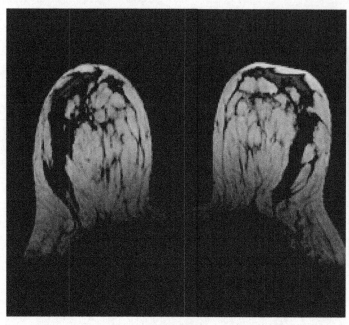
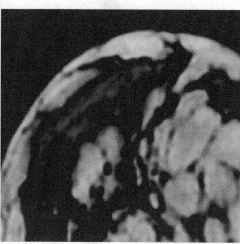

1. What is the artifact?
A. Aliasing
B. Truncation
C. Zipper
D. Chemical Shift (type 1)
E. Chemical Shift (type 2 - india ink)

2. This artifact can be seen on
A. Gradient Echo
B. Spin Echo
C. Both

3. This artifact occurs in the "?" direction
A. Phase encoding
B. Frequency Encoding
C. Both

Case 112 - Chemical Shift Artifact - Type 2 "India Ink"

Black Line Circumferential at Fat Interfaces

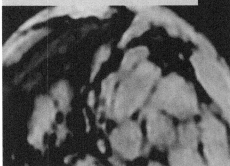

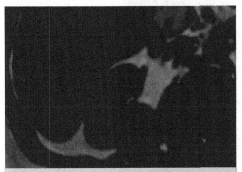

More Classic Look
- Around the Kidney on Out Phase

1. What is the artifact?
A. Aliasing
B. Truncation
C. Zipper
D. Chemical Shift (type 1)
E. **Chemical Shift (type 2 - india ink)**

2. This artifact can be seen on
A. **Gradient Echo**
B. Spin Echo
C. Both

3. This artifact occurs in the "?" direction
A. Phase encoding
B. Frequency Encoding
C. **Both**

Chemical Shift Artifact - Type 2

Artifact seen at fat - water interfaces

Essential Trivia:

- The chemical environments of fat and water are different for protons. This causes these protons to precess at different rates.

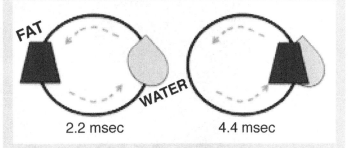

- If a spoiled GRE is performed when the protons are spinning with each other (about 4.4 msec at 1.5T) voxels containing both fat and water will cancel out producing a black line.

- This type of chemical shift artifact shows a black line in **all directions** of the fat-water interface (both the frequency-encode and phase-encode directions as it is independent of spatial encoding.

- This occurs on GRE only, as the 180 degree refocusing pulse of a spin echo sequence minimizes the phase shift.

Case 113 - MRI Physics (Case 5)

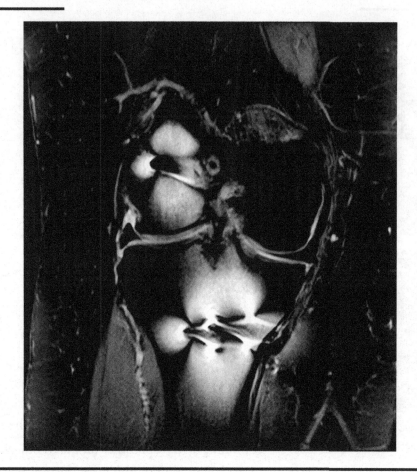

1. What causes this artifact ?
A. Field of view is too narrow
B. Abrupt change in signal
C. T2* effects
D. Overlapping signal from adjacent slices

2. The tech calls you about this artifact, what should you tell him?
A. Switch the patient to a 3T
B. Use a gradient technique instead
C. Use a STIR technique instead
D. Increase the slice gap

3. What else could be done to improve this artifact?
A. Use sequences with a lower TE
B. Use a lower bandwidth
C. Use a smaller field of view
D. Use a smaller matrix

Case 113 - Magnetic Inhomogeneity (Bad Fat-Sat)

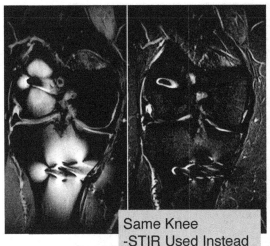

Same Knee
-STIR Used Instead

1. What causes this artifact?
A. Field of view is too narrow
B. Abrupt change in signal
C. T2* effects
D. Overlapping signal from adjacent slices

2. The tech calls you about this artifact, what should you tell him?
A. Switch the patient to a 3T
B. Use a gradient technique instead
C. Use a STIR technique instead
D. Increase the slice gap

3. What else could be done to improve this artifact?
A. Use sequences with a lower TE
B. Use a lower bandwidth
C. Use a smaller field of view
D. Use a smaller matrix

Things to Make it Better:

- The easiest fix, is to **use STIR** instead of T2FS when dealing with metal.
- Using Spin Echo - NOT Gradient
- Using Spin Echo sequences with:
  Relatively low TE,
  High bandwidth,
  Larger Field of View, and
  Higher Matrix

Metal F'd Up Your Fat Sat

Artifact mimics edema in bones

Essential Trivia:

- A metal object will become magnetized from the external field. The difference between the magnetized metal and adjacent will cause local distortions (T2*) in the magnetic field.

Why is the fat sat not working around the metal?

- As described in Case 112, Fat and Water resonate at different times. Because of this separation in frequencies, it is possible to saturate just one (and not the other).

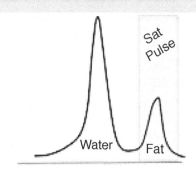

- With a magnetic field distortion (from metal), there is a precessional frequency shift. So the time targeted to the normal peak of fat misses, and you get incomplete saturation.

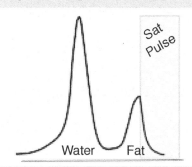

Case 114 - MRI Physics (Case 6)

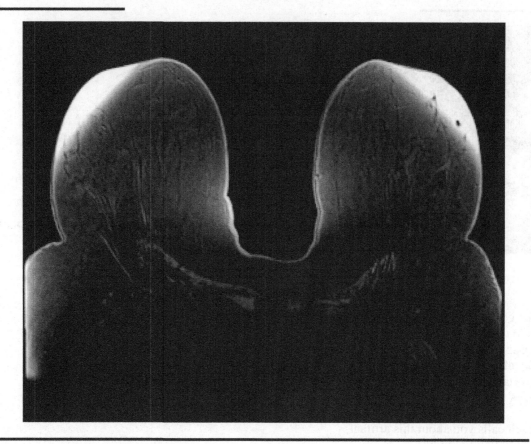

1. What causes this artifact ?
A. Field of view is too narrow
B. Proximity to the coil
C. Abrupt change in signal
D. T2* effects

2. The tech calls you about this artifact, what should you tell her?
A. Switch the patient to a 3T
B. Use a gradient technique instead
C. Use a STIR technique instead
D. Reposition the patient with additional padding between the breast and the coil

3. Is this artifact related to fat suppression technique?
A. Yup
B. Nope

4. In general, when dealing with **breast MRI** - which magnet has better fat suppression?
A. 1.5 T
B. 3 T

Case 114 - "Signal Flaring" Artifact (Coiling Burning)

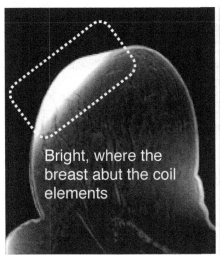

Bright, where the breast abut the coil elements

1. What causes this artifact?
A. Field of view is too narrow
B. Proximity to the coil
C. Abrupt change in signal
D. T2* effects

2. The tech calls you about this artifact, what should you tell her?
A. Switch the patient to a 3T
B. Use a gradient technique instead
C. Use a STIR technique instead
D. Reposition the patient with additional padding between the breast and the coil

3. Is this artifact related to fat suppression technique?
A. Yup
B. Nope

4. In general, when dealing with breast MRI - which magnet has better fat suppression?
A. 1.5 T
B. 3 T

Signal Flaring

Artifact creates the appearance of poor fat sat.

Essential Trivia:

- Proximity to the coil elements can cause a very bright signal (it's **not a true fat sat issue**). You see this in two main places (1) in the breasts as shown in this case, and (2) on prostate MRI when using an endorectal coil... *my God this endorectal coil, have you ever seen one of those?*

- Getting the breast away from the coil is the cure, and the easiest way to do this is with padding and repositioning.

Fat Sat in the Breast - General Points
- Most breast MRI is done with 1.5 T, because you can get a more uniform field relative to 3T. Most of the time, if there are fat sat issues the first thing breast MRI people will do is move the patient to the 1.5.

- *But Prometheus, isn't the separation of peaks better on a 3T compared to a 1.5T? Shouldn't this make it easier to fat sat?* Yes, thats true, but the inhomogeneity in the field, still make the images dirty. People who were smart enough to not go to med school (Physicists) are working on fixing this, as the improved signal to noise of a 3T offers breast imagers the chance to perform even more unnecessary biopsies.

- If the patient is already on a 1.5T, and there is still poor fat sat, "shimming" the magnet to improve inhomogeneities in the field is probably the next move.

Case 115 - MRI Physics (Case 7)

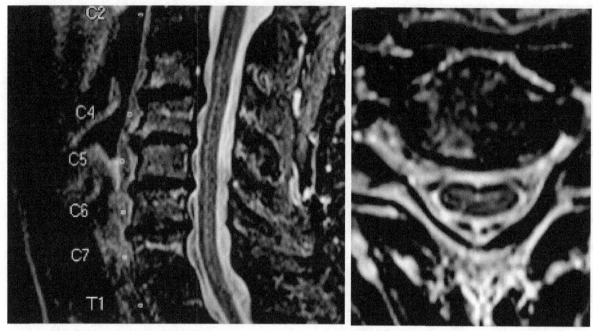

Axial - Through the cervical cord

1. Is there a syrinx?
A. Yes
B. No

2. What can you do to make this better?
A. Increase the bandwidth
B. Increase the pixel size
C. Larger Field of View
D. Increase the Matrix

3. What is the improvement pay off?
A. Increased acquisition time
B. Issues with achieving a good fat sat
C. More susceptibility artifact
D. More signal & less noise

Case 115 - Truncation Artifact (Gibbs)

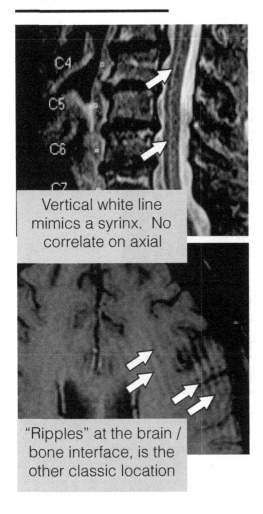

Vertical white line mimics a syrinx. No correlate on axial

"Ripples" at the brain / bone interface, is the other classic location

1. Is there a syrinx?
A. Yes
B. No

2. What can you do to make this better?
A. Increase the bandwidth
B. Increase the pixel size
C. Larger Field of View
D. Increase the Matrix

3. What is the improvement pay off?
A. Increased acquisition time
B. Issues with achieving a good fat sat
C. More susceptibility artifact
D. More signal & less noise

Gibbs / Truncation

Artifact mimics a syrinx

Essential Trivia:

- Abrupt changes in contrast gives the fourier transform ("picture making math") trouble.

- You classically see these at high contrast interfaces (skull-brain, Cord-CSF, and meniscus/fluid). The CSF-Cord interface is the most classic - mimicking a syrinx.

- If prompted I would say the cause is limited sampling of free induction decay.

- It can be seen in both the frequency encoding and phase encoding directions but is more commonly seen in the phase encoding because many times a phase encoding matrix that is smaller than the readout matrix is selected to reduce time.

- ***Making it better:***
  - Short answer = more matrix.
  - Long answer = Decreasing the transmit bandwidth or decreasing pixel size (more PE steps, less FOV, more matrix).
  - Having Adequate Receiver Bandwidth (not enough will worsen Gibbs)

- ***Improvement penalty:*** Increased acquisition time and reduced per-pixel signal to noise.

Case 116 - MRI Physics (Case 8)

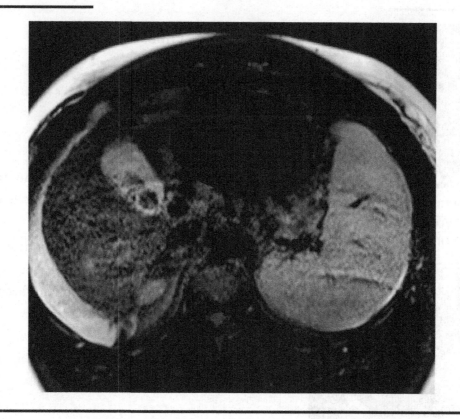

1. What is the artifact?
A. Aliasing
B. Truncation
C. Dielectric
D. Zipper
E. Herringbone

2. The tech calls you about this artifact, what should you tell her?
A. Switch the patient to a 3T
B. Use a gradient technique instead
C. Use a STIR technique instead
D. Application of dielectric pads
E. Reposition the patient

3. Which of the follow is true?
A. This is often better on a 3T
B. This is often better on a 1.5T

4. This artifact typically effects?
A. Fat people with ascites
B. Skinny people without much muscle
C. Very heavily muscled people
D. Elderly with poor bone density

Case 116 - Dielectric Effect / Standing Waves

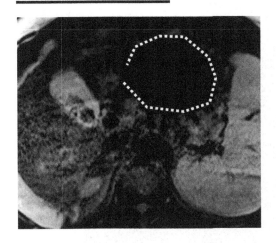

1. What is the artifact?
A. Aliasing
B. Truncation
C. Dielectric
D. Zipper
E. Herringbone

2. The tech calls you about this artifact, what should you tell her?
A. Switch the patient to a 3T
B. Use a gradient technique instead
C. Use a STIR technique instead
D. Application of dielectric pads
E. Reposition the patient

3. Which of the follow is true?
A. This is often better on a 3T
B. This is often better on a 1.5T

4. This artifact typically effects?
A. Fat people with ascites
B. Skinny people without much muscle
C. Very heavily muscled people
D. Elderly with poor bone density

DiElectric Effect

Artifact puts a black spot over the liver

Essential Trivia:

- Biologic tissues have a dielectric constant that results in reduction of wavelength by the inverse of some constant. Interactions can cause local eddy currents in the imaged tissues.

- Since RF waves are shorter at 3T - the **effects are worse with a stronger magnet.**

- You also see this worsen with large bellies, especially if they have ascites. Larger body parts (the abdomen) are primarily affected.

- Classic Look / Location: Dark signal in the central abdomen over the left lobe of the liver.

Making it better:

• Application of dielectric pads - placed between patient and anterior body array coil

• Parallel RF transmission (SENSE) - RF pulses from a set of coils; each coil sends an independent RF pulse. Gives you a longer pulse.

Case 117 - MRI Physics (Case 9)

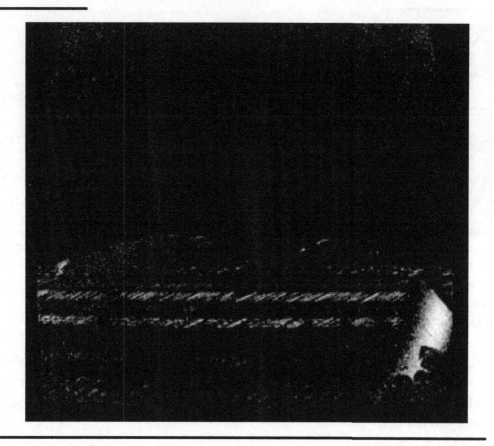

1. What is the artifact?
A. Aliasing
B. Truncation
C. Dielectric
D. Zipper
E. Herringbone

2. The tech calls you about this artifact, what should you tell him?
A. Switch the patient to a 3T
B. Decrease the pixel size
C. Close the door
D. Reposition the patient
E. Use a STIR technique instead

Case 117 - Zipper Artifact

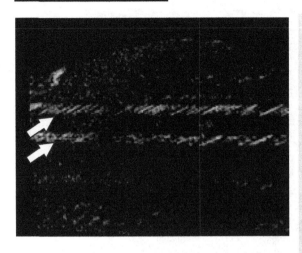

1. What is the artifact?
A. Aliasing
B. Truncation
C. Dielectric
D. Zipper
E. Herringbone

2. The tech calls you about this artifact, what should you tell him?
A. Switch the patient to a 3T
B. Decrease the pixel size
C. Close the door
D. Reposition the patient
E. Use a STIR technique instead

Zipper Artifact

Artifact creates a "zebra stripe" across the patient.

Essential Trivia:

- There are lots of random stray RF signals (radio, tv, etc...). Remember that the RF pulse is a "radio- wave."

- Anyway, if you have defective or inadequate shielding you can get a "zipper" of high signal - 1-2 pixels in width running across the image.

- This typically extends in the phase encoding direction. Although this is controversial, and not likely tested.

Classic Scenarios:
- Anesthesia left the pulse ox monitor in the room.
- The tech left the door open.

Making it better:
- Try closing the door (if it's open).
- Remove all electronic devices from the room.
- Call the tech people to repair the faulty RF shielding.

Case 118 - MRI Physics (Case 10)

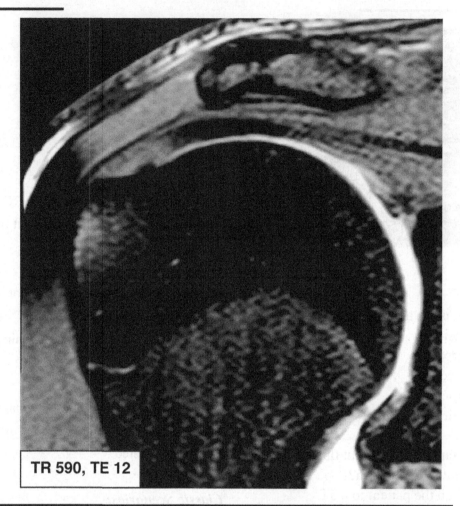

TR 590, TE 12

1. Based on the TR and TE above, what kind of sequence is this?
   A. Spin Echo T1
   B. Spin Echo T2
   C. Proton Density
   D. GRE T1 weighted
   E. GRE T2 weighted

2. Attention to the supraspinatus foot print. What other sequence would you want to check before you called this high signal tendinopathy?
   A. T1
   B. T2
   C. Proton Density
   D. GRE

3. What kinds of tissues are susceptible to this artifact?
   A. Fat
   B. Water
   C. Tightly bound collagen (tendons & cartilage)
   D. Any of these can be involved.

4. What angle must the tissue be in relationship to the main magnetic field?
   A. 15 Degrees
   B. 25 Degrees
   C. 55 Degrees
   D. 75 Degrees

Case 118 - Magic Angle

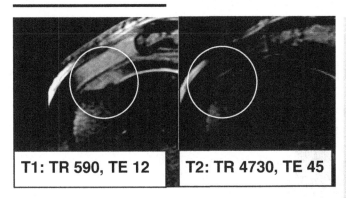

T1: TR 590, TE 12 **T2: TR 4730, TE 45**

1. Based on the TR and TE above, what kind of sequence is this?
   A. **Spin Echo T1**
   B. Spin Echo T2
   C. Proton Density
   D. GRE T1 weighted
   E. GRE T2 weighted

2. Attention to the supraspinatus foot print. What other sequence would you want to check before you called this high signal tendinopathy?
   A. T1
   B. **T2**
   C. Proton Density
   D. GRE

3. What kinds of tissues are susceptible to this artifact?
   A. Fat
   B. Water
   C. **Tightly bound collagen (tendons & cartilage)**
   D. Any of these can be involved.

4. What angle must the tissue be in relationship to the main magnetic field?
   A. 15 Degrees
   B. 25 Degrees
   C. **55 Degrees**
   D. 75 Degrees

T1 = Short TR, Short TE

T2 = Long TR, **Long TE**

PD = Long TR, Short TE

Magic Angle

Artifact creates the appearance of tendinopathy on Short TE sequences

Essential Trivia:

- This is an MSK artifact seen with tendons (and sometimes cartilage).

- You see this with short echo time (TE) sequences where the focus forms an angle of 55 degrees with the main magnetic field (magic angle phenomenon).

- This will NOT be seen in T2 sequences (with long TE).

- This phenomenon, is reduced at higher field strengths due to greater shortening of T2 relaxation times.

What is a short / long time?
- For Spin Echo:
    - Short TR < 700ms
    - Long TR > 2000 ms
    - Short TE < 25ms
    - Long TE > 60ms

- For GRE:
    - Short TR < 50ms
    - Long TR > 100 ms
    - Short TE < 5 ms
    - Long TE > 10ms

Case 119 - Nuclear Medicine Physics (Case 1)

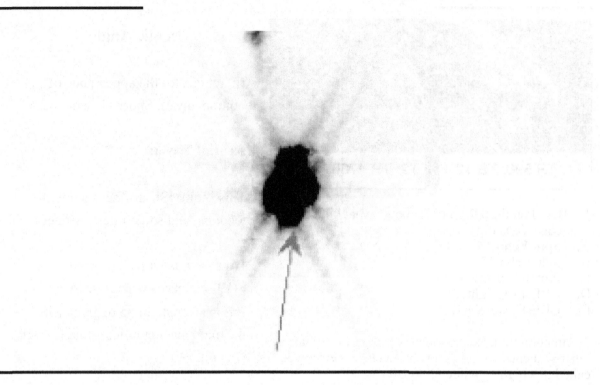

1. What causes this artifact ?
A. Wrong Gamma Energy Window
B. Septal Penetration
C. Field is not uniform
D. Image Linearity Problem
E. Center of Rotation is Off

2. What could you do to eliminate this error?
A. Switch the energy window
B. Use a higher energy collimator
C. Reset the Ion Chamber
D. Reposition the patient

3. What pattern have the collimator holes been arranged in this case?
A. Pentagonal
B. Square
C. Hexagonal
D. Heptagonal

Case 119 - Star Artifact - Septal Penetration

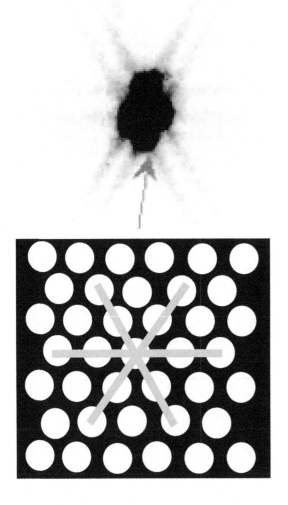

Star Artifact

This star shaped artifact can obscure underlying faint metastases

Essential Trivia:

- This occurs when the high energy photons (typically from I-131, 364 keV) break through a medium strength collimator.

- The single answer cause for this is "septal penetration"

- A thicker collimator, would reduce the artifact.

- The "star" shape, is simply a result of the arrangement of collimators, in this case a hexagonal shape.

1. What causes this artifact ?
A. Wrong Gamma Energy Window
B. Septal Penetration
C. Field is not uniform
D. Image Linearity Problem
E. Center of Rotation is Off

2. What could you do to eliminate this error?
A. Switch the energy window
B. Use a higher energy collimator
C. Reset the Ion Chamber
D. Reposition the patient

3. What pattern have the collimator holes been arranged in this case?
A. Pentagonal
B. Square
C. Hexagonal
D. Heptagonal

Case 120 - Nuclear Medicine Physics (Case 2)

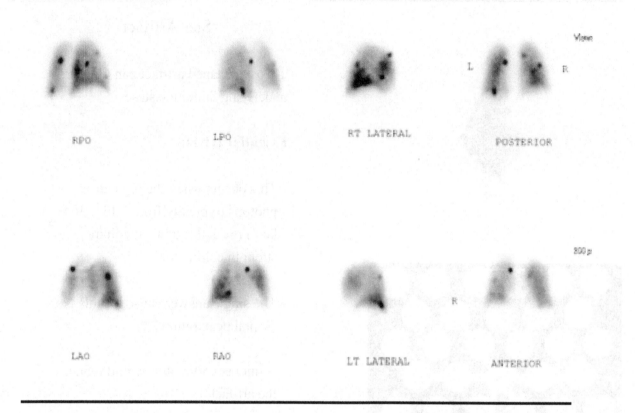

1. Is there a PE ?
A. Yup
B. Nope
C. I always read these as indeterminate

2. What causes this appearance?
A. Pulmonary Hyperemia
B. Multifocal PE
C. Clumping of the MAA
D. Shunting of MAA
E. Wrong tracer

3. What is a common cause of "pulmonary hyperemia" ?
A. Hypervascular Tumor
B. Pulmonary AVM
C. Pulmonary Embolism
D. There are no causes of pulmonary hyperemia

Case 120 - Clumped MAA

POSTERIOR

1. Is there a PE ?
A. Yup
B. **Nope**
C. I always read these as indeterminate
   ** *this is also true*

2. What causes this appearance?
A. Pulmonary Hyperemia
B. Multifocal PE
C. **Clumping of the MAA**
D. Shunting of MAA
E. Wrong tracer

3. What is a common cause of "pulmonary hyperemia" ?
A. Hypervascular Tumor
B. Pulmonary AVM
C. Pulmonary Embolism
D. **There are no causes of pulmonary hyperemia**

Clumped MAA

This artifact creates the appearance of pulmonary hyperemia.

Essential Trivia:

- MMA clumps together creating a large ball of intense signal

- MAA is very "sticky", and even the smallest amount of **blood aspirated into the syringe can cause this appearance.**

- Even though the appearance looks like "hyperemia" in the lungs, **there are no causes of pulmonary hyperemia.**

- Tumors tend to get their blood from bronchial arteries, and even then the blood to a tumor is much less than the normal pulmonary blood flow.

Case 121 - CT Physics (Case 1)

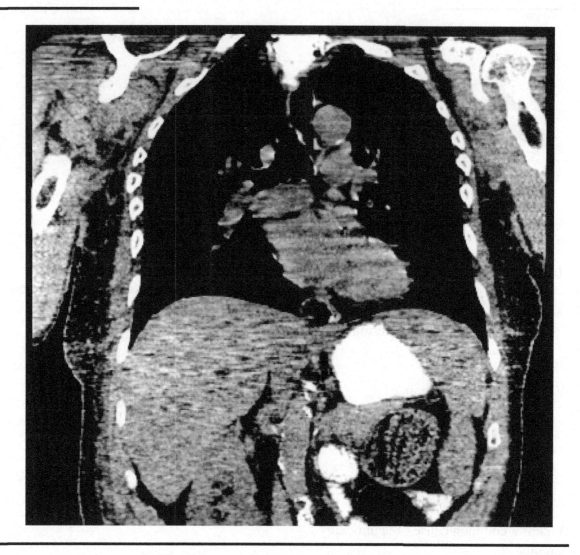

1. What causes this artifact?
A. Preferential removal of the higher energy photons
B. Preferential removal of the lower energy photons
C. The mA is set too high
D. The slices are too thin

2. What could you do to eliminate this error?
A. Turn the mA down
B. Remove the filter
C. Reposition the patient
D. Turn the kV down

3. With this artifact, is the average energy higher or lower?
A. Higher
B. Lower

Case 121 - Beam Hardening (arms are down)

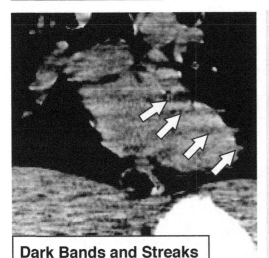

Dark Bands and Streaks

1. What causes this artifact ?
A. Preferential removal of the higher energy photons
B. Preferential removal of the lower energy photons
C. The mA is set too high
D. The slices are too thin

2. What could you do to eliminate this error?
A. Turn the mA down
B. Remove the filter
C. Reposition the patient
D. Turn the kV down

3. With this artifact, is the average energy higher or lower ?
A. Higher *Removal of lower energy photons, increases the AVERAGE energy.*
B. Lower

Beam Hardening

This artifact creates streaks and bands, obscuring lots of stuff and making "cannot exclude" a prominent phrase in the report.

Essential Trivia:

- As the x-ray beam passes through an object the lower energy photons are removed preferentially, leaving a "harder beam" with an increased average energy.

- In this case the patient's arms were left down by those lazy no good techs. X-rays which pass through the dense arms lose their lower energy photons (making them "harder"). X-rays that don't pass through the arms (the ones that pass anterior and posterior) will have a lower average energy. The result of these two groups mixing is this dark bands / streaks appearance. The tech was placed in the stocks (pillory) for this offense.

Fixing Beam Hardening:

- Increase the overall energy (turn the kV Up!)
- Filtration - Pre hardening of the beam, to remove lower energy components before it hits the patient, and/or the addition of a bow-tie filter.
- Calibration Correction - Using a phantom to allow the detector to compensate for hardening effects.
- Correct Software - An iterative correction algorithm can be used.
- Avoidance - Tilt the gantry or position the patient to avoid areas the cause hardening.

Case 122 - CT Physics (Case 2)

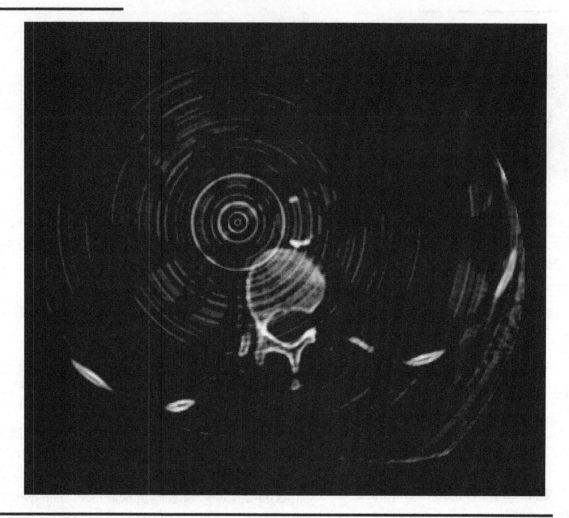

1. What is this artifact?
A. Helical Artifact
B. Spiral Artifact
C. Ring Artifact
D. Incomplete Projection Artifact

2. What causes this appearance?
A. mA is too high
B. Metal on the slice above (or below)
C. Defective Detector
D. Overscanning

Case 122 - Ring Artifact

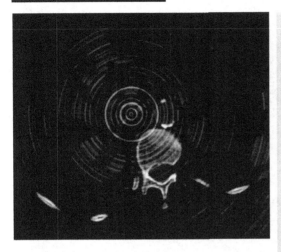

1. What is this artifact?
A. Helical Artifact
B. Spiral Artifact
C. Ring Artifact
D. Incomplete Projection Artifact

2. What causes this appearance?
A. mA is too high
B. Metal on the slice above (or below)
C. Defective Detector
D. Overscanning

Ring Artifact

This artifact creates a spiraled ring, usually on multiple slices.

Essential Trivia:

- If one of the detectors "drifts" in it's calibration a projection error will occur, which get propagated during the back projection process. The result is a ring artifact.

- This artifact is seen primarily with 3rd Generation CT scanners.

- Fixing Ring Artifact - Recalibrate your dinosaur detector, or replace the broken part.

Case 123 - Ultrasound Physics (Case 1)

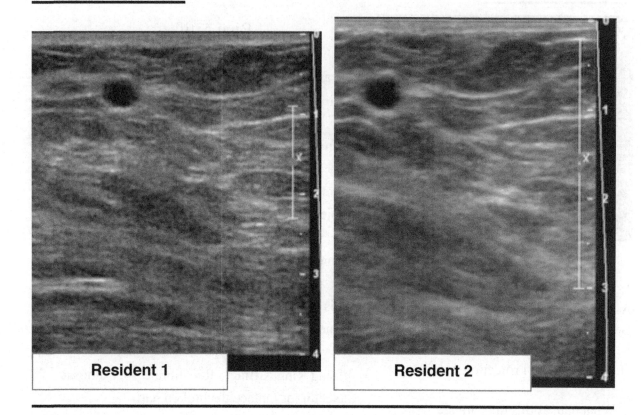

*Both Residents were placed in the stocks (pillory) for such disgraceful ultrasounding

1. What should Resident 1 have done better?
A. Turned up the gain
B. Turned down the gain
C. Centered his focal zone
D. Used a low frequency probe

2. What should Resident 2 have done better?
A. Narrowed the focal zone
B. Turned down the gain
C. Used the compound imaging feature
D. Used the harmonic imaging feature

3. Axial Resolution depends on?
A. The depth of the object you are focusing on
B. The Spatial Pulse Length
C. Time Gain Compensation
D. Receiver Focusing

Case 123 - Image Optimization - Focal Zone

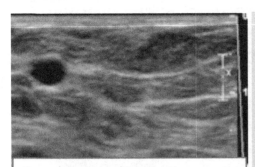

Correct Technique: Narrow focal zone, centered over the object of interest

1. What should Resident 1 have done better?
A. Turned up the gain
B. Turned down the gain
C. Centered his focal zone
D. Used a low frequency probe

2. What should Resident 2 have done better ?
A. Narrowed the focal zone
B. Turned down the gain
C. Used the compound imaging feature
D. Used the harmonic imaging feature

3. Axial Resolution depends on?
A. The depth of the object you are focusing on
B. The Spatial Pulse Length
C. Time Gain Compensation
D. Receiver Focusing

Optimizing the Image

In most mammo divisions, bad technique from a resident will result in placement in the stocks (and possible castration).

Essential Trivia:

Focal Zone (the point where the beam is most narrow, and has maximum intensity).

- Classic teaching was to place the focal zone behind the object, but that only held up for equipment that is now in the Smithsonian. Modern devices have multiple focal zones, so it's ok to land it right on the area of interest.

Resolution (the ability to resolve to adjacent objects):

- *High Frequency transducer* have high resolution but less tissue penetration, you should use them for superficial stuff.

- *Axial Resolution* - for optimal axial resolution you need the returning echoes to be separate and not overlap. The minimum required separation between two reflectors is 1/2 the spatial pulse length (SPL), otherwise the returning echoes will overlap.

- *Lateral Resolution* - this does best with a nice narrow beam (remember it's the most narrow at the focal zone). A key testable pearl is that lateral resolution worsens with depth (which makes sense because the beam diverges after the focal zone in the "far zone").

Case 124 - Ultrasound Physics (Case 2)

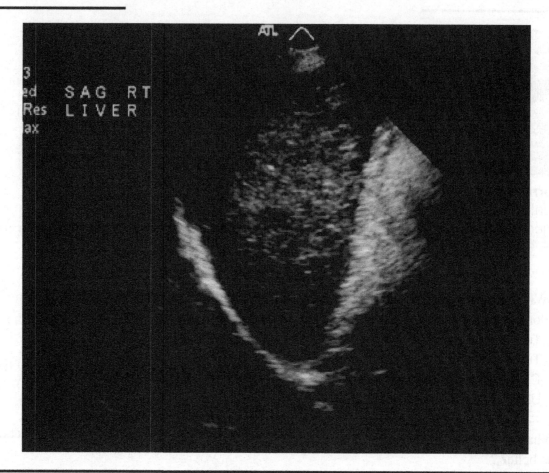

1. This artifact is caused by what "false assumption"?
A. All echoes originate from within the main beam
B. All echoes return to the transducer after a single reflection
C. The speed of sound in human tissue is constant - 1540 m/s
D. Acoustic energy is uniformly attenuated

2. Why do you put gel on people's skin before you ultrasound?
A. Makes their skin soft
B. Decreases the reflection
C. Decreases the refraction
D. Decreases the impedance

3. What factors determine refraction?
A. Speed Change and Angle of Incidence
B. Speed Change and Absorption of Sound (how much is turned to heat)
C. Frequency Change and Angle of Incidence
D. How non-specular (bumpy) the surface is

Case 124 - Mirror Image Artifact

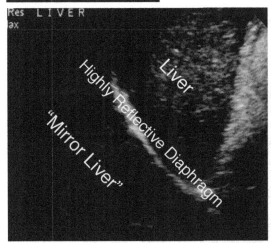

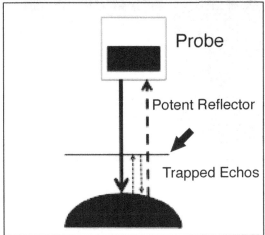

1. This artifact is caused by what "false assumption"?
A. All echoes originate from within the main beam
B. All echoes return to the transducer after a single reflection
C. The speed of sound in human tissue is constant - 1540 m/s
D. Acoustic energy is uniformly attenuated

2. Why do you put gel on people's skin before you ultrasound?
A. Makes their skin soft
B. Decreases the reflection
C. Decreases the refraction
D. Decreases the impedance

3. What factors determine refraction?
A. Speed Change and Angle of Incidence
B. Speed Change and Absorption of Sound (how much is turned to heat)
C. Frequency Change and Angle of Incidence
D. How non-specular (bumpy) the surface is

Mirror Image Artifact

Artifact generated by a repeat echo.

Essential Trivia:

- All ultrasound artifacts are the result of a violation of a display assumption (the rules the machine uses to make a picture). In this case, the assumption is that all echoes return to the transducer after a single reflection.

- In this case, the ultrasound beam passes through a highly reflective surface (the diaphragm), then gets repeatedly reflected between the back side of the reflector and the adjacent structure. This is displayed as a duplication equidistant from but deep to the strongly reflective interface.

- *Reflection:* Ultrasound energy gets reflected at a boundary between two tissues because of the differences in the acoustic impedances of the two tissues. A large difference in "stiffness" results in a large reflection of energy.

- *Impedance* is the stiffness, and is defined by the density x speed of sound in that object. Air pockets (eliminated by gel) will create a large impedance difference (lots of shadowing).

- *Refraction* is influenced by the angle of incidence and the speed change (as stated in Snells law).

Case 125 - Ultrasound Physics (Case 3)

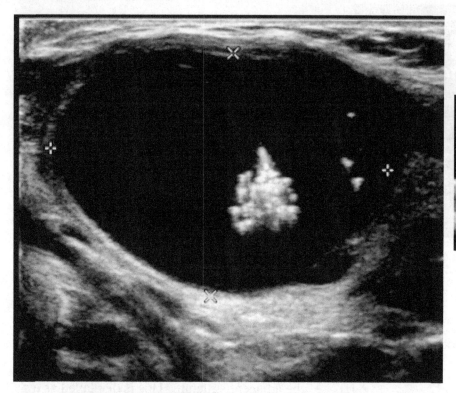
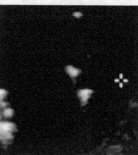

1. This artifact is caused by what "false assumption"?
A. All echoes originate from within the main beam
B. All echoes return to the transducer after a single reflection
C. The speed of sound in human tissue is constant - 1540 m/s
D. Acoustic energy is uniformly attenuated

2. What is the minimal distance needed for axial resolution?
A. One Spatial Pulse Length
B. Two Spatial Pulse Lengths
C. One Half Spatial Pulse Length
D. One Quarter Spatial Pulse Length

3. Does this thyroid nodule need a biopsy?
A. No - it's benign
B. Yes - there are no imaging features to predict benign vs malignant
C. Yes - the body division is broke

Case 125 - Comet Tail Artifact

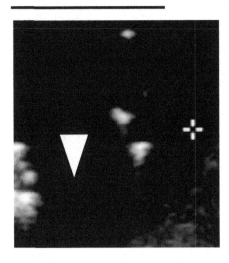

1. This artifact is caused by what "false assumption" ?
   A. All echoes originate from within the main beam
   B. **All echoes return to the transducer after a single reflection**
   C. The speed of sound in human tissue is constant - 1540 m/s
   D. Acoustic energy is uniformly attenuated

2. What is the minimal distance needed for axial resolution?
   A. One Spatial Pulse Length
   B. Two Spatial Pulse Lengths
   C. **One Half Spatial Pulse Length**
   D. One Quarter Spatial Pulse Length

3. Does this thyroid nodule need a biopsy?
   A. **No - it's benign**
   B. Yes - there are no imaging features to predict benign vs malignant
   C. Yes - the body division is broke

Comet Tail Artifact

Another Artifact generated by a repeat echo.

Essential Trivia:

- This artifact is a form of reverberation artifact. Reverberation occurs when the sound wave encounters two parallel highly reflective surfaces, the echoes generated from a primary ultrasound beam are repeatedly reflected back and forth (like a game of pong) before eventually returning to the transducer for detection. This is recorded and displayed as multiple echoes.

- This time our two parallel highly reflective surfaces are closer together which means the sequential echoes are closely spaced. The space between them may be less than 1/2 the spatial pulse length (SPL) - which as mentioned above was the minimal distance needed for axial resolution. As a result, the displayed echoes will look like a triangle, instead of linear lines.

- *Why a triangle and not a square ?* The later echoes get attenuated and have decreased amplitude. This decreased amplitude is manifested on the display as decreased width. So you get a tapering triangle (or comet tail).

- Comet Tail Artifact from micro crystals in colloid is a classic feature of this benign nodule. I would only biopsy it if the chairman was putting pressure on me to generate money for the division... uh I mean, for good patient care. You aren't gonna find cancer in it.

CASE 126 - NON-INTERPRETIVE SKILLZ (CASE 1)

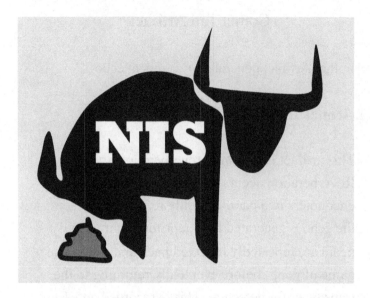

1. One of the IR fellows asks you (in front of the Attendings) to "help" out in a "big case" ? It's already past time to leave and you have boards in a week. You notice everyone in the room is suddenly staring at you. Having no other option you agree. When you enter the procedure room you are told one of the techs left, so you will be back tabling — labeling and drawing up meds. Which of the following is true?
A. It's ok to label the medications after the procedure starts.
B. You don't need to label the basins.
C. If you immediately administer something you don't have to label it.
D. Expirations dates are never necessary to write

2. Who is responsible for these stupid labeling rules?
A. The Asshole Fellow
B. The Assholes in Charge of the Section (departmental policy)
C. The Assholes in the Joint Commission
D. The Asshole Nurses - they just made this shit up to make your life miserable

3. Karma has paid a visit to the IR sweet, and the fellow has just caused a major complication with that monster TIPS Trocar. Which is true regarding administration of blood products?
A. 3 Identifiers are needed for the patient
B. The Patients Room Number is a valid identifier
C. 2 Nurses (you count as a nurse) should be involved in the verification

Case 126 - Medication Labeling and Blood

1. One of the IR fellows asks you (in front of the Attendings) to "help" out in a "big case"? It's already past time to leave and you have boards in a week. You notice everyone in the room is suddenly staring at you. Having no other option you agree. When you enter the procedure room you are told one of the techs left, so you will be back tabling — labeling and drawing up meds. Which of the following is true?
   A. It's ok to label the medications after the procedure starts.
   B. You don't need to label the basins.
   C. If you immediately administer something you don't have to label it.
   D. Expirations dates are never necessary to write

2. Who is responsible for these stupid labeling rules?
   A. The Asshole Fellow
   B. The Assholes in Charge of the Section (departmental policy)
   C. The Assholes in the Joint Commission
   D. The Asshole Nurses - they just made this shit up to make your life miserable

3. Karma has paid a visit to the IR sweet, and the fellow has just caused a major complication with that monster TIPS Trocar. Which is true regarding administration of blood products?
   A. 3 Identifiers are needed for the patient
   B. The Patients Room Number is a valid identifier
   C. 2 Nurses (you count as a nurse) should be involved in the verification

Essential Trivia - Labels:

What gets Labeled? Before the procedure starts you are supposed to label ALL the meds that are not labeled; including medicines in syringes, cups and even the fucking basins.

What if there is only one medication being used? You still have to label it.

Is there any exception to the rule? Yup – immediately administered medication (one that an authorized staff member prepares or obtains, takes directly to a patient, and administers to that patient without any break in the process).

Where are you supposed to do the labeling? In the area where medicines and supplies are set up.

What do you have to write on the labels? You better write small – Medication name, Strength, Quantity, Diluent and volume (if not apparent from the container), Expiration date when not used within 24 hours, Expiration time when expiration occurs in less than 24 hours

Exceptions to the label writing rules? You don't have to put expiration date and time – if you are doing a short procedure

Essential Trivia - Blood:

You have to use two separate indicators.

*What can **NOT** be used as identifying factor?* – Basically anything that changes – classic examples are (a) Patient's Location, or (b) Patient's Room Number

Two nurses should be involved

Case 127 - Non-Interpretive Skillz (Case 2)

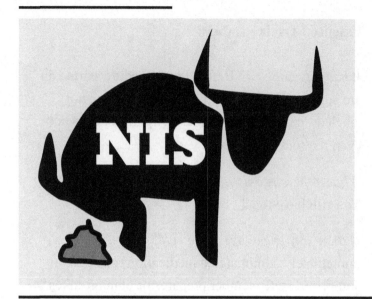

1. You assisted (watched) your attending perform a targeted biopsy of a kidney lesion. It is later revealed that the wrong kidney was targeted. Your Attending (being a veteran of academic medicine) immediately throws you under the bus - claiming you didn't follow protocol regarding the time out and site marking. Which of the following is considered correct?
A. Using a "sticky note" is valid under most circumstances
B. It's ok to mark the site once the procedure has started
C. It's optimal to involve the patient in the site marking
D. Magic markers should be used on premature infants

2. What if you are doing two procedures on the same patient?
A. You only need one time out
B. You need two time outs - but you can do them both prior to the first procedure
C. You need two time outs - one prior to the first procedure, and the second prior to the second procedure
D. Time outs are for pussies

3. Which is considered "high risk" for a wrong site event?
A. Patient undergoing general anesthesia
B. Patient having a procedure on a unilateral structure (like a nose, or a penis)
C. Patient undergoing local anesthesia

Case 127 - The Time Out / Site Marking

1. You assisted (watched) your attending perform a targeted biopsy of a kidney lesion. It is later revealed that the wrong kidney was targeted. Your Attending (being a veteran of academic medicine) immediately throws you under the bus - claiming you didn't follow protocol regarding the time out and site marking. Which of the following is considered correct?
   A. Using a "sticky note" is valid under most circumstances
   B. It's ok to mark the site once the procedure has started
   C. It's optimal to involve the patient in the site marking
   D. Magic markers should be used on premature infants

2. What if you are doing two procedures on the same patient?
   A. You only need one time out
   B. You need two time outs - but you can do them both prior to the first procedure
   C. You need two time outs - one prior to the first procedure, and the second prior to the second procedure
   D. Time outs are for pussies

3. Which is considered "high risk" for a wrong site event?
   A. Patient undergoing general anesthesia
   B. Patient having a procedure on a unilateral structure (like a nose, or a penis)
   C. Patient undergoing local anesthesia

Essential Trivia -

- General Anesthesia and Deep Sedation are Considered High Risk (patient can't correct you)

- Pre-procedural verification should be done prior the procedure

- Marking should be done with something that won't fall off / wash off during prep and dropping

- Alternatives to traditional marking are needed for Teeth, Mucosal Surfaces, or Premature infants *(the mark could cause a permanent tattoo)*.

- The Site Mark must be visible AFTER draping / prepping – in other words – near the site of the actual procedure.

- The Time Out – You need to agree on (a) Correct Patient, (b) Correct Site, and (C) Correct Procedure. Also, you have to document the time out happen.

- The Time Out - Should be done immediately prior to the procedure

- The Time Out – *What if you are doing two procedures on the same patient?* You need to perform the time out before each procedure (you can't do them both in a row at the beginning).

CASE 128 - NON-INTERPRETIVE SKILLZ (CASE 3)

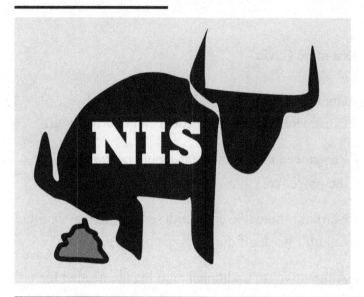

1. A 95 year old patient with widely metastatic pancreatic cancer is refusing his PET scan because he's worried about ""the radiation." Fox news ran a segment on it and he's all worked up. Which of the follow is true regarding biologic effects of ionizing radiation ?
A. A lot of the troubling data comes from the BEIR 7 report
B. The BEIR 7 report is based on modern data (not from atomic bomb survivor data)
C. There is a threshold dose for developing cancer
D. BIER 7's committee had the primary task of risk estimate for high dose human exposure (> 500 mSv).

2. Which is true ?
A. Deterministic Effects are better for cancer risk
B. Stochastic Effects are better for cancer risk
C. Depends on the type of cancer

3. The patient is still nervous even after your detailed explanation about BEIR 7 and risk models. What else might you tell him to calm his fears?
A. The typical lag period between radiation exposure and cancer diagnosis is at least 5 years, and in most cases, 1 or 2 decades or longer
B. The average background radiation dose per year is around 20mSv - a PET scan is around 10 mSv (depending on what you read).
C. Obama doesn't want him to get the PET

Case 128 - BIER 7 and Radiation Risk

1. A 95 year old patient with widely metastatic pancreatic cancer is refusing his PET scan because he's worried about ""the radiation." Fox news ran a segment on it and he's all worked up. Which of the follow is true regarding biologic effects of ionizing radiation ?
A. **A lot of the troubling data comes from the BEIR 7 report**
B. The BEIR 7 report is based on modern data (not from atomic bomb survivor data)
C. There is a threshold dose for developing cancer
D. BIER 7's committee had the primary task of risk estimate for high dose human exposure (> 500 mSv).

2. Which is true ?
A. Deterministic Effects are better for cancer risk
B. **Stochastic Effects are better for cancer risk**
C. Depends on the type of cancer

3. The patient is still nervous even after your detailed explanation about BEIR 7 and risk models. What else might you tell him to calm his fears?
A. **The typical lag period between radiation exposure and cancer diagnosis is at least 5 years, and in most cases, 1 or 2 decades or longer**
B. The average background radiation dose per year is around 20mSv - a PET scan is around 10 mSv (depending on what you read).
C. Obama doesn't want him to get the PET ** *this might also be true*

Essential Trivia -

- BEIR 7 used Atomic Bomb Survivor data, medical radiation studies, occupational radiation studies, and environmental radiation studies. *The primary source was the bomb data.*

- The primary task of the committee was to develop the best possible risk estimate for human exposure to low-dose (<100 mSv), low-LET ionizing radiation.

- The typical lag period between radiation exposure and cancer diagnosis is at least 5 years, and in most cases, the lag period may be 1 or 2 decades or longer.

- Below 10 mSv, there is no direct epidemiological data to support increased cancer risk. Although people still act like there is.

- Average natural background radiation is around 3 mSv per year

- Stochastic Effects are best thought of as "shit happens" or "bad luck" - there is no threshold ("linear-no threshold theory"). Although risky behavior increases the chance of a bad thing. This is the model used for cancer.

- Deterministic Effects are best thought of as "cause and effect". Deterministic effects are used to describe burns, cataracts, etc…. There is a described threshold / dose for those. This model does NOT work for cancer.

Case 129 - Non-Interpretive Skillz (Case 4)

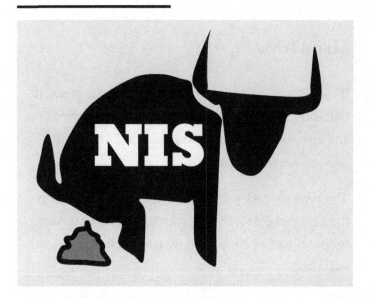

1. An experienced technologist has knowingly violated a patient safety protocol related to screening the orbits for metal. A patient was injured and now has permanent vision loss in one eye. In a "just culture" how should the situation be handled ?
A. Reckless Behavior = Punish the tech
B. Reckless Behavior = Retrain the tech
C. At Risk Behavior = Console the tech
D. Human Error = Punish the tech

2. Which is true ?
A. Mistakes are errors the occur during active problem solving
B. Slips should be corrected by "Re-Training" per Just Culture
C. Mistakes should be corrected by "Punishment" per Just Culture

3. Which is true regarding a "Human Reliability Curve" ?
A. Humans can achieve 100% Reliability ("practice makes perfect")
B. System Factors are the key to improving performance
C. Less Resources = Better Performance

Case 129 - Just Culture / Human Reliability

1. An experienced technologist has knowingly violated a patient safety protocol related to screening the orbits for metal. A patient was injured and now has permanent vision loss in one eye. In a "just culture" how should the situation be handled?
A. **Reckless Behavior = Punish the tech**
B. Reckless Behavior = Retrain the tech
C. At Risk Behavior = Console the tech
D. Human Error = Punish the tech

2. Which is true?
A. **Mistakes are errors the occur during active problem solving**
B. Slips should be corrected by "Re-Training" per Just Culture
C. Mistakes should be corrected by "Punishment" per Just Culture

3. Which is true regarding a "Human Reliability Curve"?
A. Humans can achieve 100% Reliability ("practice makes perfect") *practice makes permanent*
B. **System Factors are the key to improving performance**
C. Less Resources = Better Performance

Essential Trivia -

- Idea of a just culture is that behavior operates on a continuum of Good to Bad. Therefore certain behaviors should be punished while others should be handled with a "hug"

- Human Errors (Slips) = Console

- At Risk Behavior (Short Cut Taking) = Retrain

- Reckless Behavior (Ignoring a Critical Step) = Punish

- *Mistake* = Error that occurs during active problem solving. You choose to turn right, but should have turned left

- *Slip* = Error that occurs during automatic cognitive task. You choose to turn right, but your body turned left instead.

- Human Reliability Curves:

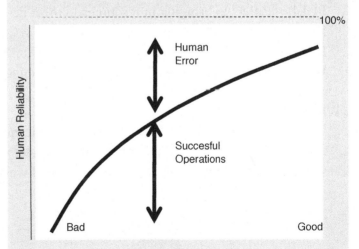

- Humans can't ever get to 100%

- More Resources / System Factors the more reliable the system becomes

Case 130 - Non-Interpretive Skillz (Case 5)

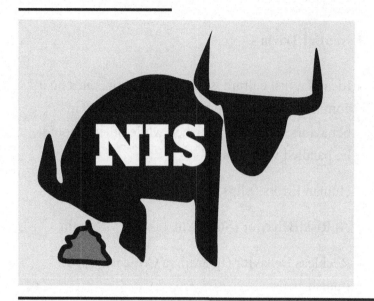

1. The Chairman has taken away everyones book / meeting funds to hire a QA officer. The QA officer previously worked in a Toyota factory and thinks the department should operate under similar principals using the "LEAN" model. Which is true?
A. LEAN principals suggest problems should be solved at a management level.
B. LEAN principals use a PULL strategy
C. LEAN principals argue against "standard work"
D. LEAN looks for ways to utilize more waste

2. Which is true ?
A. PULL = Refers to bringing in resources to meet demand
B. PUSH = Refers to "pushing" away waste
C. PULL = Refers to having resources ready prior to knowing demand
D. PUSH = Refers to "pushing" the agenda that management knows best

3. Which is true ?
A. "Kandan" refers to the idea that you should wait until you order more supplies
B. "Kandan" refers to the idea that you should not let your supplies run out
C. "Just in Time" refers to the idea that segmented workflow is best

Case 130 - LEAN

1. The Chairman has taken away everyones book / meeting funds to hire a QA officer. The QA officer previously worked in a Toyota factory and thinks the department should operate under similar principals using the "LEAN" model. Which is true?
A. LEAN principals suggest problems should be solved at a management level.
B. LEAN principals use a PULL strategy
C. LEAN principals argue against "standard work"
D. LEAN looks for ways to utilize more waste

2. Which is true ?
A. PULL = Refers to bringing in resources to meet demand
B. PUSH = Refers to "pushing" away waste
C. PULL = Refers to having resources ready prior to knowing demand
D. PUSH = Refers to "pushing" the agenda that management knows best

3. Which is true ?
A. "Kandan" refers to the idea that you should wait until you order more supplies
B. "Kandan" refers to the idea that you should not let your supplies run out
C. "Just in Time" refers to the idea Updated that segmented workflow is best

Essential Trivia -

- LEAN has a strategy that involves "engaging" the workforce. *Not just thinking problems are solved at the management level.*

- LEAN = PULL Principals

- PULL = The idea that you PULL resources to match the demand.

- PUSH = Not used in LEAN. That idea for PUSH is making the same amount regardless of demand.

- Kandan = Don't let your supplies run out, otherwise you can't do the next case and you have to wait around.

- Just in Time = Smooth Continuous Workflow. No waiting around, then getting dumped on - that's not efficient.

This vs That 1

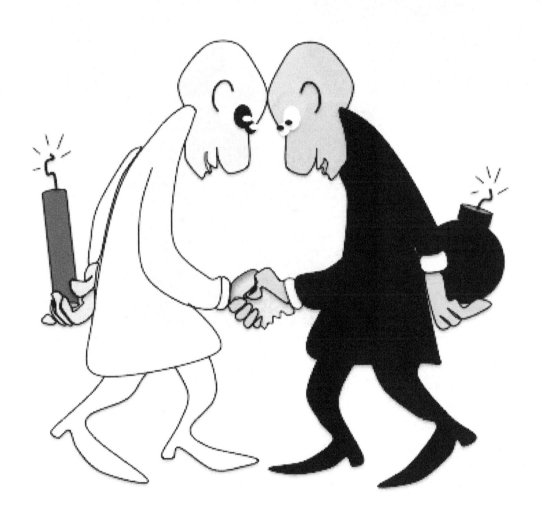

Case 1 - "Headache"

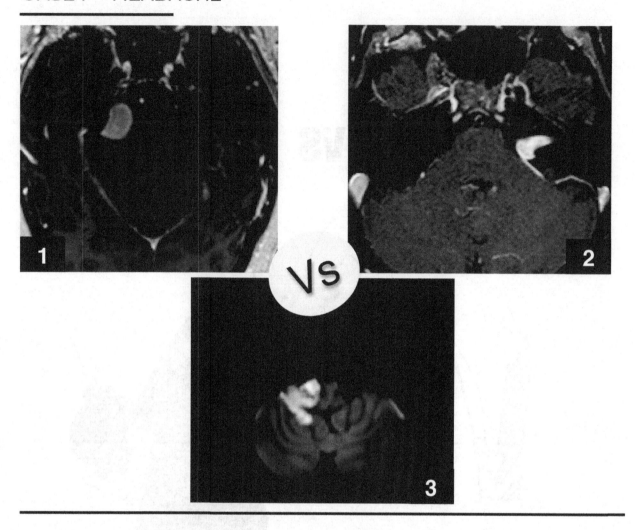

1. Which is Which ?
A. (1) Meningioma, (2) Epidermoid, (3) Schwannoma
B. (1) Epidermoid, (2) Meningioma, (3) Schwannoma
C. (1) Meningioma, (2) Schwannoma, (3) Epidermoid
D. (1) Meningioma, (2) Schwannoma, (3) Arachnoid Cyst

2. How can you tell an epidermoid from an arachnoid cyst?
A. The Epidermoid Enhances
B. The Epidermoid Restricts
C. The Epidermoid will be T2 Bright

3. How can you tell a meningioma from a schwannoma ?
A. The schwannoma will enhance more homogeneously
B. The schwannoma will calcify more
C. The schwannoma will invade the IAC

This vs That

Case 1 - Cerebellopontine Angle ("CPA") Masses

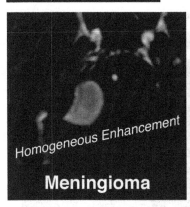
Homogeneous Enhancement
Meningioma

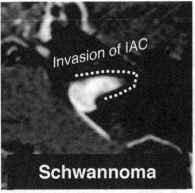
Invasion of IAC
Schwannoma

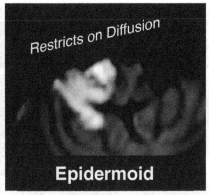
Restricts on Diffusion
Epidermoid

1. Which is Which ?
A. (1) Meningioma, (2) Epidermoid, (3) Schwannoma
B. (1) Epidermoid, (2) Meningioma, (3) Schwannoma
C. (1) Meningioma, (2) Schwannoma, (3) Epidermoid
D. (1) Meningioma, (2) Schwannoma, (3) Arachnoid Cyst

2. How can you tell an epidermoid from an arachnoid cyst?
A. The Epidermoid Enhances
B. The Epidermoid Restricts
C. The Epidermoid will be T2 Bright

3. How can you tell a meningioma from a schwannoma ?
A. The schwannoma will enhance more homogeneously
B. The schwannoma will calcify more
C. The schwannoma will invade the IAC

Meningioma vs Schwannoma

- Both enhance, but the meningioma tends to do it more homogeneously.

- Both can calcify, but the meningioma tends to do it more often.

- The Schwannoma tends to invade the IAC. This can be also be shown with a non-contrast CT - with a widened "trumpet shaped" pours acousticus

Epidermoid vs Arachnoid Cyst

- Both are T2 Bright (iso-intense to CSF)
    - There is a zebra called a "white epidermoid" that is dark on T2 - but this is not gonna show up on a multiple choice test, it's too obscure, even for this test.

- ONLY Epidermoid will be dirty - but not black on FLAIR (the CSF in the arachnoid cyst will suppress)

- **ONLY Epidermoid will restrict on Diffusion**

Case 2 - "Ugly Baby"

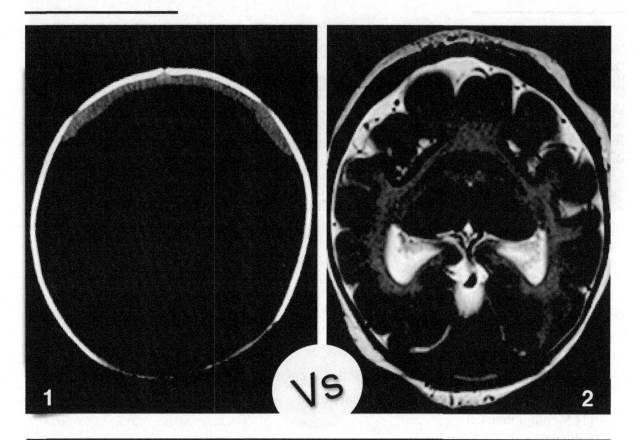

1. Which is Which ?
A. (1) Lobar Holoprosencephaly, (2) Alobar Holoprosencephaly
B. (1) Lobar Holoprosencephaly, (2) Semi-lobar Holoprosencephaly
C. (1) Alobar Holoprosencephaly, (2) Semi-lobar Holoprosencephaly
D. (1) Semi-lobar Holoprosencephaly, (2) Alobar Holoprosencephaly

2. What is classically absent in Lobar Holoprosencephaly?
A. The thalamus
B. The cerebellum
C. The septum pellucidum
D. The falx

3. What is the most common genetic abnormally associated with Holoprosencephaly?
A. Trisomy 21
B. Trisomy 18
C. Trisomy 13
D. DiGeorge Syndrome

CASE 2 - "HOLOPROSENCEPHALY SPECTRUM"

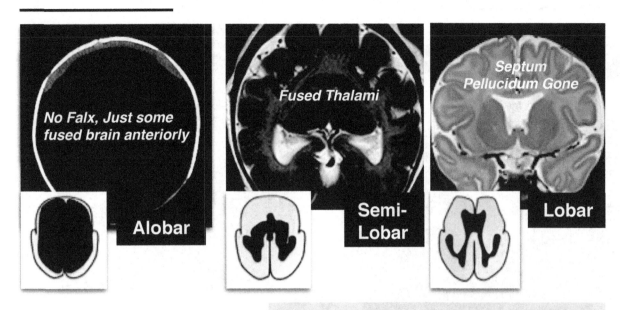

1. Which is Which ?
A. (1) Lobar Holoprosencephaly, (2) Alobar Holoprosencephaly
B. (1) Lobar Holoprosencephaly, (2) Semi-lobar Holoprosencephaly
C. **(1) Alobar Holoprosencephaly, (2) Semi-lobar Holoprosencephaly**
D. (1) Semi-lobar Holoprosencephaly, (2) Alobar Holoprosencephaly

2. What is classically absent in Lobar Holoprosencephaly?
A. The thalamus
B. The cerebellum
C. **The septum pellucidum**
D. The falx

3. What is the most common genetic abnormally associated with Holoprosencephaly?
A. Trisomy 21
B. Trisomy 18
C. **Trisomy 13**
D. DiGeorge Syndrome

What do they have in common?
These are all midline cleavage errors. The brain is supposed to have two hemispheres.

How does the cleavage normally go down?
Remember that the corpus colosseum forms front to back? Well, the cleavage occurs just in the opposite way - back to front — *sorta sounds like a rap song.* The most mild forms will have a cleaved posterior a and fused anterior.

Lobar *(mild):*
- Just Think Absent Septum Pellucidum
- If there is a fusion, it's gonna be Anterior/Inferior

Semi-Lobar *(Probably retarded, but not a monster):*
- Just Think Fusion of the Thalami
- Olfactory bulbs are trashed - don't bother to stop and smell the roses
- Posterior brain should be normal

Lobar *(Possibly a one eyed cyclops monster):*
- Just think single big ventricle with an **absent falx**
- **Cortical mantle is present**

Case 3 - Epilepsy (demonic possession)

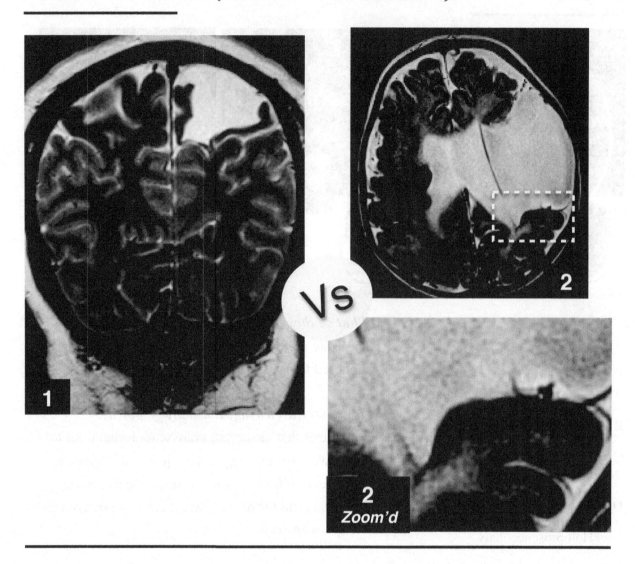

1. Which is Which ?
A. (1) Open Lip Schizencephaly (2) Porencephaly
B. (1) Closed Lip Schizencephaly (2) Porencephaly
C. (1) Porencephaly, (2) Open Lip Schizencephaly
D. (1) Porencephaly, (2) Closed Lip Schizencephaly

2. How do you distinguish Schizencephaly from Porencephaly
A. Porencephaly patient's parents won't have insurance
B. Schizencephaly - the cleft should enhance
C. Schizencephaly - the cleft should restrict
D. Schizencephaly - the cleft should be lined with grey matter

Case 3 - Open Lip Schizencephaly vs Porencephaly

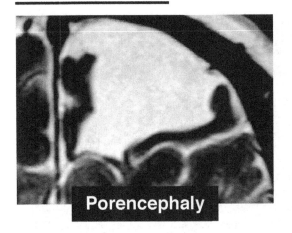
Porencephaly

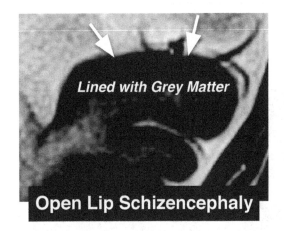
Lined with Grey Matter
Open Lip Schizencephaly

1. Which is Which ?
A. (1) Open Lip Schizencephaly (2) Porencephaly
B. (1) Closed Lip Schizencephaly (2) Porencephaly
C. (1) Porencephaly, (2) Open Lip Schizencephaly
D. (1) Porencephaly, (2) Closed Lip Schizencephaly

2. How do you distinguish Schizencephaly from Porencephaly
A. Porencephaly patient's parents won't have insurance ** *actually the schizencephaly kid is more likely to have uninsured parents - as there is a known association with abandoned children and use of "street drugs" during pregnancy.*
B. Schizencephaly - the cleft should enhance
C. Schizencephaly - the cleft should restrict
D. Schizencephaly - the cleft should be lined with grey matter

Schizencephaly:

Migrational disorder that results in a **grey matter lined cleft** that will extend through the entire hemisphere.

It comes in two main flavors:
(1) *Closed Lip* - cleft walls appose each other
  - more common in bilateral cases
(2) *Open Lip* - cleft walls are separated by CSF
  - more common in unilateral cases

Highly Testable Associations:
- Optic Nerve Hypoplasia (30%)
- Absent Septum Pellucidum (70%)

Porencephaly

This is basically an in-utero stroke resulting in encephalomalacia. The **cleft will be lined with white matter.**

CASE 4 - DECREASED LEVEL OF CONSCIOUSNESS

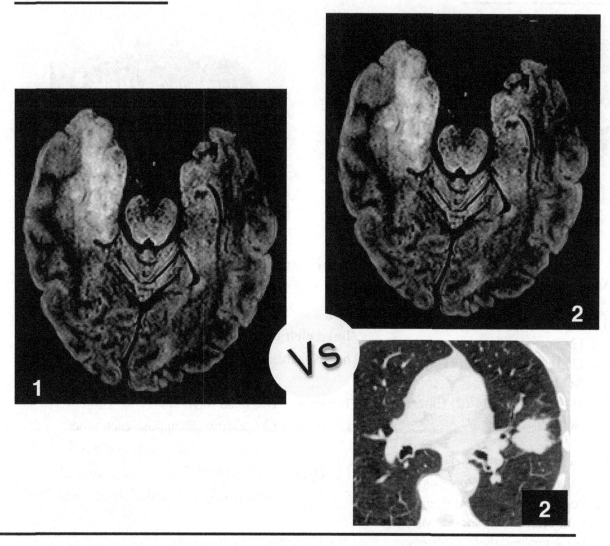

1. Which is Which ?
A. (1) Herpes Encephalitis, (2) Also Herpes Encephalitis - incidental lung CA
B. (1) Herpes Encephalitis, (2) Zinc Toxicity
C. (1) Herpes Encephalitis, (2) Limbic Encephalitis
D. (1) Herpes Encephalitis, (2) Toxoplasmosis

2. Which is the "most sensitive" sequence for diagnosis of case 1?
A. T2
B. T1
C. FLAIR
D. Diffusion

3. How can you distinguish Herpes Encephalitis from an MCA infarct?
A. Herpes will NOT restrict Diffusion, the stroke will
B. Herpes will be bright on FLAIR, the stroke will not
C. The MCA stroke will commonly involve the basal ganglia, Herpes will not
D. The MCA stroke will spare the grey-white interface, Herpes will not

This vs That 9

Case 4 - HSV Encephalitis vs Limbic Encephalitis

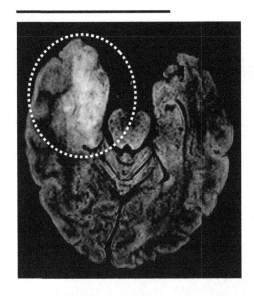

1. Which is Which ?
A. (1) Herpes Encephalitis, (2) Also Herpes Encephalitis - incidental lung CA
B. (1) Herpes Encephalitis, (2) Zinc Toxicity
C. (1) Herpes Encephalitis, (2) Limbic Encephalitis
D. (1) Herpes Encephalitis, (2) Toxoplasmosis

2. Which is the "most sensitive" sequence for diagnosis of case 1?
A. T2
B. T1
C. FLAIR
D. Diffusion

3. How can you distinguish Herpes Encephalitis from an MCA infarct?
A. Herpes will NOT restrict Diffusion, the stroke will
B. Herpes will be bright on FLAIR, the stroke will not
C. The MCA stroke will commonly involve the basal ganglia, Herpes will not
D. The MCA stroke will spare the grey-white interface, Herpes will not

HSV Encephalitis:

- Serious business, and potentially fatal

- Swollen (unilateral or bilateral) medial temporal lobe, which will be T2 bright.

- Earliest sign is actually restricted diffusion – related to vasogenic edema.

- Blooming on gradient means it's bleeding (common in adults, rare in neonate form).

- **Spares the basal ganglia** *(distinguishes it from MCA stroke).*

Limbic Encephalitis:

- Paraneoplastic syndrome that looks alot like HSV, - often involving the mesial temporal lobes, with bright signal on T2.

- It's bilateral about 60%

- Tends to have a less acute time course compared to HSV

- HSV is more likely to have a fever (although cancer can cause one)

- Small cell lung CA is the classic cause

Case 5 - Headache

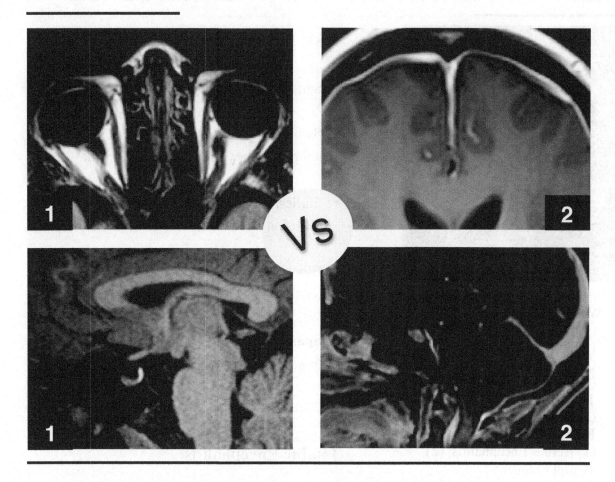

1. Which is Which ?
A. (1) Intracranial Hypertension (2) Intracranial Hypotension
B. (1) Intracranial Hypotension (2) Intracranial Hypertension

2. Dural Venous Sinuses Do What with What ?
A. Shrink with Hypertension, Expand with Hypotension
B. Shrink with Hypotension, Expand with Hypertension
C. Always stay constant in volume

3. What do you think Case 1 looks like?
A. Skinny 70 year old woman
B. Fat teenage boy
C. 45 Year old homeless man (with terrible BO)
D. Fat Middle Aged Woman

Case 5 - Intracranial Hyper vs HypoTension

Monro-Kellie Doctrine:

The Monro-Kellie doctrine is the idea that the head is a closed shell, and that the three major components: (1) brain, (2) blood – both arterial and venous, and (3) CSF, are in a state of dynamic equilibrium. As the volume of one goes up, the volume of another goes down.

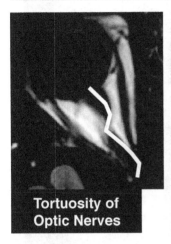
Tortuosity of Optic Nerves

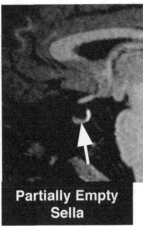
Partially Empty Sella

Intracranial Hypertension

Findings follow the equilibrium idea:
- Ventricles become slit like,
- Pituitary shrinks (partially empty sella),
- Venous sinuses appear compressed.
- Vertical tortuosity of the optic nerves and flattening of the posterior sclera.

Pseudotumor Cerebri: Classic scenario of a fat middle aged women with a headache.

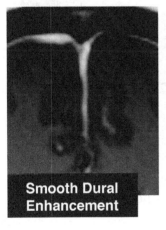
Smooth Dural Enhancement

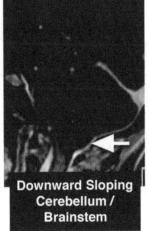
Downward Sloping Cerebellum / Brainstem

Intracranial Hypotension

Findings follow the equilibrium idea:
- Volume of venous blood will increase to maintain the equilibrium.
- The result is **meningeal engorgement (enhancement)**, distention of the dural venous sinuses **(concave appearance of the transverse sinus)**, prominence of the intracranial vessels and
- Engorgement of the pituitary.
- The **development of subdural hematoma and hygromas is also a classic look** (again, compensating for lost volume).

1. Which is Which ?
A. **(1) Intracranial Hypertension (2) Intracranial Hypotension**
B. (1) Intracranial Hypotension (2) Intracranial Hypertension

2. Dural Venous Sinuses Do What with What ?
A. **Shrink with Hypertension, Expand with Hypotension**
B. Shrink with Hypotension, Expand with Hypertension
C. Always state constant in volume

3. What do you think Case 1 looks like?
A. Skinny 70 year old woman
B. Fat teenage boy
C. 45 Year old homeless man (with terrible BO)
D. **Fat Middle Aged Woman**

This vs That 12

Case 6 - IV Drug User... Also Likes Unprotected Sex With Multiple Anonymous Partners

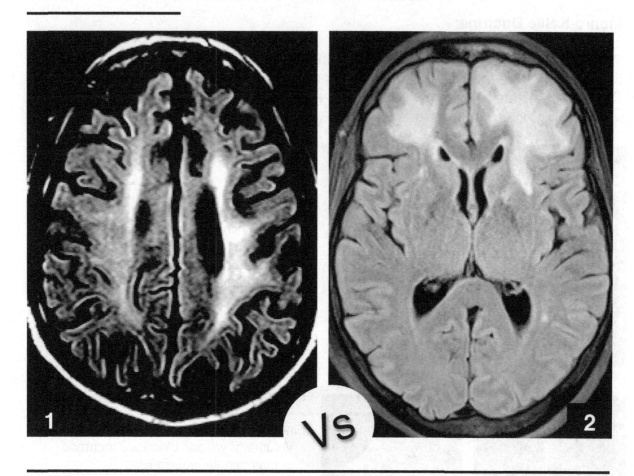

1. Which is Which ?
A. (1) HIV Encephalitis, (2) Progressive Multifocal Leukoencephalopathy (PML)
B. (1) Progressive Multifocal Leukoencephalopathy (PML), (2) HIV Encephalitis

2. How do you tell these two apart?
A. HIV Encephalitis will be asymmetric
B. PML will involve the cortical U Fibers
C. PML will have normal T1 signal
D. HIV lesions will enhance

Case 6 - HIV Encephalitis vs PML

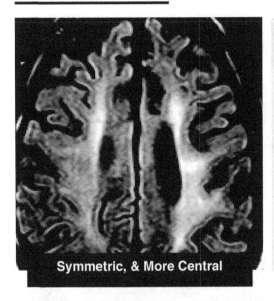

Symmetric, & More Central

HIV Encephalitis

- This is actually pretty common and affects about 50% of AIDS patients.
- CD4 < 200.
- What you are going to see is **symmetric** increased T2 / FLAIR signal in the deep white matter.
- **T1 will be normal**.
- These tend to **spare the subcortical U-fibers** (PML will involve them).

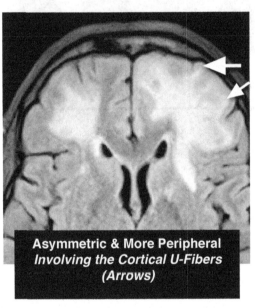

Asymmetric & More Peripheral
Involving the Cortical U-Fibers
(Arrows)

PML

- This is caused by the JC virus.
- CD4 less than 50.
- **Asymmetric** T2/FLAIR hyperintensities out of proportion to mass effect - buzzword
- **Corresponding T1 hypointensity** (remember HIV was T1 normal)
- The lesions have a **predilections for the subcortical U-fibers.**

1. Which is Which ?
A. (1) HIV Encephalitis, (2) Progressive Multifocal Leukoencephalopathy (PML)
B. (1) Progressive Multifocal Leukoencephalopathy (PML), (2) HIV Encephalitis

2. How do you tell these two apart?
A. HIV Encephalitis will be asymmetric
B. PML will involve the cortical U Fibers
C. PML will have normal T1 signal
D. HIV lesions will enhance

Case 7 - Mom Thinks Vaccines Cause Autism

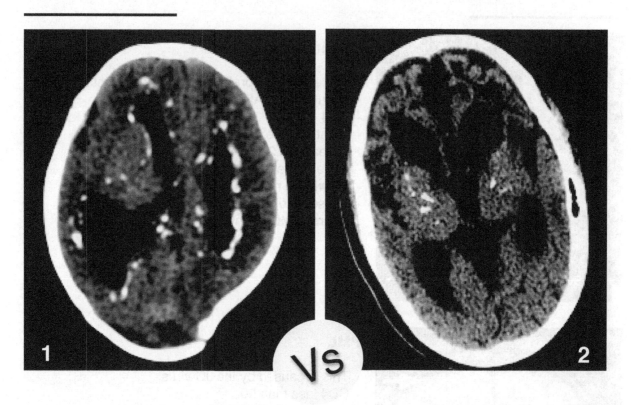

1. Which is Which ?
A. (1) CMV (2) Toxoplasmosis
B. (1) Toxoplasmosis, (2) CMV

2. How do you tell these two apart?
A. Toxo is more common
B. Toxo famously has polymicrogyria
C. Toxo has hydrocephalus
D. CMV famously has brain atrophy in the frontal lobes
E. CMV has less calcifications - more ischemia / Vasculopathy

3. Which of the follow is true?
A. HSV targets the same locations within the brain - regardless of virus subtype (I or II)
B. Rubella has more calcifications than other TORCHS
C. HIV tends to cause brain atrophy (frontal lobe)
D. CMV classically spares the germinal matrix

Case 7 - TORCH -- CMV vs Toxoplasmosis

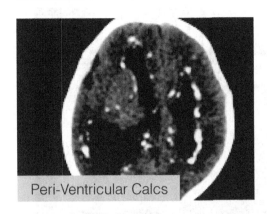

Peri-Ventricular Calcs

CMV:

- This is the most common TORCH (by far!, it's 3x more common than Toxo – which is the second most common).
- It likes the germinal matrix and causes periventricular tissue necrosis.
- Classically **Periventricular calcifications**.
- CMV has the highest association with **polymircogyria** .

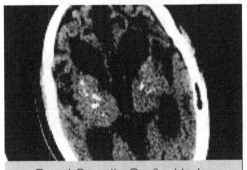

Basal Ganglia Ca^{+2} + Hydro

Toxo:

- This is the second most common TORCH. It's seen in women who clean up cat shit.
- The calcification pattern is more random, and affects the basal ganglia (like most other TORCH infections).
- The most likely test question = **hydrocephalus**.

CNS TORCH - What you need to remember

- **CMV** = *Most Common, Periventricular Calcifications, Polymicrogyria*
- **Toxo** = *Hydrocephalus, Basal Ganglia Calcifications*
- **Rubella** = *Vasculopathy / Ischemia. High T2 signal - Less Calcifications*
- **HSV** = *Hemorrhagic Infarct, and lead to bad encephalomalcia (hydranencephaly)*
- **HIV** = *Brain Atrophy in frontal lobes*

---

1. Which is Which ?
A. **(1) CMV (2) Toxoplasmosis**
B. (1) Toxoplasmosis, (2) CMV

2. How do you tell these two apart?
A. Toxo is more common
B. Toxo famously has polymicrogyria
C. **Toxo has hydrocephalus**
D. CMV famously has brain atrophy in the frontal lobes
E. CMV has less calcifications - more ischemia / Vasculopathy

3. Which of the follow is true?
A. HSV targets the same locations within the brain - regardless of virus subtype (I or II)
B. Rubella has more calcifications than other TORCHS
C. **HIV tends to cause brain atrophy (frontal lobe)**
D. CMV classically spares the germinal matrix

Case 8 - Headache

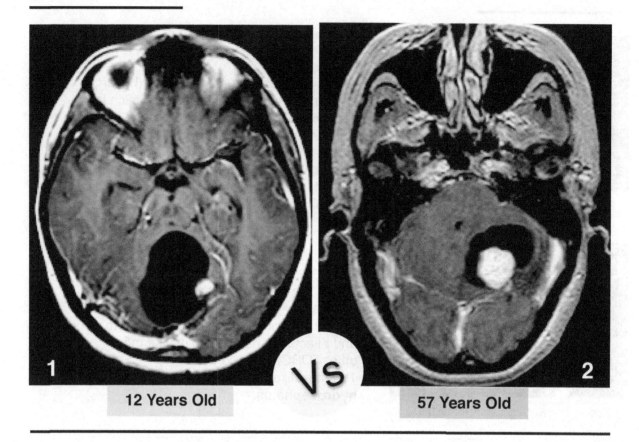

1 — 12 Years Old vs 2 — 57 Years Old

1. Which is Which ?
A. (1) Pilocytic Astrocytoma (2) Oligodendroglioma
B. (1) Hemangioblastoma (2) Pilocytic Astrocytoma
C. (1) Pilocytic Astrocytoma, (2) Hemangioblastoma
D. (1) Central Neurocytoma, (2) Xanthogranuloma

2. Which is true ?
A. Pilocystic Astrocystomas are seen more with NF 2
B. Pilocystic Astrocystomas are seen more with NF 1
C. Pilocystic Astrocytomas are WHO Grade 4
D. Pilocystic Astrocystomas rarely arise from midline structures

3. Which is true ?
A. Hemangioblastomas are seen with Tuberous Sclerosis
B. Hemangioblastomas are seen with Von Hippel Lindau
C. Hemangioblastomas are seen with NF 2
D. Hemangioblastomas are seen with Gorlin Syndrome

Case 8 - Posterior Fossa Cyst with A Nodule - Pilocystic Astrocytoma vs Hemangioblastoma

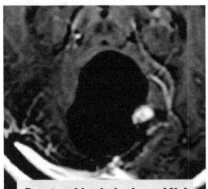

Cyst + Nodule in a Kid

Pilocystic Astrocytoma:

- Most common primary brain tumor of childhood.
- They are WHO 1 - although they do demonstrate enhancement (just the nodule). *This is an important exception to the rule that low grade intra-axial things don't enhance.*
- Classically in midline structures (optic nerve/chiasm) and cerebellum.
- **NF-1** Patients get these in the optic nerve bilaterally
- The syndromic (NF1) optic gliomas are pilocystic astrocytoma - WHO 1, and have a good prognosis.
- The sporadic optic nerve gliomas are GBMs (WHO 4) and they fucking destroy you.

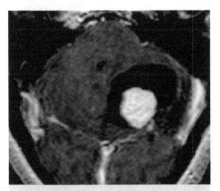

Cyst + Nodule in an Adult

Hemangioblastoma:

- Most common posterior fossa mass in a young adult.
- About 50% of patients with **VHL** get these
- About 25% of the time you see one of these, the patient has VHL.
- Remember you can also get these things in your spine.
- Because they happen more in VHL patients a testable association is the pheochromocytoma
- *Polycythemia is seen in 20% of cases*

1. Which is Which ?
A. (1) Pilocytic Astrocytoma (2) Oligodendroglioma
B. (1) Hemangioblastoma (2) Pilocytic Astrocytoma
C. (1) Pilocytic Astrocytoma, (2) Hemangioblastoma
D. (1) Central Neurocytoma, (2) Xanthogranuloma

2. Which is true ?
A. Pilocystic Astrocystomas are seen more with NF 2
B. Pilocystic Astrocystomas are seen more with NF 1
C. Pilocystic Astrocytomas are WHO Grade 4
D. Pilocystic Astrocystomas rarely arise from midline structures

3. Which is true ?
A. Hemangioblastomas are seen with Tuberous Sclerosis
B. Hemangioblastomas are seen with Von Hippel Lindau
C. Hemangioblastomas are seen with NF 2
D. Hemangioblastomas are seen with Gorlin Syndrome

Case 9 - "Gotta Bump On My Neck"

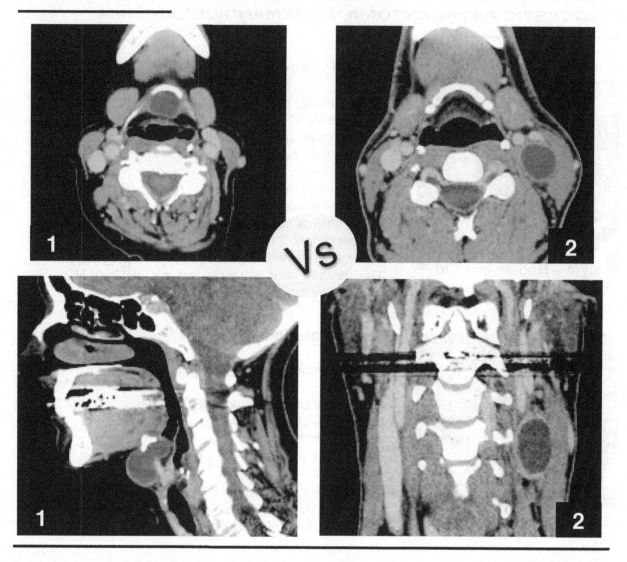

1. Which is Which ?
A. (1) Thyroglossal Duct Cyst (2) Brachial Cleft Cyst
B. (1) Brachial Cleft Cyst (2) Thyroglossal Duct Cyst

2. Is there anything else #2 could be?
A. Nope - it's in a classic location
B. Could be a floor of the mouth cancer met… but only if he's old and smokes
C. Could be a floor of the mouth cancer met, even in a younger non-smoker
D. Could be a peri-tonsillar abscess - probably should drain it.

3. You scroll through #1 and notice some solid components. What is the patient at risk for?
A. Neck Hematoma
B. Hypothyroidism
C. Thyroid Storm
D. Papillary CA

Case 9 - Cystic Neck Mass
- Brachial Cleft Cyst vs Thyroglossal Duct Cyst

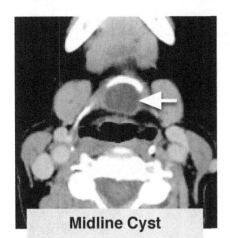

Midline Cyst

Thyroglossal Duct Cyst

- Most common **midline** congenital neck mass

- Found along the tract left by the thyroid gland after descent from the foramen cecum at the tongue base

- The main thing to know (other than its midline position) is that it can get cancer — usually **p**apillary "the **p**opular" subtype. If you see solid components, it has to get a cancer workup.

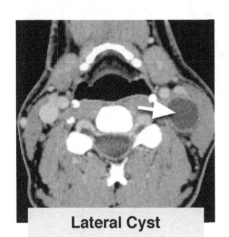

Lateral Cyst

Brachial Cleft Cyst

- There are a bunch of types - but type II is by far the most common and makes up like 95%.

- They can mimic a necrotic level 2 lymph node.

- The most important thing to remember is that in an adult with a new neck mass (unless it's midline, or clearly a goiter) they have SCC nodal mets until proven otherwise. Why? Because HPV related floor of the mouth cancer can (and does) occur in people in their 20s. The idea that only old smokers get mouth cancer is incorrect.

1. Which is Which ?
A. (1) Thyroglossal Duct Cyst (2) Brachial Cleft Cyst
B. (1) Brachial Cleft Cyst (2) Thyroglossal Duct Cyst

2. Is there anything else #2 could be?
A. Nope - it's in a classic location
B. Could be a floor of the mouth cancer met... but only if he's old and smokes
C. Could be a floor of the mouth cancer met, even in a younger non-smoker
D. Could be a peri-tonsillar abscess - probably should drain it.

3. You scroll through #1 and notice some solid components. What is the patient at risk for?
A. Neck Hematoma
B. Hypothyroidism
C. Thyroid Storm
D. Papillary CA

This vs That 20

Case 10 - "My Ear Hurts"

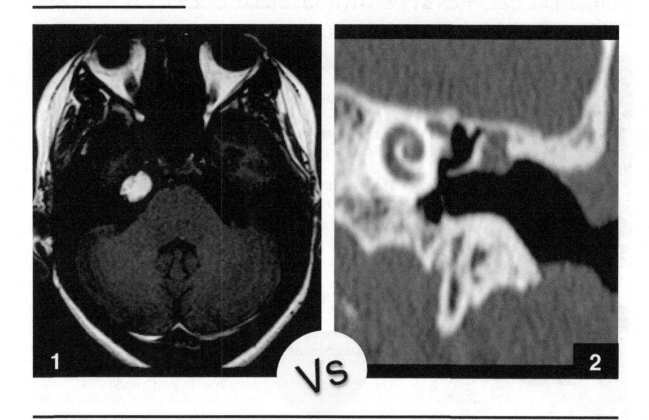

1. Which is Which ?
A. (1) Cholesteatoma (2) Cholesterol Granuloma,
B. (1) Cholesterol Granuloma, (2) Cholesteatoma

2. The pathology is #2 likely started at ?
A. Pars Flaccida
B. Pars Tensa

3. What is true about these two pathologies on Diffusion Weighted Imaging?
A. (1) Will Restrict, (2) Will NOT Restrict
B. (1) Will Restrict, (2) Will Also Restrict
C. (1) Will NOT Restrict, (2) Will Restrict
D. (1) Will NOT Restrict, (2) Will Also NOT Restrict

Case 10 - "Cholesteatoma vs Cholesterol Granuloma"

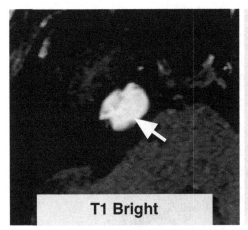

T1 Bright

Cholesterol Granuloma

- The most common primary petrous apex lesion.

- Mechanism is likely obstruction of the air cell, with repeated cycles of hemorrhage and inflammation leading to expansion and bone remodeling.

- On MRI it's gonna be T1 and T2 bright. The **bright T1** signal makes it unique.

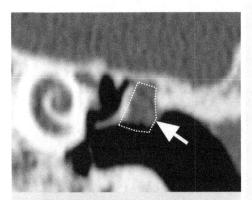

Soft tissue in the "Attic" / Epitympanum. There is erosion of the scutum

Cholesteatoma

- This is basically an epidermoid (ectopic epithelial tissue).

- This one is an acquired type (pars flaccida - from the upper floppy part of the ear drum).

- In the petrous apex they are more likely to be congenital.

- They are typically slow growing, and produce bony changes similar to cholesterol granuloma.

- The difference is their MRI findings; **T1 dark**, T2 bright, **and restricted diffusion.**

1. Which is Which ?
A. (1) Cholesteatoma (2) Cholesterol Granuloma,
B. (1) Cholesterol Granuloma, (2) Cholesteatoma

2. The pathology is #2 likely started at ?
A. Pars Flaccida
B. Pars Tensa

3. What is true about these two pathologies on Diffusion Weighted Imaging?
A. (1) Will Restrict, (2) Will NOT Restrict
B. (1) Will Restrict, (2) Will Also Restrict
C. (1) Will NOT Restrict, (2) Will Restrict
D. (1) Will NOT Restrict, (2) Will Also NOT Restrict

Case 11 - "Hoarseness"

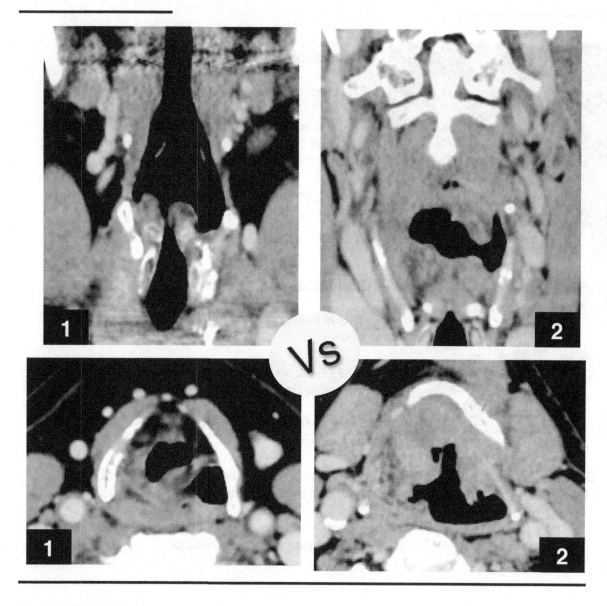

1. Which is Which ?
A. (1) Vocal Cord Paralysis (2) Vocal Cord Tumor
B. (1) Vocal Cord Tumor (2) Vocal Cord Paralysis

2. In the setting of left sided vocal cord paralysis, the "next step" is ?
A. Brain MRI
B. NM Bone Scan
C. CT Abd and Pelvis
D. CT Chest

3. Which of the following has the BEST prognosis?
A. Supraglottic CA
B. Glottic CA
C. Infraglottic CA

Case 11 - Ventricle Dilation - Cancer vs Paralysis

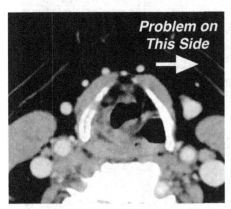

Paralysis = Same Side Dilation

Vocal Cord Paralysis

- The vast majority of cases are secondary to problems with the recurrent laryngeal nerve (which innervates nearly all the laryngeal muscles

- When it's left sided you need to look at the AP window next - for a mass compressing the recurrent laryngeal nerve.

- There are Two Key Imaging Features:
  - (1) Atrophy of the Thyroarytenoid muscle which makes up the bulk of the true cord
  - (2) Dilation of the Laryngeal Ventricle — on the same side as the paralyzed cord.

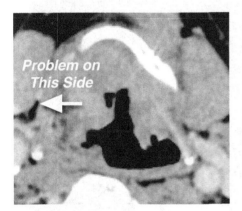

Mass = Other Side Dilation

Laryngeal CA

- The role of the Radiologist is to help stage

- Laryngeal cancers are subdivided into (a) supraglottic, (b) glottic, and (c) subglottic types.

- Glottic SCC has the best outcome (least lymphatics), and is the most common (60%)

- Subglottic is the least common (5%), and can be clinically silent till you get nodes

- The laryngeal ventricle will dilate with a cancer, but this time it's gonna be on the opposite side.

1. Which is Which ?
A. (1) Vocal Cord Paralysis (2) Vocal Cord Tumor
B. (1) Vocal Cord Tumor (2) Vocal Cord Paralysis

2. In the setting of left sided vocal cord paralysis, the "next step" is ?
A. Brain MRI
B. NM Bone Scan
C. CT Abd and Pelvis
D. CT Chest

3. Which of the following has the BEST prognosis?
A. Supraglottic CA
B. Glottic CA
C. Infraglottic CA

Case 12 - "Bump on My Finger"

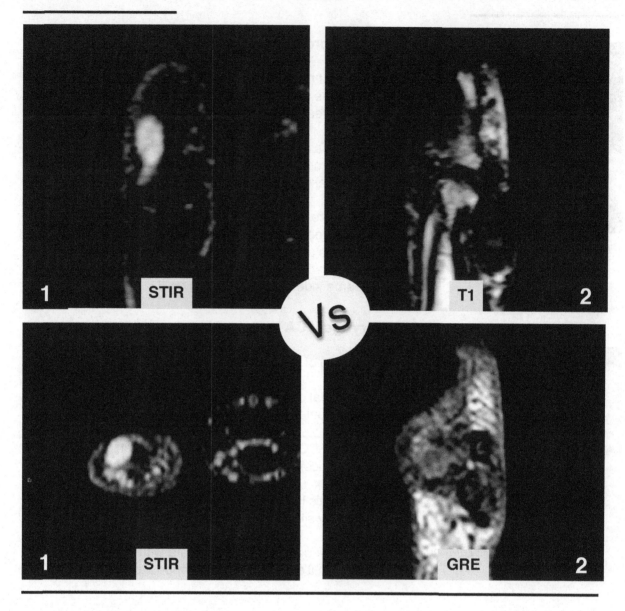

1. Which is Which ?
A. (1) Glomus (2) Fibroma
B. (1) Giant Cell Tumor (2) Glomus
C. (1) Glomus, (2) Giant Cell Tumor
D. (1) Fibroma, (2) Giant Cell Tumor

2. How do you tell them apart?
A. Glomus is T2 Dark
B. Fibroma is T2 Bright
C. Giant Cell Tumor will Bloom on Gradient
D. Glomus will only enhance peripherally.

Case 12 - Finger Masses - Glomus vs GCT of Tendon

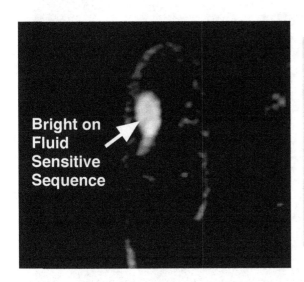

Glomus (Glomangioma)

- Benign Vascular Tumor (best thought of as a hamartoma).

- Almost always found in the finger

- Classic Imaging Features:
  - T2 BRIGHT
  - AVID contrast enhancement

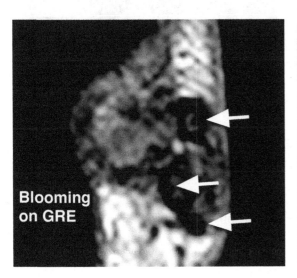

Giant Cell Tumor (of the tendon)

- Benign lesion arising from the tendon sheath.

- It is basically PVNS.

- They favor the palmar tendons

- Classic Imaging Features:
  - T1 and T2 Dark (just like a fibroma)
  - GRE - Blooms (fibromas won't bloom)

1. Which is Which ?
A. (1) Glomus (2) Fibroma
B. (1) Giant Cell Tumor (2) Glomus
C. (1) Glomus, (2) Giant Cell Tumor
D. (1) Fibroma, (2) Giant Cell Tumor

2. How do you tell them apart?
A. Glomus is T2 Dark
B. Fibroma is T2 Bright
C. Giant Cell Tumor will Bloom on Gradient
D. Glomus will only enhance peripherally.

Case 13 - "Shoulder Pain"

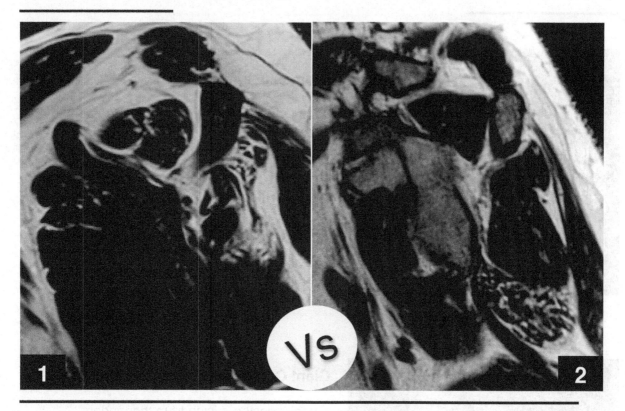

1. A mass would have to be centered where to cause the atrophy pattern in "1" ?
A. Suprascapular Notch
B. Spinoglenoid Notch
C. Quadrilateral Space
D. Brachial Plexus

2. A mass would have to be centered where to cause the atrophy pattern in "2" ?
A. Suprascapular Notch
B. Spinoglenoid Notch
C. Quadrilateral Space
D. Brachial Plexus

3. Which muscle(s) are innervated by the axillary nerve ?
A. Supraspinatous
B. Infraspinatous
C. Teres Minor
D. Teres Major
E. Subscapularis
F. "A & B"

This vs That 27

Case 13 - Innervation of the Rotator Cuff

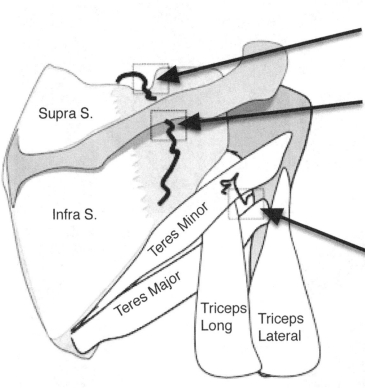

Suprascapular Notch:
- Suprascapular Nerve traveling to the Surpraspinatus
- A hit here will de-innervate both the Supra S. and the Infra S.

Spinoglenoid Notch:
- Suprascapular Nerve traveling to the Infraspinatous
- A hit here will de-innervate only the Infra S.

Quadrilateral Space
- Axillary Nerve traveling to the Teres Minor
- A hit here will de-innervate the Teres Minor

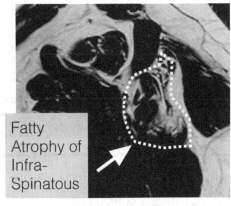

Fatty Atrophy of Infra-Spinatous

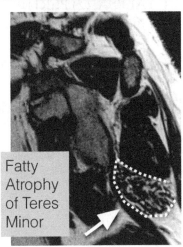

Fatty Atrophy of Teres Minor

1. A mass would have to be centered where to cause the atrophy pattern in "1" ?
   A. Suprascapular Notch
   B. Spinoglenoid Notch
   C. Quadrilateral Space
   D. Brachial Plexus

2. A mass would have to be centered where to cause the atrophy pattern in "2" ?
   A. Suprascapular Notch
   B. Spinoglenoid Notch
   C. Quadrilateral Space
   D. Brachial Plexus

3. Which muscle(s) are innervated by the axillary nerve ?
   A. Supraspinatous
   B. Infraspinatous
   C. Teres Minor
   D. Teres Major
   E. Subscapularis
   F. "A & B"

Case 14 - "Shoulder Pain"

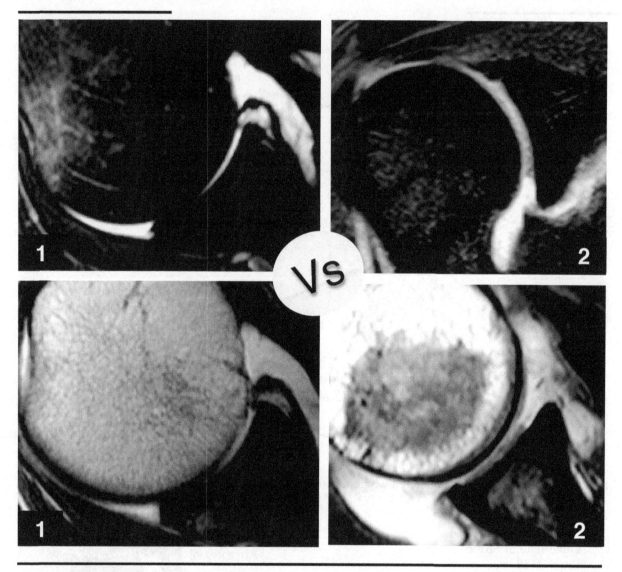

1. Which is Which ?
A. (1) ALPSA, (2) PERTHES
B. (1) PERTHES, (2) GLAD
C. (1) GLAD, (2) ALPSA
D. (1) Bony Bankart, (2) GLAD

2. Which of the following is typically NOT association with shoulder instability?
A. Bankart
B. ALPSA
C. PERTHES
D. GLAD

Case 14 - Glenoid Labrum - Alphabet Soup — PERTHES vs GLAD

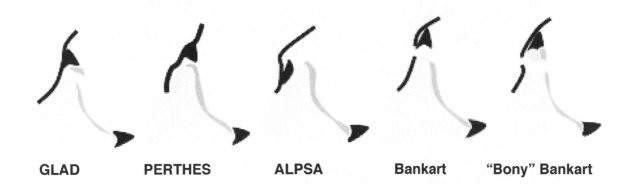

GLAD | PERTHES | ALPSA | Bankart | "Bony" Bankart

Least Severe → Most Severe

GLAD:
- Impaction injury with a cartilage defect.
- There will be an associated superficial anterior inferior labral tear
- NOT associated with underlying instability

PERTHES:
- Lifting of the anterior inferior labrum off the edge of the glenoid, with medial displacement of the sleeve periosteum
- You have loss of the normal stabilizing effects of the inferior glena-humeral

ALPSA:
- **A**nterior **L**abral **P**eriosteal **S**leeve **A**vulsion.
- The anterior inferior labral is torn off the glenoid but remains stuck to the periosteum.
- It can heal in this folded off position - requiring surgery to fix.

Bankart:
- This is defined by disruption of the periosteum.
- This can be cartilage or bony - depending on how much is banged off.
- Remember this is usually from anterior dislocation (& has a matching hill-sacks).

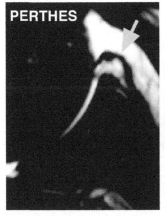

Lifted Labrum, with Displacement of the Sleeve Periosteum

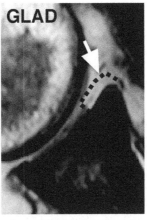

Cartilage Defect with Detached Labrum

1. Which is Which?
A. (1) ALPSA, (2) PERTHES
B. (1) PERTHES, (2) GLAD
C. (1) GLAD, (2) ALPSA
D. (1) Bony Bankart, (2) GLAD

2. Which of the following is typically NOT association with shoulder instability?
A. Bankart
B. ALPSA
C. PERTHES
D. GLAD ** *aren't you glad it's just a glad.*

This vs That 30

Case 15 - Arm Pain

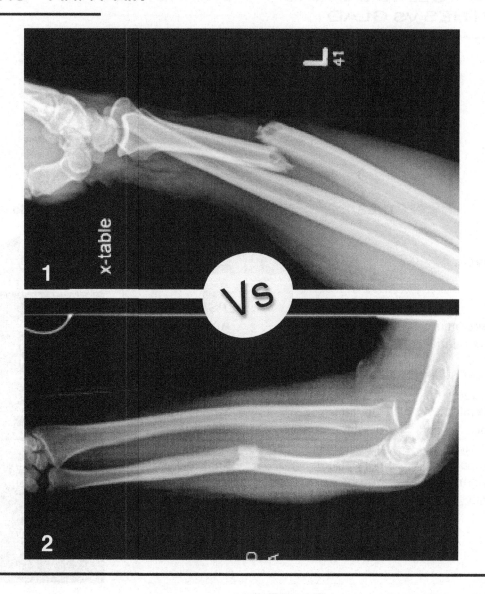

1. Which is Which ?
A. (1) Galeazzi Fx, (2) Monteggia Fx
B. (1) Monteggia Fx, (2) Galeazzi Fx

2. What The F' is an "Essex- Lopresti" Fx ?
A. Comminuted fracture of the radial head with a dislocation at the DRUJ
B. Comminuted fracture of the proximal ulnar with a dislocation at the DRUG
C. Fracture of the ulnar shaft with dislocation of the radial head
D. Fracture of the distal radius with dislocation of the DRUJ

Case 15 - Eponymous Fractures

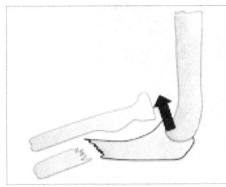

Monteggia Fracture (MUGR)

- Fracture of the Ulna + Radial Head Dislocation
- The direction in which the apex of the ulnar fracture points is the same direction as the radial head dislocation (usually anterior)
- Fracture classification is based on the direction of radial dislocation (usually anterior).

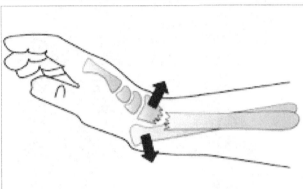

Galeazzi Fracture (MUGR)

- Fracture of the Distal Radius + DRUJ (distal-radial ulnar joint) Dislocation
- Classification is based on dorsal vs volar displacement of the distal radius

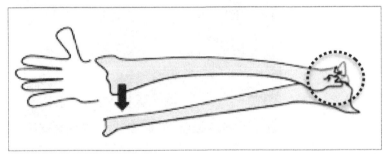

Essex-Lopresti

- Comminuted Fracture of Radial Head + DRUJ Dislocation

1. Which is Which?
A. (1) Galeazzi Fx, (2) Monteggia Fx
B. (1) Monteggia Fx, (2) Galeazzi Fx

2. What The F' is an "Essex-Lopresti" Fx?
A. Comminuted fracture of the radial head with a dislocation at the DRUJ
B. Comminuted fracture of the proximal ulnar with a dislocation at the DRUG
C. Fracture of the ulnar shaft with dislocation of the radial head
D. Fracture of the distal radius with dislocation of the DRUJ

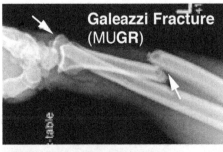

Galeazzi Fracture (MUGR)

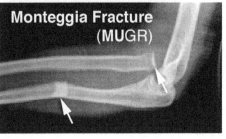

Monteggia Fracture (MUGR)

This vs That 32

Case 16 - Cough

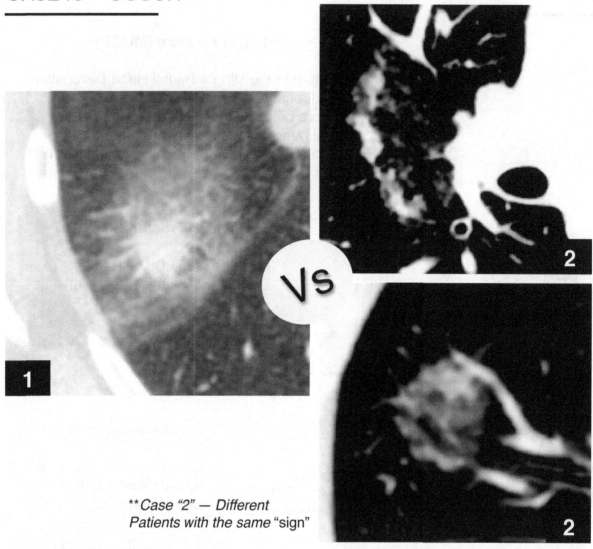

Case "2" — Different Patients with the same "sign"

1. Which is Which ?
A. (1) Halo Sign , (2) Reverse Halo (Atoll) Sign
B. (1) Reverse Halo (Atoll) Sign, (2) Halo Sign

2. What is the classic single answer diagnosis for #1 ?
A. Cryptogenic Organized Pneumonia (COP)
B. Angioinvasive Aspergillosis
C. Sarcoid
D. Pulmonary Lymphoma

3. What is the classic single answer diagnosis for #2 ?
A. Cryptogenic Organized Pneumonia (COP)
B. Angioinvasive Aspergillosis
C. Sarcoid
D. Pulmonary Lymphoma

Case 16 - Halo Signs - Halo vs Reverse Halo (Atoll)

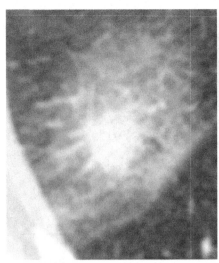
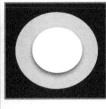

Halo

- Consolidative opacity - with a ground glass halo

- The ground glass part is suppose to represent the hemorrhage / invasion into surrounding tissue

- It has a DDx in real life. But on multiple choice it's **Invasive Aspergillosis** (or other bad fungal infections).

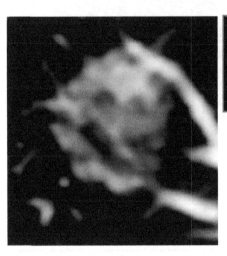

Reverse Halo (Atoll)

- Central ground glass with rim of consolidate opacity.

- It has a DDx in real life. But on multiple choice it's **Organizing Pneumonia (COP).** *Cryptogenic when cause not known.

- Classic causes of organizing pneumonia include drugs (amiodarone), & collagen vascular disease.

1. Which is Which ?
A. (1) Halo Sign , (2) Reverse Halo (Atoll) Sign
B. (1) Reverse Halo (Atoll) Sign, (2) Halo Sign

2. What is the classic single answer diagnosis for #1 ?
A. Cryptogenic Organized Pneumonia (COP)
B. Angioinvasive Aspergillosis
C. Sarcoid
D. Pulmonary Lymphoma

3. What is the classic single answer diagnosis for #2 ?
A. Cryptogenic Organized Pneumonia (COP)
B. Angioinvasive Aspergillosis
C. Sarcoid
D. Pulmonary Lymphoma

Case 17 - Cough

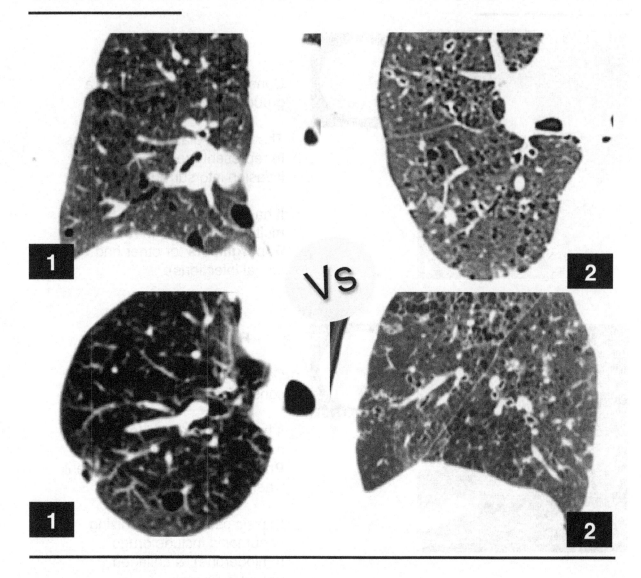

1. Which is Which ?
A. (1) Lymphangiomyomatosis (LAM), (2) Langerhans cell histiocytosis (LCH)
B. (1) Langerhans cell histiocytosis (LCH), (2) Lymphangiomyomatosis (LAM)

2. Which of the follow is true?
A. LAM has thick walled cysts
B. LCH has thin walled cysts
C. LCH is seen more in people who smoke
D. LAM has a strict lower lobe predominance
E. LCH has an association with tuberous sclerosis

3. Which of the following classically spares the costophrenic angles ?
A. Hypersensitivity Pneumonitis
B. LAM
C. NSIP
D. UIP

Case 17 - Cystic Lung Disease - LAM vs LCH

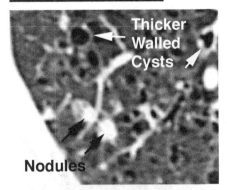
Thicker Walled Cysts
Nodules

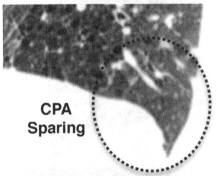
CPA Sparing

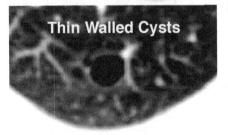
Thin Walled Cysts

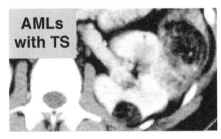
AMLs with TS

Pulmonary Langerhans Cell Histiocytosis (LCH)

- Young Adult (20-30s) Smokers

- Starts out with upper lobe predominant centrilobular nodules - which then cavitate into bizarre thick walled cysts.

- *Thick Walled Cysts + Nodules - upper lobe predominant

- Sparing of the costophrenic angles - only seen with LCH and Hypersensitivity Pneumonitis

- Resolves about 50% of the time, if they quit smoking.

Lymphangiomyomatosis (LAM)

- Women of child bearing age

- Association with Tuberous Sclerosis *(gamesmanship is to show an AML of the kidney first)*

- *Thin walled cysts, diffuse distribution

- They are known to develop chylothorax

1. Which is Which ?
A. (1) Lymphangiomyomatosis (LAM), (2) Langerhans cell histiocytosis (LCH)
B. (1) Langerhans cell histiocytosis (LCH), (2) Lymphangiomyomatosis (LAM)

2. Which of the follow is true?
A. LAM has thick walled cysts
B. LCH has thin walled cysts
C. LCH is seen more in people who smoke
D. LAM has a strict lower lobe predominance
E. LCH has an association with tuberous sclerosis

3. Which of the following classically spares the costophrenic angles ?
A. Hypersensitivity Pneumonitis
B. LAM
C. NSIP
D. UIP

This vs That 36

Case 18 - Cough

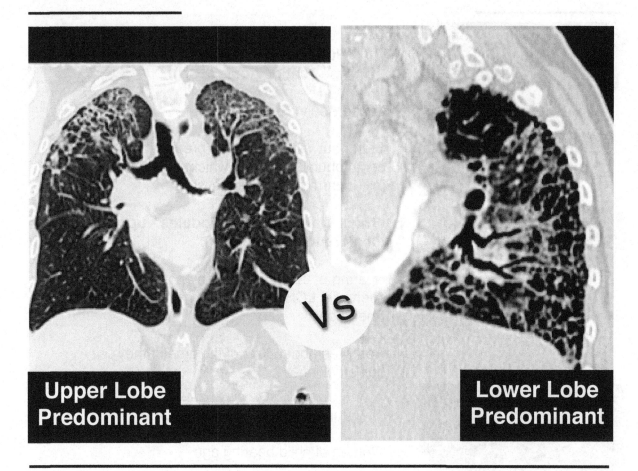

1. Which of the following has an upper lobe predominance ?
A. Asbestosis
B. Rheumatoid Lung
C. Ankylosing Spondylitis
D. Sarcoid

2. Which of the following has a lower lobe predominance ?
A. CF
B. RB-ILD
C. Primary Ciliary Dyskinesia
D. Silicosis

3. Which of the following has a lower lobe predominance ?
A. Primary Lung Cancer
B. Progressive Massive Fibrosis
C. Emphysema (Centrilobular)
D. Scleroderma

Case 18 - Upper vs Lower Lobe Distribution

Upper Lobe Predominant	Lower Lobe Predominant
Most inhaled stuff (not asbestosis). Coal Workers, and Silicosis. This includes progressive massive fibrosis.	Asbestosis ** *the exception to the upper lobe predominant rule for inhaled crap.*
CF	Primary Ciliary Dsykinesia
RB-ILD *(remember it has an association with smoking)*	Most Interstitial Lung Diseases (UIP, NSIP, DIP)
Centrilobular Emphysema	Panlobular Emphysema (Alpha 1)
Ankylosing Spondylitis	Rheumatoid Lung
Sarcoid	Scleroderma (associated with NSIP)
Most Primary Lung Cancers *(more exposure to air born toxins - cigarette smoke etc...)*	Most Hematogenously Spread Metastatic Cancers *(more blood flow to the bases)*

1. Which of the following has an upper lobe predominance ?
A. Asbestosis
B. Rheumatoid Lung
C. Ankylosing Spondylitis
D. Sarcoid

2. Which of the following has a lower lobe predominance ?
A. CF
B. RB-ILD
C. Primary Ciliary Dyskinesia
D. Silicosis

3. Which of the following has a lower lobe predominance ?
A. Primary Lung Cancer
B. Progressive Massive Fibrosis
C. Emphysema (Centrilobular)
D. Scleroderma

Case 19 - Cough

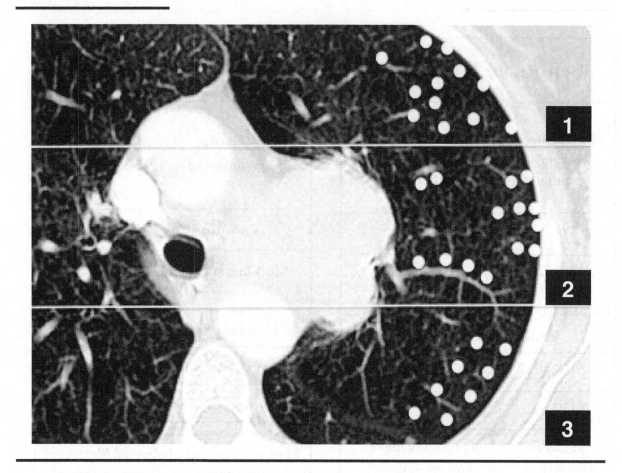

1. Which distribution of nodules is which ?
A. (1) Random, (2) Centrilobular, (3) Perilymphatic
B. (1) Random, (2) Perilymphatic, (3) Centrilobular
C. (1) Perilymphatic, (2) Centrilobular, (3) Random
D. (1) Centrilobular, (2) Random, (3) Perilymphatic

2. Which of the following classically has a perilymphatic distribution ?
A. Sarcoid
B. Hypersensitivity Pneumonitis
C. Endobronchial Infection
D. Hematogenous Spread of Cancer

3. Which of the following classically has a centrilobular distribution ?
A. Sarcoid
B. Systemic Fungal Infection
C. Hypersensitivity Pneumonitis
D. Lymphangitic Spread of Cancer

Case 19 - Nodule Patterns

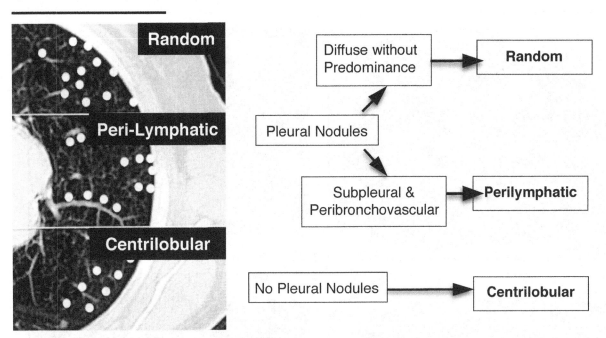

Perilymphatic	Random	Centrilobular
Sarcoid — *Most Classic*	Miliary TB - *Most Classic*	Hypersensitivity Pneumonitis - *Most Classic*
Silicosis	Disseminated Fungal Infection	Resp Bronchiolitis (RB-ILD)
Lymphangetic Spread CA	Hematogenous Spread CA	Infectious Diseases (Endobronchial Spread)

1. Which distribution of nodules is which ?
A. (1) Random, (2) Centrilobular, (3) Perilymphatic
B. (1) Random, (2) Perilymphatic, (3) Centrilobular
C. (1) Perilymphatic, (2) Centrilobular, (3) Random
D. (1) Centrilobular, (2) Random, (3) Perilymphatic

2. Which of the following classically has a perilymphatic distribution ?
A. Sarcoid
B. Hypersensitivity Pneumonitis
C. Endobronchial Infection
D. Hematogenous Spread of Cancer

3. Which of the following classically has a centrilobular distribution ?
A. Sarcoid
B. Systemic Fungal Infection
C. Hypersensitivity Pneumonitis
D. Lymphangitic Spread of Cancer

This vs That 40

Case 20 - Belly Pain

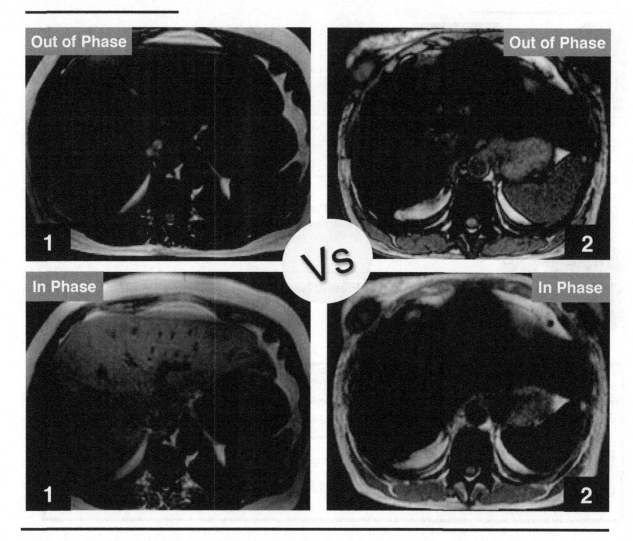

1. Which is which ?
A. (1) Hepatic Steatosis (2) Hemochromatosis
B. (1) Hemochromatosis (2) Hepatic Steatosis

2. Which should be acquired first ?
A. Out of phase imaging
B. In phase imaging
C. Makes no difference

3. Iron causes a signal drop out by?
A. Causing T2* effects
B. Elongates T1 signal
C. Increasing local eddy currents in the imaged tissues
D. Worsening sample size limitations

Case 20 - Signal Drop-Out; Fatty Liver vs Iron Liver

Physics Crash Course

- When iron is present in high concentrations it essentially becomes a small magnet ("Iron is Paramagnetic"). The presence of a magnet within the magnet changes the field surrounding it (makes the field dirty). This results in a shortening of lots of stuff, the most testable is due to T2 star (remember those are the ones from a non-uniform field). An easy way to think about this is if you had a totally uniform field T2 would equal T2*.

- The longer you wait to image something, the more noticeable the effects of T2* are going to be. Think about two runners at the starting line, one is fat & one is from Kenya. If you took a picture 0.5 seconds into the race they would be close together, but if you waited 10 seconds the distance between them would be huge. T2* is the Kenyan and Iron laden livers have more T2*…. so the longer the echo time, the darker iron looks (why it's dark on in-phase, which is traditionally done later - as shown below).

- Lets briefly review in and out of phase imaging. This is basically two gradient sequences done with different echo times, based on the precession speed of water and fat (which are different). At different echo times fat and water can be seen on opposite sides (out of phase), or perfectly lined up (in phase). When opposed, the signals drop out. This is why fat drops out on out of phase imaging.

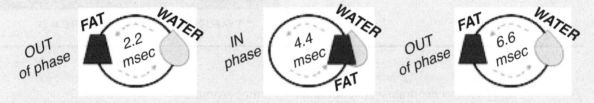

- Now, because this lining up and not lining up is occurring over and over again (every 2.2 msec at 1.5T) you can wait and do the out of phase at 6.6msec. BUT, if you do that, and you are dealing with an iron laden liver the T2* effects will be even more pronounced (the Kenyan runner will be way away) and will not be able to tell if you have signal drop out from fat, or signal drop out from iron.

1. Which is which ?
A. **(1) Hepatic Steatosis (2) Hemochromatosis**
B. (1) Hemochromatosis (2) Hepatic Steatosis
Fat dark on OUT of phase, Iron dark on IN phase

2. Which should be acquired first ?
A. **Out of phase imaging**
B. In phase imaging
C. Makes no difference

3. Iron causes a signal drop out by?
A. **Causing T2* effects**
B. Elongates T1 signal
C. Increasing local eddy currents in the imaged tissues
D. Worsening sample size limitations

Case 21 - Bronze Skin

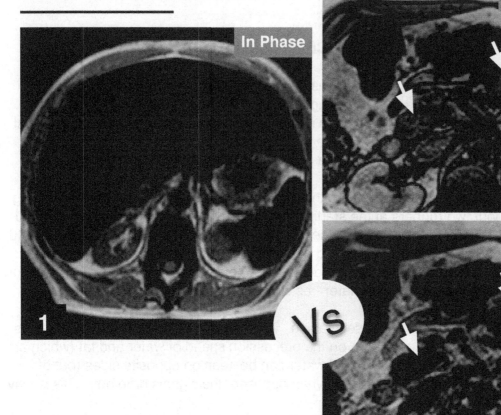

** Arrows on Pancreas

1. Which is which ?
A. (1) Primary Hemochromatosis (2) Secondary Hemochromatosis
B. (1) Secondary Hemochromatosis (2) Primary Hemochromatosis

2. How can you tell them apart ?
A. The liver is involved in primary but not secondary
B. The pancreas is involved in secondary but not primary
C. The spleen is involved in secondary but not primary

3. What "internal control" can be used to evaluate for iron overload in the liver?
A. The pancreas
B. The paraspinal muscles
C. The vertebral bodies
D. The large bowel

4. How is iron quantification accomplished?
A. Using Spin Echo Sequences with a specific TR
B. A double inversion protocol is done, with a specific TI
C. GRE Sequences with progressively longer echo times
D. It's done with diffusion set at varying B_0 values.

Case 21 - Hemochromatosis - Primary vs Secondary

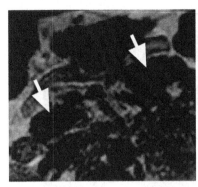

Signal Drop out in Pancreas

Primary

- Autosomal Recessive Condition
- Seen mostly in white Europeans
- You see the manifestations later in women, because they self treat by having bloody periods
- It can cause cirrhosis, heart failure, arthritis, bronze skin, and pancreas failure ("bronze diabetes")
- On Imaging:
  - The liver signal **drops out** (darkens) **on** delayed sequences - typically **in phase**)
  - The **liver will be darker than the paraspinal muscles** (which is never normal).
  - Pancreas can be involved (**P**ancreas for **P**rimary)
  - Spleen is spared.

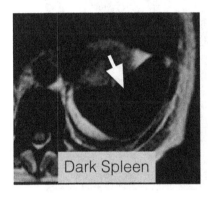

Dark Spleen

Secondary

- From frequent blood transfusions (usually)
- All the same stuff from primary (drop out on in phase, liver darker than spine muscles) PLUS you have a dark spleen. **S**pleen for **S**econdary.

1. Which is which ?
A. (1) Primary Hemochromatosis (2) Secondary Hemochromatosis
B. **(1) Secondary Hemochromatosis (2) Primary Hemochromatosis**

2. How can you tell them apart ?
A. The liver is involved in primary but not secondary
B. The pancreas is involved in secondary but not primary
C. **The spleen is involved in secondary but not primary**

3. What "internal control" can be used to evaluate for iron overload in the liver?
A. The pancreas
B. **The paraspinal muscles**
C. The vertebral bodies
D. The large bowel

4. How is iron quantification accomplished?
A. Using Spin Echo Sequences with a specific TR
B. A double inversion protocol is done, with a specific TI
C. **GRE Sequences with progressively longer echo times** ** *more drop out with progressive echo time*
D. It's done with diffusion set at varying B_0 values.

This vs That 44

Case 22 - Hepatitis C - AFP Rising

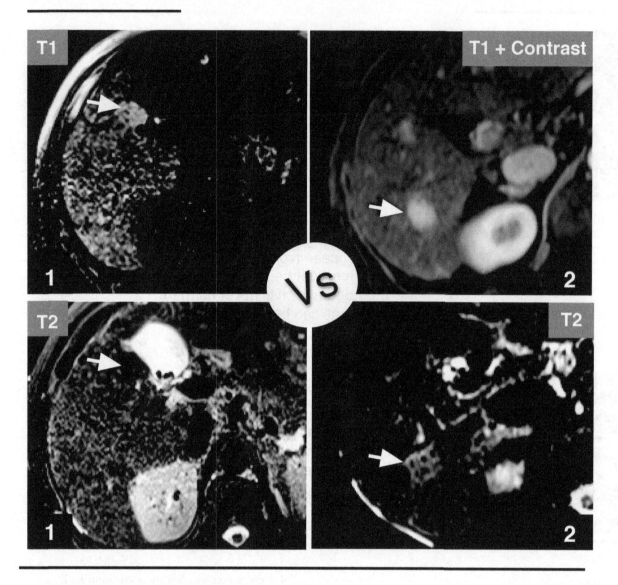

1. Which is which ?
A. (1) Regenerative Nodule (2) Dysplastic Nodule
B. (1) Dysplastic Nodule, (2) HCC
C. (1) Dysplastic Nodule, (2) Regenerative Nodule

2. How can you tell them apart ?
A. Dysplastic Nodules are T2 Bright
B. Regenerative Nodules enhance
C. HCC is T2 Bright

3. What if you saw large (4cm) enhancing nodules in a patient with Budd Chiari ?
A. They are cancer until proven otherwise
B. Probably benign

Case 22 - Liver Nodules

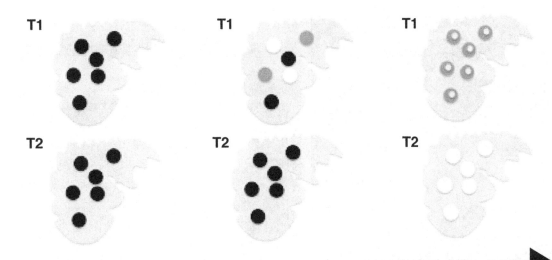

Regenerative Nodule → **Dysplastic Nodule** → **HCC**

Regenerative:
- Most Common Cirrhosis Associated Nodule
- Usually numerous
- Histologically their function is normal, they are just scarred up
- T2; DARK
- T1: Variable - but think about them being T1 dark
- C+: Enhance the same as liver

Dysplastic:
- Progressive architectural derangement on histology
- T2: Dark - especially when low grade. The higher grade ones will have mildly increased signal
- T1: Variable - but **think about them being T1 Bright**
- C+: Enhance the same as liver

HCC:
- **T2: BRIGHT**
- T1: Hypointense with internal foci of isointense signal
- Signal Drop out on In-out of phase imaging (**internal fat**) - makes them more likely to be HCCs
- C+: Intense early enhancement

1. Which is which ?
A. (1) Regenerative Nodule (2) Dysplastic Nodule
B. (1) Dysplastic Nodule, (2) HCC
C. (1) Dysplastic Nodule, (2) Regenerative Nodule

2. How can you tell them apart ?
A. Dysplastic Nodules are T2 Bright
B. Regenerative Nodules enhance
C. HCC is T2 Bright

3. What if you saw large (4cm) enhancing nodules in a patient with Budd Chiari ?
A. They are cancer until proven otherwise
B. Probably benign

Budd Chiari Nodules

Large Multiple Nodules in Budd Chiari livers are characteristic of regenerative nodules (hyperplastic). They can enhance, but don't washout out quickly like an HCC.

Case 23 - Belly Pain

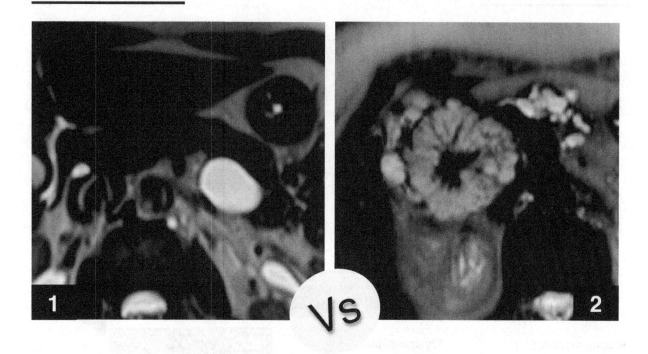

1. Which is which ?
A. (1) Serous Cystadenoma (2) Mucinous Cystic Neoplasm (MCN)
B. (1) Mucinous Cystic Neoplasm (MCN) (2) Serous Cystadenoma
C. (1) Solid Pseudopapillary Neoplasm (SPN), (2) Serous Cystadenoma

2. Generally Speaking ...
A. Serous Cystadenoma is seen in grandmas, MCNs are seen in moms
B. MCNs are seen in grandmas, Serous Cystadenoma is seen in moms
C. SPNs are seen in teenage asian boys

3. Which is true ?
A. Serous Cystadenoma is malignant until proven otherwise
B. MCNs are usually in the body/tail
C. SPNs do NOT enhance
D. MCNs have no malignant potential

Case 23 - Cystic Pancreatic Lesions-

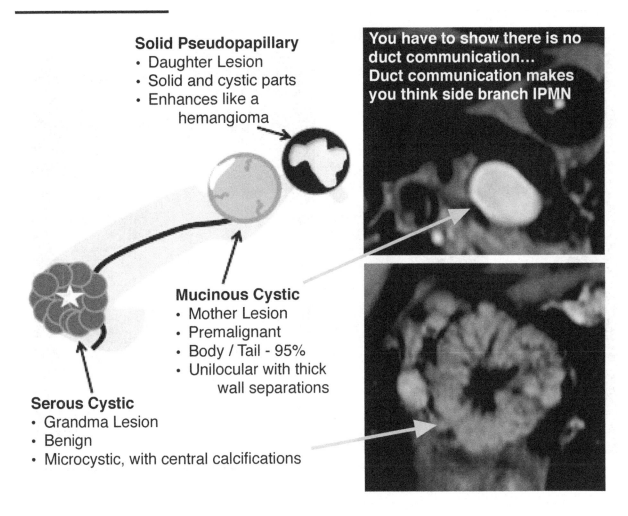

1. Which is which?
A. (1) Serous Cystadenoma (2) Mucinous Cystic Neoplasm (MCN)
B. (1) Mucinous Cystic Neoplasm (MCN) (2) Serous Cystadenoma
C. (1) Solid Pseudopapillary Neoplasm (SPN), (2) Serous Cystadenoma

2. Generally Speaking ...
A. Serous Cystadenoma is seen in grandmas, MCNs are seen in moms
B. MCNs are seen in grandmas, Serous Cystadenoma is seen in moms
C. SPNs are seen in teenage asian boys ** *asian or african american teenage girls*

3. Which is true?
A. Serous Cystadenoma is malignant until proven otherwise
B. MCNs are usually in the body/tail
C. SPNs do NOT enhance
D. MCNs have no malignant potential

This vs That 48

Case 24 - Belly Pain

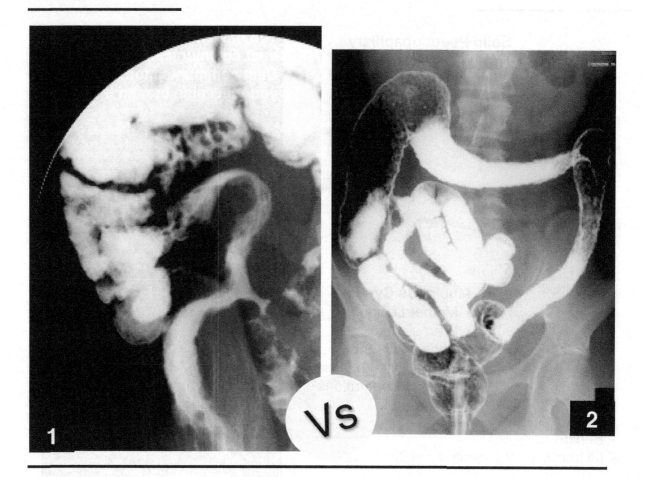

1. Which is which ?
A. (1) Crohns (2) Ulcerative Colitis
B. (1) Ulcerative Colitis (2) Crohns

2. Ulcerative colitis "always" involves the ?
A. Terminal Ileum
B. Splenic Flexure
C. Rectum
D. Small Bowel

3. Which is true ?
A. Primary Sclerosing Cholangitis is more common with Crohns
B. Gall Stones are more common with Crohns
C. Fistula are more common with UC
D. Crohns has a higher malignant risk compared to UC
E. UC has a malignant risk (higher than gen pop) when limited to the rectum only

Case 24 - Inflammatory Bowel Disease

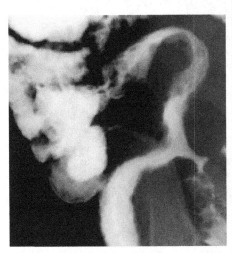

Epic String Sign - Strictured TI

Crohns

- Typically seen in a young adult (15-30), but has a second smaller peak 60-70.
- Discontinuous involvement of the entire GI tract (mouth -> asshole).
- Stomach, usually involves antrum (Ram's Horn Deformity).
- Small bowel is involved 80% of the time, with the terminal ileum almost always involved (Marked Narrowing = String Sign).
- After surgery the "neo-terminal ileum" will frequently be involved.
- Complications include fistulae, abscess, gallstones, fatty liver, and sacroiliitis.

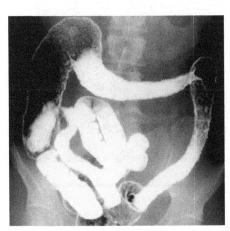

Ahaustral - Lead Pipe Colon

Ulcerative Colitis

- Similar dual peak age breakdown
- Involves the rectum 95% of the time, and has retrograde progression.
- Terminal ileum is involved 5-10% of the time via backwash ileitis (wide open appearance).
- It is continuous and does not "skip" like Crohns.
- It is associated with Colon Cancer, Primary Sclerosing Cholangitis, and Arthritis (similar to Ankylosing Spondylitis).
- Cancer risk is only above general population when disease progresses to the splenic flexure.
- On Barium, it is said that the colon is ahaustral, with a diffuse granular appearing mucosa. "Lead Pipe" is the buzzword (shortened from fibrosis).

1. Which is which ?
A. (1) Crohns (2) Ulcerative Colitis
B. (1) Ulcerative Colitis (2) Crohns

2. Ulcerative colitis "always" involves the ?
A. Terminal Ileum
B. Splenic Flexure
C. Rectum
D. Small Bowel

3. Which is true ?
A. Primary Sclerosing Cholangitis is more common with Crohns
B. Gall Stones are more common with Crohns
C. Fistula are more common with UC
D. Crohns has a higher malignant risk compared to UC
E. UC has a malignant risk (higher than gen pop) when limited to the rectum only ** *only when it extends past the splenic flexure.*

This vs That 50

Case 25 - Belly Pain

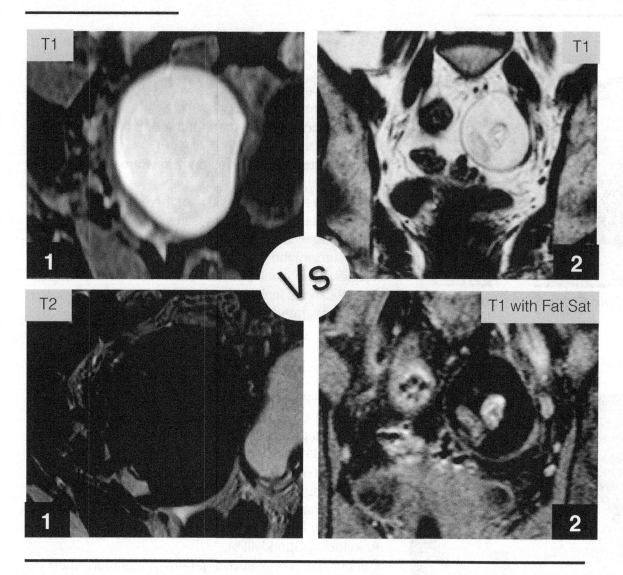

1. Which is which ?
A. (1) Endometrioma (2) Hemorrhagic Cyst
B. (1) Hemorrhagic Cyst (2) Endometrioma
C. (1) Dermoid, (2) Endometrioma
D. (1) Endometrioma, (2) Dermoid

2. Which is the correct rare malignant transformation pairing?
A. Endometrioma -> Clear Cell CA, Dermoid -> Adenocarcinoma
B. Endometrioma -> Clear Cell CA, Dermoid -> Squamous Cell CA
C. Endometrioma -> Squamous Cell CA, Dermoid -> Adenocarcinoma
D. Endometrioma -> Transitional Cell CA, Dermoid -> Squamous Cell CA

Case 25 - Ovarian Mass - MRI Differential

	T1	T1FS	T2	
	○	○	● (gray)	**Endometrioma**
	○	● (black)	○	**Dermoid**

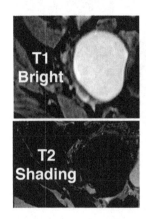

Endometrioma

- A known cause of pelvic pain
- T1 Bright (from blood), Fat Sat don't do shit, **T2 will be dark.** This is the so called *"shading sign"*
- They can become cancer (clear cell), but it's rare. If they are big (like 9cm) and seen in an older women - then they are at higher risk.

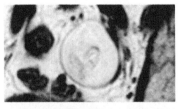
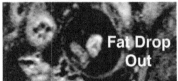

Dermoid

- Most common ovarian neoplasm in patients < 20.
- Hyperechoic solid mural nodule - is classic on ultrasound
- T1 & T2 Bright (from fat), and **will suppress on fat sat**.
- They can become cancer (squamous), but it's rare. Risk factors are similar - large size, and advanced patient age.
- Bilateral about 10% of the time.

1. Which is which ?
A. (1) Endometrioma (2) Hemorrhagic Cyst
B. (1) Hemorrhagic Cyst (2) Endometrioma
C. (1) Dermoid, (2) Endometrioma
D. (1) Endometrioma, (2) Dermoid

2. Which is the correct rare malignant transformation pairing?
A. Endometrioma -> Clear Cell CA, Dermoid -> Adenocarcinoma
B. Endometrioma -> Clear Cell CA, Dermoid -> Squamous Cell CA
C. Endometrioma -> Squamous Cell CA, Dermoid -> Adenocarcinoma
D. Endometrioma -> Transitional Cell CA, Dermoid -> Squamous Cell CA

Case 26 - Stinky Breath

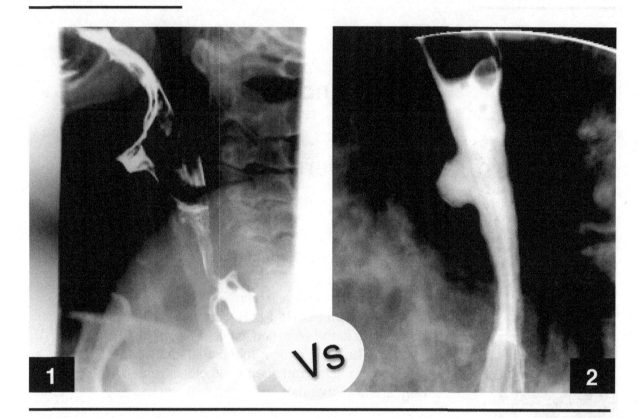

1. Which is which?
A. (1) Killian Jamieson Diverticulum (2) Zenker Diverticulum
B. (1) Traction Diverticulum (2) Zenker Diverticulum
C. (1) Epiphrenic Diverticulum (2) Killian Jamieson Diverticulum
D. (1) Zenker Diverticulum (2) Traction Diverticulum

2. Most likely cause?
A. (1) Esophageal motor disorder (failure of cricopharyngeus muscle to relax), (2) Granulomatous Disease
B. (1) Granulomatous Disease, (2) Esophageal motor disorder failure of cricopharyngeus muscle to relax),

3. Where does the Zenker Diverticulum occur?
A. Just Above the cricopharyngeus muscle
B. Lateral to the suspensory ligaments of the esophagus inserting on the cricoid cartilage
C. Killian's Triangle (Dehiscence)
D. Just above the gastroesophageal junction

Case 26 - Esophageal Diverticula

Zenker Diverticulum

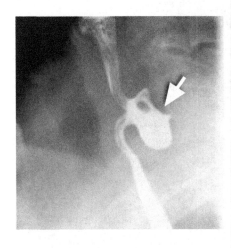

- These are the posterior ones
- They occur between the oblique and horizontal fibers of the esophageal wall, known as a Killian dehiscence or triangle.
- If the cricopharyngeus muscle refuses to relax, a lot of pressure is generated - this results in herniation through the weak Killian Triangle.
- Why won't it just relax? Most people say that it's from a hypertrophied morphology secondary to chronic reflux.
- Just remember **reflux -> Killian Dehiscence.**
- These things are classified as "pulsion" diverticulum (*The Round Kind*).
- A true pulsion diverticulum contains no muscle in their walls) with a peristaltic contraction.

Traction Diverticulum

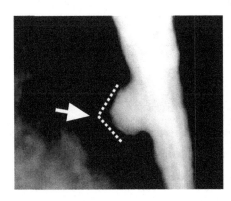

- *The Triangle Kind*
- Historically these were caused by TB - and that's probably still the case outside the US. Other inflammatory disease (Histo) or radiation can do it as well. Think about it as a scarring / tethering.

1. Which is which ?
A. (1) Killian Jamieson Diverticulum (2) Zenker Diverticulum
B. (1) Traction Diverticulum (2) Zenker Diverticulum
C. (1) Epiphrenic Diverticulum (2) Killian Jamieson Diverticulum
D. (1) Zenker Diverticulum (2) Traction Diverticulum

2. Most likely cause?
A. (1) Esophageal motor disorder (failure of cricopharyngeus muscle to relax), (2) Granulomatous Disease
B. (1) Granulomatous Disease, (2) Esophageal motor disorder failure of cricopharyngeus muscle to relax),

3. Where does the Zenker Diverticulum occur?
A. Just Above the cricopharyngeus muscle
B. Lateral to the suspensory ligaments of the esophagus inserting on the cricoid cartilage
C. Killian's Triangle (Dehiscence)
D. Just above the gastroesophageal junction

Case 27 - Decided to have "One More", To Try and Save the Marriage

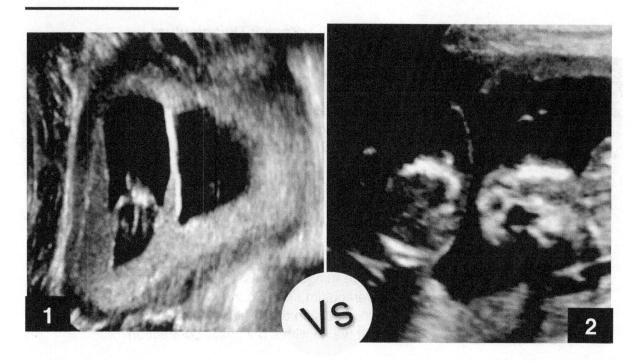

1. Which is which ?
A. (1) Monochorionic (2) Dichorionic
B. (1) Dichorionic (2) Monochorionic

2. Which one of these would be susceptible to "Twin-Twin Transfusion" Syndrome ?
A. (1)
B. (2)

3. Which of the following is true regarding the Umbilical Artery Systolic / Diastolic Ratio ?
A. The ratio should increase with gestational age
B. The ration should always be more than 3 at 34 weeks
C. High Resistance patterns are seen with IUGR
D. Reversed diastolic flow is associated with favorable outcomes

4. Which of the following is true regarding Fetal Middle Cerebral Artery Assessment ?
A. The fetal MCA should be low resistance, with normal antegrade flow in diastole
B. Checking fetal MCA resistance is done for the workup of fetal anemia & twin-twin transfusion
C. Fetal MCA S/D Ratio should always be lower than the Umbilical Artery S/D ratio

Case 27 - Twins - Placenta Morphology

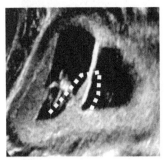
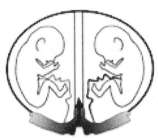

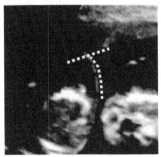
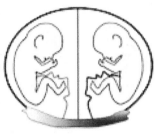

Twin-Peak Sign:

- A beak-like tongue between the two membranes of a dichorionic (*2 placentas*) diamniotic (*2 sacs*) fetuses.
- This excludes a monochorionic pregnancy.
- This is the good one.

T - Sign:

- This is essentially the absence of the twin peak sign. You don't see chorion between membrane layers.
- **T sign = monochorionic** *(1 placenta)* pregnancy.
- These are susceptible to lots of bad things from "blood sharing" - including twin-twin transfusion.

1. Which is which?
A. (1) Monochorionic (2) Dichorionic
B. **(1) Dichorionic (2) Monochorionic**

2. Which one of these would be susceptible to "Twin-Twin Transfusion" Syndrome?
A. (1)
B. **(2)**

3. Which of the following is true regarding the Umbilical Artery Systolic / Diastolic Ratio?
A. The ratio should increase with gestational age
B. The ration should always be more than 3 at 34 weeks
C. **High Resistance patterns are seen with IUGR**
D. Reversed diastolic flow is associated with favorable outcomes

4. Which of the following is true regarding Fetal Middle Cerebral Artery Assessment?
A. The fetal MCA should be low resistance, with normal antegrade flow in diastole
B. **Checking Fetal MCA resistance is done for the workup of fetal anemia & twin-twin transfusion**
C. Fetal MCA S/D Ratio should always be lower than the Umbilical Artery S/D ratio

Fetal Doppler Trivia

- **Umbilical Artery:**
  - The ratio of systolic to diastolic pressure (S/D) should decrease with age.
  - **The general rule is 2-3 at 32 weeks.** The ratio should not be more than 3 at 34 weeks.
  - Elevation should make you think IUGR or pre-eclampsia

- **MCA S/D Ratio:**
  - Usually done to monitor anemia (from a variety of causes)
  - **Normal Fetal MCA is high resistance.** If it turns low resistance the head is attempting to "spare itself" — thats bad.
  - As a general rule the MCA S/D should always be higher than the umbilical one

Case 28 - NICU Baby... Probably Named "Miracle"

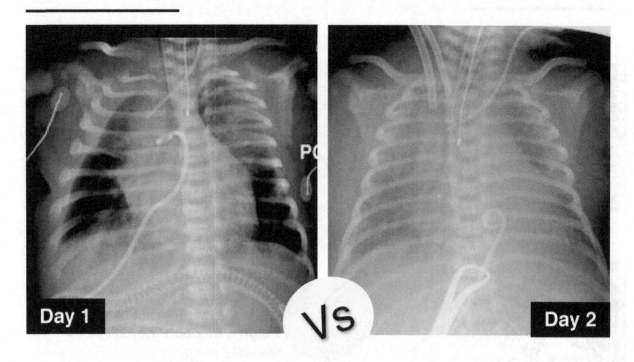

1. What happened to his lungs on Day 2?
A. He developed full on pulmonary edema - tell the intern to give him lasix
B. He developed bilateral interstitial pneumonia - tell the intern to give him ABx
C. This is normal given the procedure he had in the interval (between Day 1 & 2)

2. What is the "primary risk" of the therapy shown in "Day 2" ?
A. Pneumonia
B. NEC
C. Intracranial Hemorrhage
D. Anastomotic Breakdown

3. What is the reason a daily CXR is done after this therapy ?
A. Look for catheter migration (in or out)
B. Detection of subtle pneumonia
C. Detection of interstitial pulmonary edema
D. Because all health care resources are free and unlimited.

Case 28 - ECMO

ECMO
(Extracorporeal Membrane Oxygenation)

- ECMO is a cardiopulmonary bypass technique used to support patients with severe respiratory or cardiac failure (usually both) unresponsive to conventional ventilatory support.

- The standard indications for the use of ECMO include meconium aspiration (for which it actually has pretty good outcomes), primary pulmonary hypertension, congenital diaphragmatic hernia, and the most common reason in the US which is the desire to run the NICU bill up as high as possible to burden the parents not only with the inevitable death of their child but also with an un-payable multi-million dollar bill, which will then add to the rising cost of health care and the need to reduce physician salaries (while at the same time raising hospital administrator salaries).

- The main role of the radiologist when reading these daily NICU films is to **check for catheter migration** - both in and out. The carotid catheter should terminate over the arch, and the jugular catheter should terminate over the right atrium.

- Generalized lung opacification (**white out) is typical and expected** when the patient is placed on ECMO - as shown on this case. This occurs because of the changes in pulmonary hemodynamics and physiology from the abrupt change in airway pressure. Remember the lungs are getting bypassed.

- Systemic anticoagulation is required for ECMO. Additionally, there is a known continuous consumption of platelets that occurs in these patients. These two factors make the baby **high risk for hemorrhage**. As a result, these kids get daily head ultrasounds to monitor for this complication (plus the risk of stroke from having their jugular and carotid ligated on one side).

1. What happened to his lungs on Day 2?
A. He developed full on pulmonary edema - tell the intern to give him lasix
B. He developed bilateral interstitial pneumonia -tell the intern to give him ABx
C. This is normal given the procedure he had in the interval (between Day 1 & 2)

2. What is the "primary risk" of the therapy shown in "Day 2" ?
A. Pneumonia
B. NEC
C. Intracranial Hemorrhage
D. Anastomotic Breakdown

3. What is the reason a daily CXR is done after this therapy ?
A. Look for catheter migration (in or out)
B. Detection of subtle pneumonia
C. Detection of interstitial pulmonary edema
D. Because all health care resources are free and unlimited.

Case 29 - NICU Baby... Also Named "Miracle"

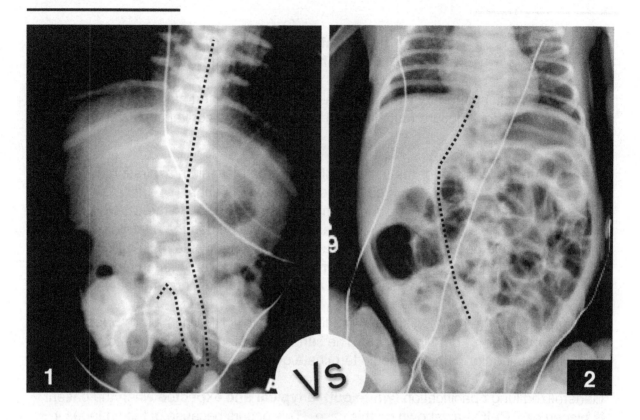

1. Which is Which ?
A. (1) Umbilical Arterial Catheter, (2) Umbilical Venous Catheter
B. (1) Umbilical Venous Catheter, (2) Umbilical Arterial Catheter

2. How can you tell them apart?
A. The venous catheter first goes down, then up
B. The arterial catheter first goes down, then up

3. Which is true about positioning of Umbilical Arterial Catheters ?
A. L1 is the ideal location
B. It should always be above the renals (T6-T10)
C. It should always be below the renals (L3-L5)
D. It can be above (T68-T10) or below (L3-L5) the renals

Case 29 - Umbilical Catheters

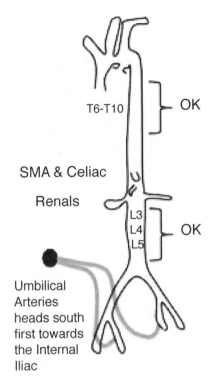

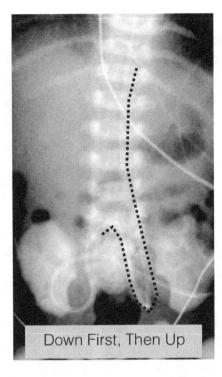

Down First, Then Up

UAC

- In order to avoid placement into (and thrombosis of) aortic branches, the catheter should be either in a high position (T6-T10) above the celiac, mesenteric and renal arteries or in a low position (L3-L5) below the inferior mesenteric artery.

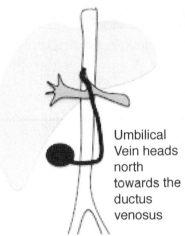

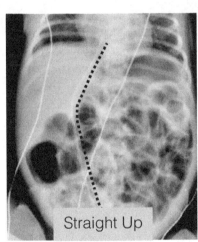

Straight Up

UVC

- Position at the right atrium is ideal.

- Placement in the left portal vein can cause a liver infarct

1. Which is Which?
A. (1) Umbilical Arterial Catheter, (2) Umbilical Venous Catheter
B. (1) Umbilical Venous Catheter, (2) Umbilical Arterial Catheter

2. How can you tell them apart?
A. The venous catheter first goes down, then up
B. The arterial catheter first goes down, then up

3. Which is true about positioning of Umbilical Arterial Catheters?
A. L1 is the ideal location
B. It should always be above the renals (T6-T10)
C. It should always be below the renals (L3-L5)
D. It can be above (T6-T10) or below (L3-L5) the renals

Case 30 - Cardiac Workup

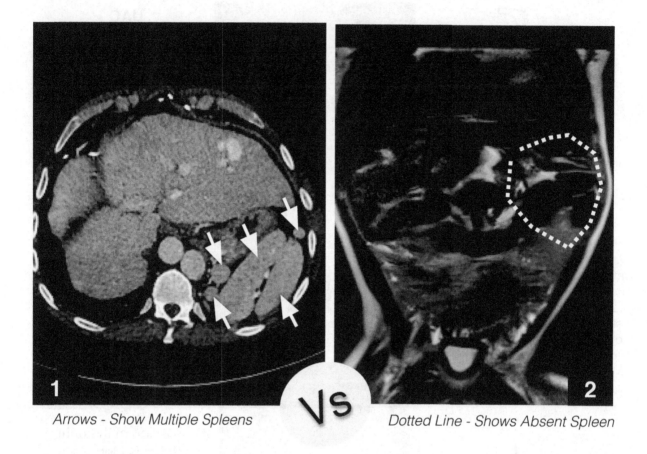

Arrows - Show Multiple Spleens Vs Dotted Line - Shows Absent Spleen

1. Which will have more cardiac malformations ?
A. (1)
B. (2)

2. Which is true regarding the IVC positioning ?
A. (1) will have azygous continuation of the IVC, (2) will have reversed aortic/IVC position
B. (1) will have reversed aortic/IVC position, (2) will have azygous continuation of the IVC

3. Which is true regarding lung fissures ?
A. (1) will have two left fissures, (2) will have one right fissure
B. (1) will have one right fissure, (2) will have two left fissures

Case 30 - Heterotaxia Syndromes

UVC

- The major game played on written tests is "left side vs right side."

- *So what the hell does that mean?*

  - I like to start in the lungs. The right side has two fissures (major and minor). The left side has just one fissure. So if I show you a CXR with two fissures on each side, (a left sided minor fissure), then the patient has two right sides. Thus the term "bilateral right sidedness."

  - *What else is a right sided structure?* The liver. So, these patients won't have a spleen (the spleen is a left sided structure). The opposite is true, bilateral left sided patients have polysplenia.

  - *What about the IVC?* Its usually a right sided structure, so it flips in a bilateral right sided situation.

Bilateral Right Sided	Bilateral Left Sided
Two Fissures in the Left Lung	One Fissure in the Right Lung
Asplenia	Polysplenia
Increased Cardiac Malformations	Less Cardiac Malformations
Reversed Aorta / IVC	Azygous Continuation of the IVC

1. Which will have more cardiac malformations ?
A. (1)
B. (2)

2. Which is true regarding the IVC positioning ?
A. (1) will have azygous continuation of the IVC, (2) will have reversed aortic/IVC position
B. (1) will have reversed aortic/IVC position, (2) will have azygous continuation of the IVC

3. Which is true regarding lung fissures ?
A. (1) will have two left fissures, (2) will have one right fissure
B. (1) will have one right fissure, (2) will have two left fissures

Case 31 - Hip Pain / Limp

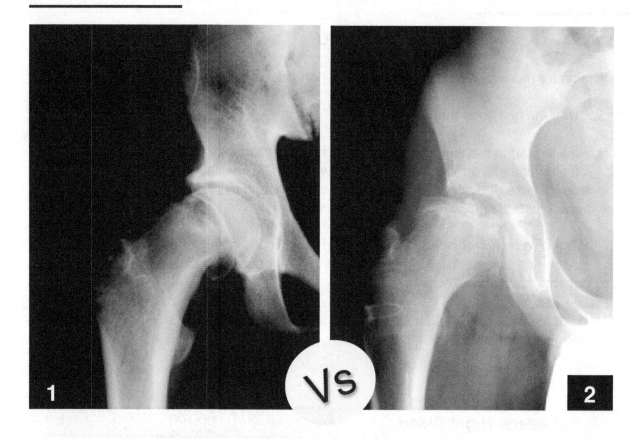

1. Which is Which ?
A. (1) SCFE, (2) Perthes,
B. (1) Perthes, (2) Development Dysplasia
C. (1) SCFE, (2) Development Dysplasia
D. (1) Development Dysplasia, (2) Perthes

2. Which is true about the classic age for these ?
A. (1) Around 6, (2) Around 12
B. (1) Around 12 (2) Around 6

3. Which of these is bilateral more often?
A. (1)
B. (2)

4. Which is true regarding the treatment of SCFE?
A. You should relocate it first, then pin it
B. You should just pin it, don't relocate it
C. You should never pin it… just relocate it

Case 31 - The Pediatric Hip - SCFE vs Perthes

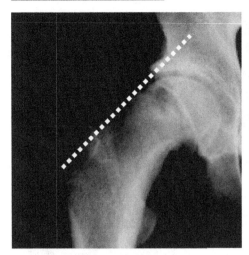

"Klein's Line" - Should intersect the femoral head... this one clearly doesn't

Slipped Capital Femoral Epiphysis (SCFE)

- This is a **type 1 salter harris**,
- Unlike most SH1s, this guy has a bad prognosis if not fixed.
- The classic history is *fat black adolescent* (age 12-15) with hip pain.
- It's bilateral in 1/3 of cases (both hips don't usually present at same time).
- The **frog leg view** is the money - think about this view on "next step" type questions.
- They pin these to stop further slippage, but they do NOT move the epiphysis back into place (supposedly that causes AVN and chondrolysis).

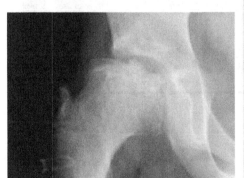

Flattened collapsed femoral Head, with widened femoral

Legg-Calve-Perthes

- This is AVN of the proximal femoral epiphysis.
- Favors white males around age 5-8.
- It's bilateral about 10% of the time.
- The subchondral lucency (crescent sign) is best seen on a frog leg.
- Other early signs include an asymmetric small ossified femoral epiphysis.
- MRI has more sensitivity. The sequella of a collapsed femoral head is easier to see. Loss of normal bright T1 marrow.

1. Which is Which ?
A. (1) SCFE, (2) Perthes,
B. (1) Perthes, (2) Development Dysplasia
C. (1) SCFE, (2) Development Dysplasia
D. (1) Development Dysplasia, (2) Perthes

2. Which is true about the classic age for these ?
A. (1) Around 6, (2) Around 12
B. (1) Around 12 (2) Around 6

3. Which of these is bilateral more often?
A. (1)
B. (2)

4. Which is true regarding the treatment of SCFE?
A. You should relocate it first, then pin it
B. You should just pin it, don't relocate it
C. You should never pin it... just relocate it

Case 32 - Belly Pain

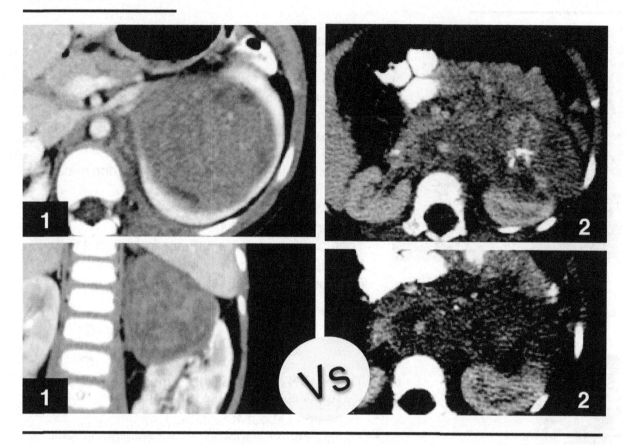

1. Which is Which ?
A. (1) Wilms, (2) Neuroblastoma
B. (1) Neuroblastoma, (2) Wilms

2. Which is true ?
A. Neuroblastoma has a better prognosis when it occurs in the chest (versus the abdomen)
B. Wilms tumors calcify more than Neuroblastoma
C. Wilms tumors are seen in a younger population compared to neuroblastoma
D. You can NOT be born with a neuroblastoma
E. If you can't decided between adrenal hemorrhage vs neuroblastoma on ultrasound - the next best step should be biopsy.

3. What is true about Neuroblastoma "Stage 4S" ?
A. Seen in an older population (age 4 and up)
B. Has distal mets to the skin, liver, and bone marrow and has the worst prognosis
C. Has distal mets to the skin, liver, and bone cortex and has an excellent prognosis
D. Has distal mets to the skin, liver, and bone marrow and has an excellent prognosis

Case 32 - Classic Pediatric Tumors - Neuroblastoma vs Wilms

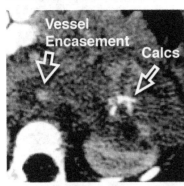

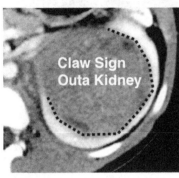

Neuroblastoma

- *Staging Trivia:* Crossing the Midline is bad
- *Prognosis Trivia:* Thoracic Primary does better than Abdomen Primary
- *Staging & Prognosis Trivia:* Stage 4S is Bone MARROW, Liver, and Skin - it's seen in kids < 1 year old and has a pretty good prognosis.

Wilms

- "Solid Renal Tumor of Childhood"
- Lots of Associations: Omphaloceles, Hepatoblastomas, Beckwith Weidemann (Overgrowth Syndromes)
- There are two Wilms Variants, the essential trivia is:
    - Clear Cell — Likes to Met to Bones
    - Rhabdoid - Terrible Prognosis, associated with high grade brain tumors

Neuroblastoma	**Wilms**
Usually less than 2 (you can have it in utero)	Usually around age 4 (NEVER before 2 months)
Calcifies like 90%	Calcification is rare
Encases Vessels	Invades Vessels
Poorly Marginated	Well Circumscribed
Mets to Bone	Does NOT usually met to bone *(exception is the wilms variant 'clear cell' - which loves bone).*

1. Which is Which ?
A. **(1) Wilms, (2) Neuroblastoma**
B. (1) Neuroblastoma, (2) Wilms

2. Which is true ?
A. **Neuroblastoma has a better prognosis when it occurs in the chest (versus the abdomen)**
B. Wilms tumors calcify more than Neuroblastoma
C. Wilms tumors are seen in a younger population compared to neuroblastoma
D. You can NOT be born with a neuroblastoma
E. If you can't decided between adrenal hemorrhage vs neuroblastoma on ultrasound - the next best step should be biopsy.

3. What is true about Neuroblastoma "Stage 4S" ?
A. Seen in an older population (age 4 and up)
B. Has distal mets to the skin, liver, and bone marrow and has the worst prognosis
C. Has distal mets to the skin, liver, and bone cortex and has an excellent prognosis
D. **Has distal mets to the skin, liver, and bone marrow and has an excellent prognosis**

Case 33 - Belly Pain

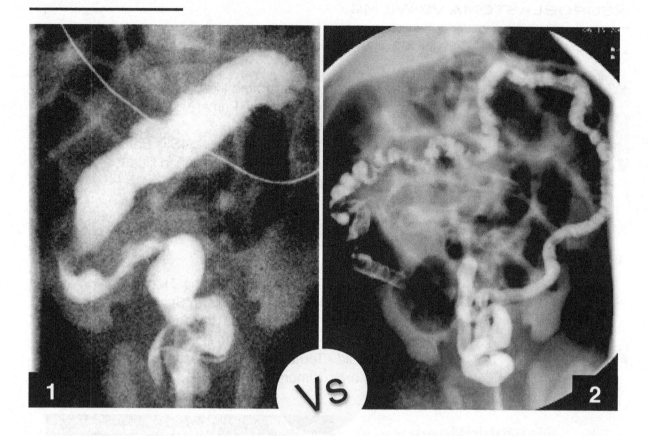

1. Which is Which ?
A. (1) Small Left Colon Syndrome, (2) Hirschsprung
B. (1) Colonic atresia, (2) Small Left Colon Syndrome
C. (1) Hirschsprung Disease, (2) Meconium Ileus

2. Which is true ?
A. Small left colon is seen in the children of diabetic mothers
B. Meconium Ileus is not specific to any diagnosis, (it's seen with multiple entities)
C. In Hirschsprungs - the rectum is bigger than the sigmoid colon
D. Ileal Atresia is typically a failure to cannulate

3. Which of the following can be "cured" with an enema?
A. Hirschsprung Disease
B. Small Left Colon Syndrome
C. Ileal Atresia
D. Acting Like a Huge Asshole

Case 33 - Low Obstruction in a Neonate

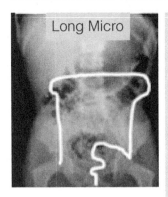
Long Micro

Enema Finding = Long Micro Colon

- **Meconium Ileus** – ONLY in patients with CF. The pathology is the result of tenacious meconium causing obstruction of the distal ileum. *Contrast will reach ileal loops*, and demonstrate multiple filling defects (meconium).
- This can be addressed with an enema.

- **Distal Ileal Atresia** - This is the result of intrauterine vascular insult. *Contrast will NOT reach ileal loops.*
- This needs surgery.

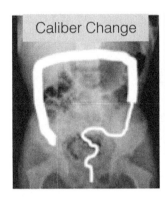
Caliber Change

Enema Finding = Caliber Change

- *Small Left:* Transient "Functional" obstruction, seen in babies of diabetic mothers, or moms who got Mag Sulfate (for eclampsia)

- **Hirschsprung:** The rectum (poop bucket) should always be bigger than sigmoid colon. In Hirschsprungs it is NOT. *"Recto-Sigmoid Ration < 1"*
- Another key finding is a sawtooth appearance of the rectum.
- Dx is from biopsy.

1. Which is Which ?
A. (1) Small Left Colon Syndrome, (2) Hirschsprung
B. (1) Colonic atresia, (2) Small Left Colon Syndrome
C. (1) Hirschsprung Disease, (2) Meconium Ileus

2. Which is true ?
A. Small left colon is seen in the children of diabetic mothers
B. Meconium Ileus is not specific to any diagnosis, (it's seen with multiple entities) ** *only CF*
C. In Hirschsprungs - the rectum is bigger than the sigmoid colon ** *S>R*
D. Ileal Atresia is typically a failure to cannulate ** *It's a vascular insult (usually)*

3. Which of the following can be "cured" with an enema?
A. Hirschsprung Disease
B. Small Left Colon Syndrome
C. Ileal Atresia
D. Acting Like a Huge Asshole * *Although an enema is often therapeutic, there is no cure for this condition*

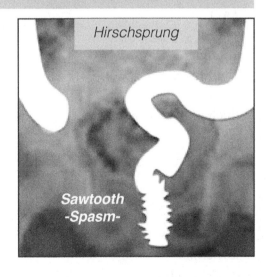

Case 34 - I Told the ED I Only Read These as Intermediate, There is really No Point In Ordering The Study, But Here it is... They Never Listen.

"PowerScribe Intermediate"

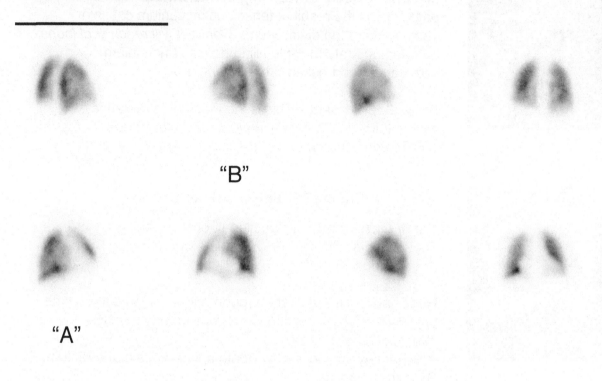

"B"

"A"

1. Which projection is "A"
A. RAO
B. LAO
C. Anterior
D. Right Lateral

2. Which projection is "B"
A. LPO
B. RPO
C. Posterior
D. Right Lateral

3. How big are the MAA particles for the perfusion part of the VQ?
A. 5 Microns
B. 100 Microns
C. 250 Microns
D. 1000 Microns

Case 34 - VQ Anatomy & Trivia

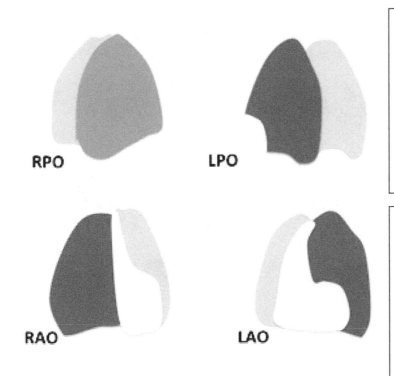

RPO vs LPO:

The posterior views look very similar. Just Remember the heart shadow is on the left (mostly), so look for the faint attenuation of tracer (white) outline of the heart. The right posterior oblique view won't have it.

RAO vs LAO:

I like to think of the anterior oblique views as "almost a CXR." You can see a lot more heart shadow compared to a posterior oblique view.

I use the same thinking about the heart to distinguish R vs L. The LAO has a larger heart shadow (tracer attenuation) than the right.

1. Which projection is "A"
A. RAO
B. LAO
C. Anterior
D. Right Lateral

2. Which projection is "B"
A. LPO
B. RPO
C. Posterior
D. Right Lateral

3. How big are the MAA particles for the perfusion part of the VQ?
A. 5 Microns
B. 100 Microns
C. 250 Microns
D. 1000 Microns

A capillary is about 10 micrometers. You need your particles to stay in the lung, so they can't be smaller than that. You don't want them to be so big they block arterioles (150 micrometers).

This vs That 70

Case 35 - Renal Transplant

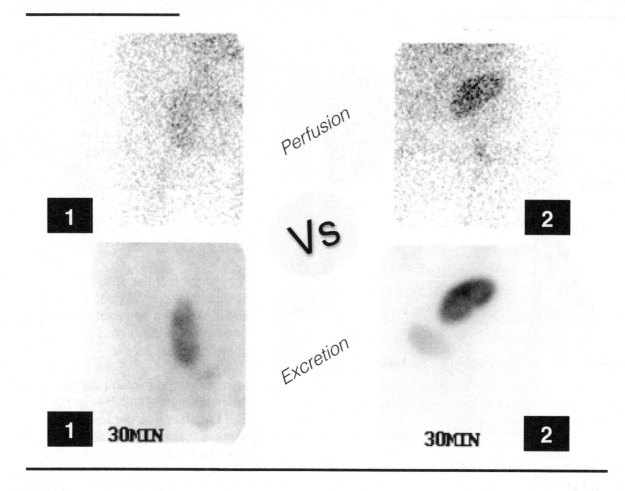

1. Which is Which?
A. (1) Cyclosporin Toxicity, (2) ATN
B. (1) Acute Rejection, (2) ATN
C. (1) ATN, (2) Acute Rejection
D. (1) ATN, (2) Cyclosporin Toxicity

2. How does one distinguish ATN from Cyclosporin Toxicity?
A. Flow
B. Perfusion
C. Excretion
D. How long post op they are

3. You get a DMSA scan to evaluate for pyelonephritis. Which of the following is true?
A. Scar and Pyelo Look totally different on DMSA
B. The critical organ for both MAG-3 and DMSA is the bladder
C. Gentamicin does NOT cause problems with DMSA scans
D. Areas of infection appear "cold" (photopenic) on DMSA

Case 35 - Renal Transplant - Related Trivia:

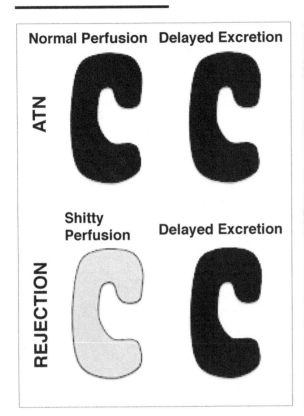

ATN vs Rejection

ATN:
- Usually in the first week after transplant, and is more common in cadaveric donors.
- There will be preserved renal perfusion with delayed excretion in the renal parenchyma
- ATN usually gets better.
- ***Cyclosporin toxicity*** can also look like ATN (normal perfusion, with retained tracer) but will **NOT be seen in the immediate post op period.**

Rejection
- Will have poor perfusion, and delayed excretion.
- A chronically rejected kidney won't really take up the tracer.

1. Which is Which ?
A. (1) Cyclosporin Toxicity, (2) ATN
B. (1) Acute Rejection, (2) ATN
C. (1) ATN, (2) Acute Rejection
D. (1) ATN, (2) Cyclosporin Toxicity

2. How does one distinguish ATN from Cyclosporin Toxicity ?
A. Flow
B. Perfusion
C. Excretion
D. How long post op they are

3. You get a DMSA scan to evaluate for pyelonephritis. Which of the following is true?
A. Scar and Pyelo Look totally different on DMSA
B. The critical organ for both MAG-3 and DMSA is the bladder
C. Gentamicin does NOT cause problems with DMSA scans
D. Areas of infection appear "cold" (photopenic) on DMSA

DMSA

- Tc-DMSA - is cortically bound, and used for structure more than function.
- The critical organ is the kidney (different than MAG-3 - which is the bladder).

- ***Pyelo vs Scar:*** It's all timing. Both are photopenic (cold), but scar is a chronic finding and pyelo is acute. "Clinical Correlation"

- Nephrotoxic drugs like Gentamicin & Cisplatinum are known to inhibit the uptake of DMSA.

Case 36 - History Withheld

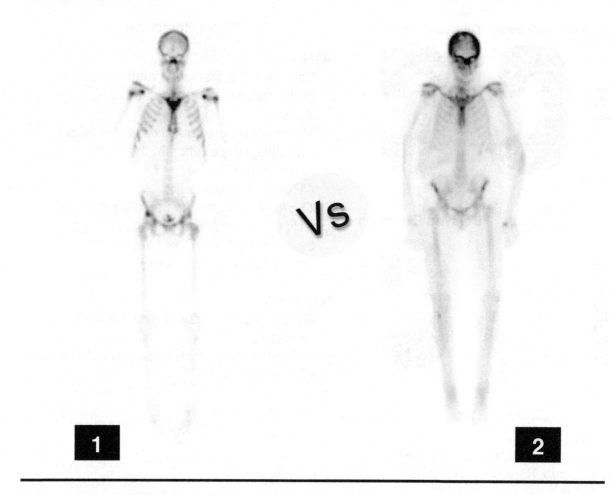

1. Which is Which ?
A. (1) Normal (2) Diffuse Mets - "Superscan"
B. (1) Diffuse Mets "Superscan", (2) Normal
C. (1) Hyperparathyroidism "Superscan", (2) Diffuse Mets "Superscan"

2. How does one distinguish a "metabolic" vs "metastatic" Superscan ?
A. Extremity Involvement (intensity)
B. Tracer in the bladder
C. Skull Involvement (intensity)
D. They can't be distinguished on the scan, you need blood work

3. Tracer in bone on which of the following is NORMAL?
A. MIBG
B. I-131
C. Octreotide
D. Gallium

Case 36 - Superscan(s)

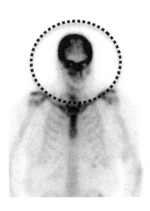

"Metabolic Super Scan"

- You don't see the kidneys (seen in both types).
- The **skull seems unusually hot.**
- Classic multiple choice answer is = Hyperparathyroidism
- Other things that can do this: renal osteodystrophy, pagets, or severe thyrotoxicosis.

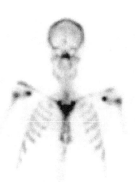

"Metastatic Super Scan"

- You don't see the kidneys (seen in both types).
- The **skull takes up tracer just like the other bones**
- Classic multiple choice answer = Breast or Prostate CA

---

1. Which is Which ?
A. (1) Normal (2) Diffuse Mets - "Superscan"
B. (1) Diffuse Mets "Superscan", (2) Normal
C. **(1) Hyperparathyroidism "Superscan", (2) Diffuse Mets "Superscan"**

2. How does one distinguish a "metabolic" vs "metastatic" Superscan ?
A. Extremity Involvement (intensity)
B. Tracer in the bladder
C. **Skull Involvement (intensity)**
D. They can't be distinguished on the scan, you need blood work

3. Tracer in bone on which of the following is NORMAL ?
A. MIBG
B. I-131
C. Octreotide
D. **Gallium** * *"Poor man's bone scan"*

BAD BONES

The metastatic super scan is not unique to Tc MDP. Remember thyroid CA and Neuroblastoma will go to bones.

It is **NEVER** normal to see bone uptake on:

MIBG
Octreotide
I-131

This vs That

Case 37 - Terrorists have ATTACKED!!

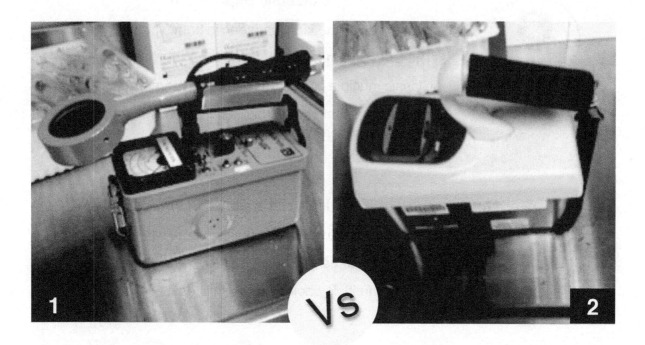

1. Which is Which ?
A. (1) Geiger Muller Counter (2) Ion Chamber
B. (1) Ion Chamber, (2) Gieger Muller Counter

2. Which of these devices would you want to use for higher doses (the terrorist attack) ?
A. (1)
B. (2)

3. Hospital administration needs someone to assist the National Guard in checking the radiation levels after Al-Qaeda attacked the hospital with a "dirty bomb." The Chairman called down and asked your Attending to do it, but your attending thinks it would be a good learning experience for you… the Trainee. On the way to ground zero, you encounter a smiling medical student (who is wearing one of those dorky short white coats). You ask him if he would like a good learning experience. He says yes out of fear (secretly he hates learning, he only went into medicine to keep his Indian parents from disowning him). You hand him device "1", and he enters the radioactive room. The device clicks once, then stops. What does this mean ?
A. He is probably gonna die of acute radiation poisoning.
B. He is totally gonna be fine.

Case 37 - Tools that Techs Use (and doctors don't) but are for some reason testable.

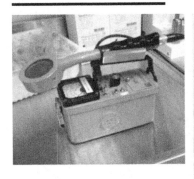

*Very Sensitive
*Problems with High Levels

"Geiger-Mueller Counter"

- *How it works:* It has a gas filled chamber, with a HIGH voltage applied from an anode to cathode. Radiation causes the conduction of an electric current, which can be measured.

- A single ionization can result in a *"Townsend Avalanche"*, which *really increases the sensitivity.* The downside of this is that it takes time to dissipate.

- **Dead Time** - The GM Counter can get over-run by high levels because of the need for things to dissipate. If the meter clicks once then stops… that means it's flooded, and it's probably *dead time* - for the person holding the probe.

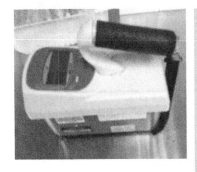

*Less Sensitive
*No Problems with High Levels

"Ionization Chamber"

- *How it works:* It has a gas filled chamber, with a LOW voltage applied from an anode to cathode. Radiation causes the conduction of an electric current, which can be measured.

- Because of the low voltage applied it has no avalanche effect and is therefore less sensitive at very low levels. The upside is that it does not encounter "dead time" tissues, and it superior for very high levels of radiation (like Dirty Bombs).

1. Which is Which ?
A. (1) Geiger Muller Counter (2) Ion Chamber
B. (1) Ion Chamber, (2) Gieger Muller Counter

2. Which of these devices would you want to use for higher doses (the terrorist attack) ?
A. (1)
B. (2)

3. Hospital administration needs someone to assist the National Guard in checking the radiation levels after Al-Qaeda attacked the hospital with a "dirty bomb." The Chairman called down and asked your Attending to do it, but your attending thinks it would be a good learning experience for you… the Trainee. On the way to ground zero you encounter a smiling medical student (who is wearing one of those dorky short white coats). You ask him if he would like a good learning experience. He says yes out of fear (secretly he hates learning, he only went into medicine to keep his Indian parents from disowning him). You hand him device "1", and he enters the radioactive room. The device clicks once, then stops. What does this mean ?
A. He is probably gonna die of acute radiation poisoning.
B. He is totally gonna be fine.

This vs That 76

CASE 38 - THERE ARE TWO PACKAGES TO CHECK IN

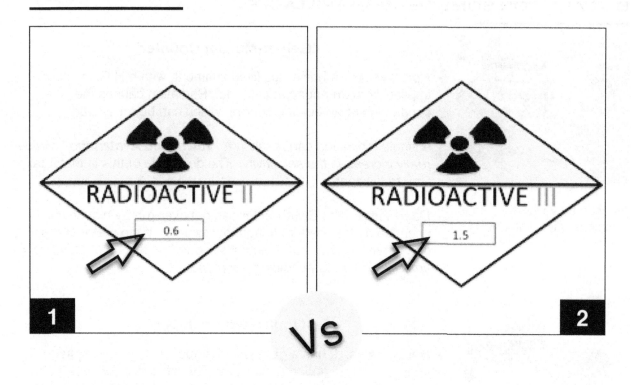

1. Which is true ?
A. No special instructions are needed for a "Yellow II" package
B. The surface dose rate of a "Yellow III" should not exceed 200 mrem/hr
C. Packages should be checked in within 5 hours of receipt
D. A "common carrier" is a truck that carries different kinds of radiopharmaceuticals

2. What is that square box under the word "radioactive" ? (I put an arrow on it)
A. It's the dose of the pharmaceutical (in mCu)
B. It's the surface dose at the time of check in ("Check Index")
C. It's the surface dose at the time of shipping ("Shipping Index")
D. It's the dose at 1 meter at the time of shipping ("Transportation Index")

3. Which is true ?
A. The T.I. for "1" should not exceed 1 mR per hour
B. The T.I. for "2" should not exceed 1 mR per hour
C. If the allowable limit is exceeded, you only need to contact the NRC
D. There is a Yellow 1.

Case 38 - Receiving Radioactive Material

Testable Trivia:

- *Whose job is it to check in the package ?* - A Tech... not a Radiologist

- *Who will be tested on obscure trivia applicable to a task they have never done, and will never do ?* - The Radiologist

- *How long do you have to check in the package ?* 3 hours

- *What are the limits?* There are 3 classes. "White 1", "Yellow 2', and "Yellow 3." Yes, I said "Yellow 3," these assholes couldn't just pick another color. There is no "Yellow 1"

  Limits are as follows:
  - **White 1:** No special handling, surface dose rate < 0.5 mrem/hr, 1 meter 0 mrem/hr
  - **Yellow 2:** Surface dose rate < 50 mrem/hr, 1 meter < 1 mrem/hr
  - **Yellow 3:** Surface dose rate < 200 mrem/hr, 1 meter < 10 mrem/hr

- The box under the word radiation is for the "transportation index," This is the dose rate measured at 1 meter **at the time of shipping.**

  Limits are as follows:
  - **White 1:** There is no T.I. because the rate at 1 meter will be so low.
  - **Yellow 2:** The T.I. is < 1.0 mR per hour.
  - **Yellow 3:** The T.I. is > 1.0 mR per hour.

- If the package is over the limit you have to contact (1) NRC, and (2) the Shipper

- "Common Carrier" is someone who caries both radioactive packages and regular stuff

---

1. Which is true ?
A. No special instructions are needed for a "Yellow II" package
B. The surface dose rate of a "Yellow III" should not exceed 200 mrem/hr
C. Packages should be checked in within 5 hours of receipt
D. A "common carrier" is a truck that carries different kinds of radiopharmaceuticals

2. What is that square box under the word "radioactive" ? (I put an arrow on it)
A. It's the dose of the pharmaceutical (in mCu)
B. It's the surface dose at the time of check in ("Check Index")
C. It's the surface dose at the time of shipping ("Shipping Index")
D. It's the dose at 1 meter at the time of shipping ("Transportation Index")

3. Which is true ?
A. The T.I. for "1" should not exceed 1 mR per hour
B. The T.I. for "2" should not exceed 1 mR per hour
C. If the allowable limit is exceeded, you only need to contact the NRC
D. There is a Yellow 1.

Case 39 - Shit! I Dropped It....

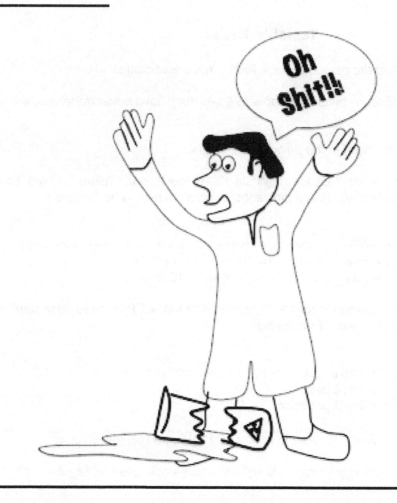

1. Which of the following is true, regarding major vs minor spills ?
A. Activity level greater than 10 mCi of Tc-99m is considered a major spill.
B. Activity level greater than 100 mCi of Tl-201 is considered a major spill.
C. Activity level greater than 1 mCi of In-111, is considered to represent a major spill.
D. Activity level greater than 1 mCi of Ga-67, is considered to represent a major spill.

2. Which of the following is true?
A. You should clean up a major spill, then call the Radiation Safety Officer (RSO) to Check your work
B. You should let the RSO clean up the major spills

3. Which is true ?
A. Agreement states can have less strict rules than the National Agency
B. Agreement states can be more strict than the National Agency

Case 39 - Radiation Safety / Contamination

Testable Trivia:

- The "NRC" is the governing body that has been charged with the task of enforcing all these various directives. It is possible for individual states to reach an agreement with the Federal Government to enforce these rules on their own. These are called **"Agreement States"**, and the main thing to know is that they **can be more strict, but not less strict** than the national agency.

- Spills can be broken into major and minor spills

  - **Major Spills:**
    - Activity level greater than 100 mCi of Tc-99m is considered a major spill.
    - Activity level greater than 100 mCi of Tl-201 is considered a major spill.
    - Activity level greater than 10 mCi of In-111, is considered to represent a major spill.
    - Activity level greater than 10 mCi of Ga-67, is considered to represent a major spill.
    - Activity level greater than 1 mCi of I-131 is considered to constitute a major spill.

- Radiation Safety Officer (RSO) needs to be notified immediately when a major spill occurs, to direct the decontamination process. You can clean up the Minor Spills Major Spills are cleaned under the direction of the RSO.

1. Which of the following is true?
A. Activity level greater than 10 mCi of Tc-99m is considered a major spill.
B. Activity level greater than 100 mCi of Tl-201 is considered a major spill.
C. Activity level greater than 1 mCi of In-111, is considered to represent a major spill.
D. Activity level greater than 1 mCi of Ga-67, is considered to represent a major spill.

2. Which of the following is true?
A. You should clean up a major spill, then call the Radiation Safety Officer (RSO) to Check your work
B. You should let the RSO clean up the major spills

3. Which is true ?
A. Agreement states can have less strict rules than the National Agency
B. Agreement states can be more strict than the National Agency

Case 40 - More Stuff Techs Do

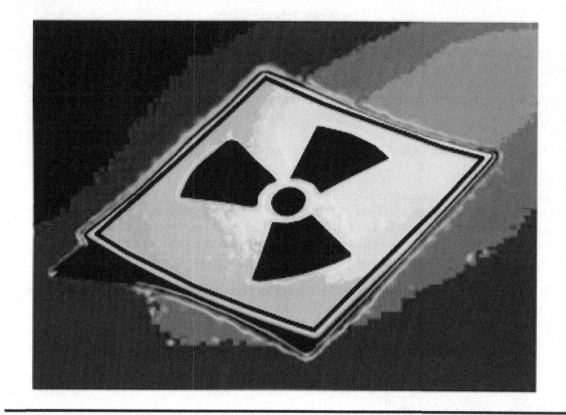

1. Which is Which ?
A. Radionuclide Purity = How much Al is in the Tc, Chemical Purity = How much Mo is in the Tc, Radiochemical Purity = How much Free Tc
B. Radionuclide Purity = How much Mo is in the Tc, Chemical Purity = How much Al is in the Tc, Radiochemical Purity = How much Free Tc
C. Radionuclide Purity = How much Free Tc, Chemical Purity = How much Al is in the Tc, Radiochemical Purity = How much Mo is in the Tc

2. Which of the following is true?
A. You test Chemical Purity with pH paper
B. You test Radionuclide Purity with Thin Layer Chromatography
C. You test Radiochemical Purity with a Dose Calibrator

3. Which is of the follow is true regarding Radionuclide Purity ?
A. The limit is 0.15 microcuries of Mo per 1 millicurie of Tc
B. The limit is 0.15 millicuries of Mo per 1 millicurie of Tc
C. The limit is 0.15 millicuries of Mo per 1 microcurie of Tc

Case 40 - Tc Purity

Tc^{99} is produced from a "generator" of Molybdenum (which has a much longer half life than Tc). The generator is basically a tube with Moly stuck to Aluminum walls. As the Moly breaks down into Tc it becomes less sticky. If you run water over it, the Tc will wash off the Aluminum column. Because of this process, there is the potential to have contamination from both Moly, and washed off Aluminum. This is tested for, and therefore you are likely to be tested on how it's tested for.

Vocab	What is it?	Tested?	Limit?
Radionuclide Purity	How much Mo in the Tc ?	Tested in a dose calibrator with lead shields;	0.15 **micro**curies of Mo per 1 **milli**curie of Tc
Chemical Purity	How much Al in the Tc ?	Tested with pH paper	< 10 **micro**grams Al per 1ml
Radiochemical Purity	How much Free Tc?	Tested with Thin Layer Chromotography	• 95% $Na^{99m}TcO_4$ • 92% for ^{99m}Tc sulfur colloid (MAA) • 91% for all other Tc radiopharmaceuticals

1. Which is Which ?
A. Radionuclide Purity = How much Al is in the Tc, Chemical Purity = How much Mo is in the Tc, Radiochemical Purity = How much Free Tc
B. Radionuclide Purity = How much Mo is in the Tc, Chemical Purity = How much Al is in the Tc, Radiochemical Purity = How much Free Tc
C. Radionuclide Purity = How much Free Tc, Chemical Purity = How much Al is in the Tc, Radiochemical Purity = How much Mo is in the Tc

2. Which of the following is true?
A. You test Chemical Purity with pH paper
B. You test Radionuclide Purity with Thin Layer Chromatography
C. You test Radiochemical Purity with a Dose Calibrator

3. Which is of the follow is true regarding Radionuclide Purity ?
A. The limit is 0.15 microcuries of Mo per 1 millicurie of Tc
B. The limit is 0.15 millicuries of Mo per 1 millicurie of Tc
C. The limit is 0.15 millicuries of Mo per 1 microcurie of Tc

Case 41 - Labels on The Axis of a Graph are a Luxury

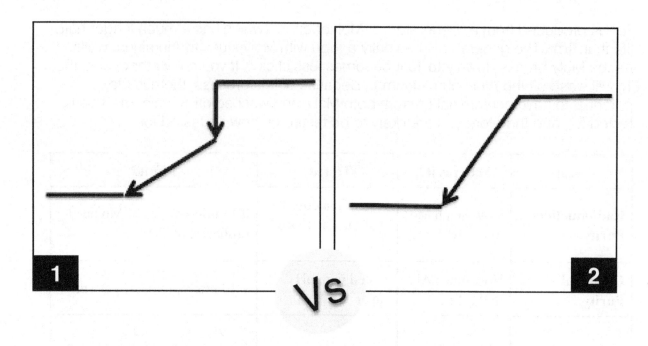

1. Which is Which ?
A. "1" is Beta Plus "2" is Beta Minus
B. "1" is Beta Plus, "2" is Electron Capture
C. "1" is Beta Minus, "2" is Beta Plus
D. "1" is Electron Capture, "2" is Beta Plus

2. Which of the following is true?
A. Beta Minus is seen with Neutron Excess
B. Beta Plus is seen with Neutron Excess
C. Electron Capture is seen with Neutron Excess

3. Which of the following is true?
A. Beta Plus occurs in the setting of insufficient energy (less than 1.02 MeV)
B. Beta Plus occurs in the setting of insufficient energy (less than 511 keV)
C. Electron Capture occurs in the setting of insufficient energy (less than 1.02 MeV)
D. Electron Capture occurs in the setting of insufficient energy (less than 511 keV)

4. What is the best shield against a beta emitter?
A. Lead
B. Plastic

CASE 41 - TRANSMUTATION GRAPHS / TRIVIA

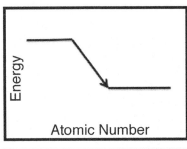

Beta Minus Decay

- Seen with <u>Neutron Excess</u>.
- A neutron is converted to a proton, then emits an electron (beta particle) and antineutrino.
- Worthless for imaging, but can harm DNA.
- *Used for Radionucleotide Therapy* with 32P, 89Sr, 90Y, 131I, and 153Sm

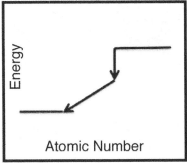

Beta Plus Decay

- Seen with <u>Proton Excess</u> (Neutron Deficiency).
- A proton is "transformed" into a neutron. **(Trivia to know= you need 1.02MeV for this to occur)**
- A positron (beta particle) is then emitted which collides into a real electron. The mutual destruction emits two 511 keV photons which come out 180 degrees apart.
- *Used for PET*

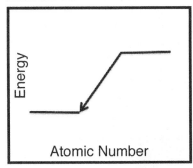

Electron Capture

- Also Seen with <u>Proton Excess</u> (Neutron Deficiency).
- This occurs in the setting of insufficient energy (remember beta plus needs 1.02MeV).
- A proton eats (captures) an electron and then turns into a neutron. The neutron (formerly a proton) then burps (emits) characteristic radiation
- *Used for most Diagnostic Imaging*

1. Which is Which ?
A. "1" is Beta Plus "2" is Beta Minus
B. "1" is Beta Plus, "2" is Electron Capture
C. "1" is Beta Minus, "2" is Beta Plus
D. "1" is Electron Capture, "2" is Beta Plus

2. Which of the following is true?
A. Beta Minus is seen with Neutron Excess
B. Beta Plus is seen with Neutron Excess
C. Electron Capture is seen with Neutron Excess

3. Which of the following is true?
A. Beta Plus occurs in the setting of insufficient energy (less than 1.02 MeV)
B. Beta Plus occurs in the setting of insufficient energy (less than 511 keV)
C. Electron Capture occurs in the setting of insufficient energy (less than 1.02 MeV)
D. Electron Capture occurs in the setting of insufficient energy (less than 511 keV)

4. What is the best shield against a beta emitter?
A. Lead * *(NOT LEAD because it will create Bremmstahlung x-rays).*
B. Plastic

Case 42 - I Just Look At the Color Pictures

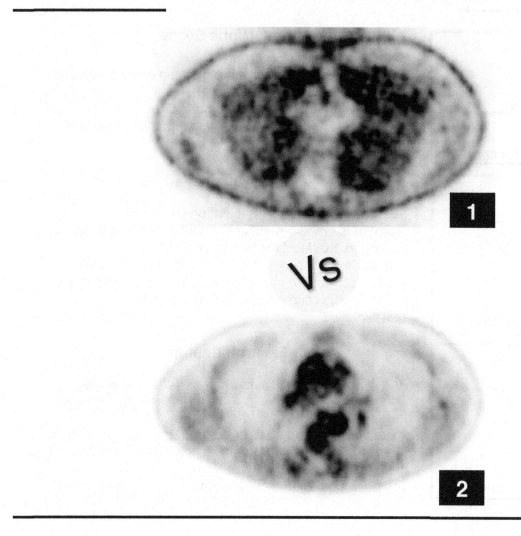

1. Which is Which ?
A. "1" is Uncorrected, "2" is Corrected
B. "1" is Corrected, "2" is Uncorrected

2. Is PET Attenuation depth dependent ?
A. Yes, it's depth dependent - just like CT
B. No, it's depth independent

3. Which is true regarding a Pacemaker ?
A. It will look HOT on the corrected PET
B. It will look HOT on the uncorrected PET
C. It will look COLD on both corrected & uncorrected

Case 42 - Attenuation Correction

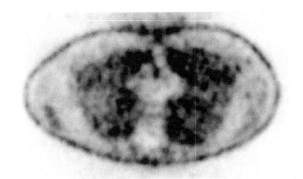

Uncorrected
- DARK Skin
- DARK Lungs

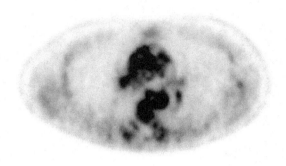

Corrected
- LIGHT Skin
- LIGHT Lungs

Attenuation Correction

- The CT part of PET-CT is performed for two main reasons: (1) so that you can see where things are and (2) for attenuation correction.

- Attenuation correction is a correction for the different levels of attenuation a photon might undergo as it tries to get out of the body to the detector. Think about traveling through bone vs traveling through lung.

- The classic trick is the pacemaker (metal) making something appear really really hot – when attenuation is corrected for. This is why you always look at the uncorrected data, when reading a PET.

1. Which is Which ?
A. "1" is Uncorrected, "2" is Corrected
B. "1" is Corrected, "2" is Uncorrected

2. Is PET Attenuation depth dependent ?
A. Yes, it's depth dependent - just like CT
B. No, it's depth independent

3. Which is true regarding a Pacemaker ?
A. It will look HOT on the corrected PET
B. It will look HOT on the uncorrected PET
C. It will look COLD on both corrected & uncorrected

Case 43 - Eval for Rupture

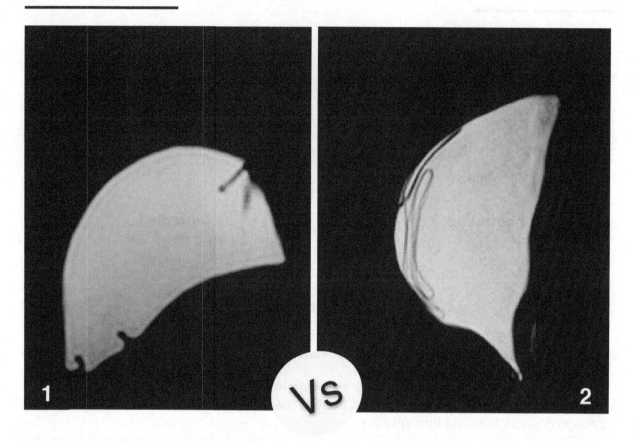

1. Which is Which ?
A. "1" is Intra Capsular Rupture "2" is Extra Capsular Rupture
B. "1" is Extra Capsular Rupture, "2" is Intra Capsular Rupture
C. "1" is an example of "Radial Folds", "2" is Intra Capsular Rupture
D. "1" is Intra Capsular Rupture, "2" is an example of "Radial Folds"

2. Which of the following is true?
A. You can have isolated intra capsular rupture, but you cannot have isolated extra capsular rupture
B. You can have isolated extra capsular rupture, but you cannot have isolated intra capsular rupture
C. You can have isolated intra and extra capsular rupture

3. What is the typical sequence for evaluating implants ?
A. Heavy T1 weighting with Fat Sat
B. Heavy T2 weighting with Fat Sat
C. Heavy T2 weighting with both Fat and Water Sat
D. Diffusion

Case 43 - Implant Rupture

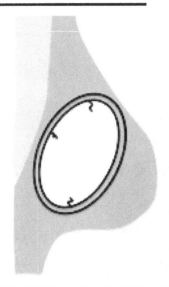
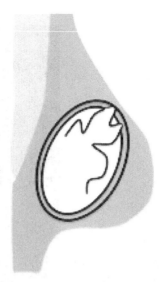
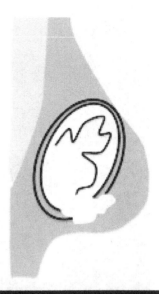

Radial Folds	**Intracapsular Rupture:**	**Extra & Intracapsular**
- Guys like squishy boobs. The bigger and the squishier the better. - Therefore, implants are not bound tightly - so they can be squishy. - Because they are loosely bound the shell in-folds creating radial folds - **The folds always attach to the shell*** - The **folds are thicker** than a rupture, because they represent both layers.	- The "capsule" is not part of the implant. It's the fibrous coat your body makes (the outer black line in my diagram). - Silicone can rupture through the shell of the implant, but stay confined inside the fibrous coat - this is intra-capsular rupture. - The classic sign is the floating **"linguine"** - as in these case.	- You can NOT have isolated extra capsular silicone. It has to make it through the implant shell first. - Silicone outside the capsule can create a "snow storm" look on ultrasound. It can also infiltrate lymph nodes and do the same (snow storm nodes).

1. Which is Which ?
A. "1" is Intra Capsular Rupture "2" is Extra Capsular Rupture
B. "1" is Extra Capsular Rupture, "2" is Intra Capsular Rupture
C. "1" is an example of "Radial Folds", "2" is Intra Capsular Rupture
D. "1" is Intra Capsular Rupture, "2" is an example of "Radial Folds"

2. Which of the following is true?
A. You can have isolated intra capsular rupture, but you cannot have isolated extra capsular rupture
B. You can have isolated extra capsular rupture, but you cannot have isolated intra capsular rupture
C. You can have isolated intra and extra capsular rupture

3. What is the typical sequence for evaluating implants ?
A. Heavy T1 weighting with Fat Sat
B. Heavy T2 weighting with Fat Sat
C. Heavy T2 weighting with both Fat and Water Sat - "Silicone Sequences" are usually heavily T2-weighted, with both fat and water suppression. Silicone will be bright white on these sequences
D. Diffusion

Case 44 - Male Mammogram (Ugh, the Horror)

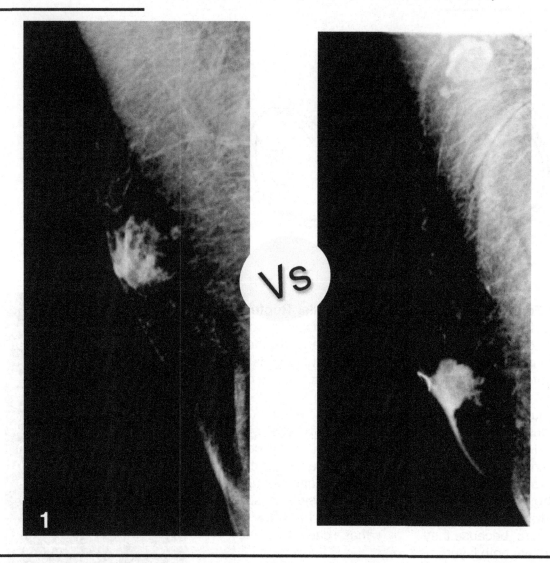

1. Which is Which ?
A. "1" is Gynecomastia "2" is Pseudo - Gynecomastia
B. "1" is Gynecomastia "2" is Breast CA
C. "1" is Breast CA "2" is Gynecomastia

2. Which of the following is true?
A. Males who have had gender reassignment (on hormones) should get screening mammograms
B. BRCA 1 is more common than BRCA 2 - in men with breast CA
C. Klinefelter patients have increased risk for Breast CA.
D. Gynecomastia is typically eccentric to the nipple

Case 44 - The Male Breast

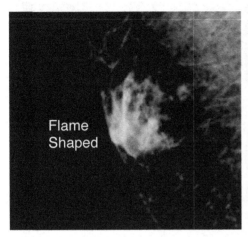

Gynecomastia

- This is a non-neoplastic enlargement of the epithelial and stromal elements in a man's breast

- Just think flame shaped, behind nipple, bilateral but asymmetric, and can be painful.

- Associated with a variety of conditions (spironolactone, psych meds, marijuana, alcoholic cirrhosis, testicular cancer).

- NEVER evaluate it on ultrasound. Always get a mammogram. It will look scary on US - don't let this trick you.

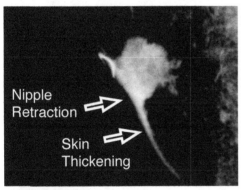
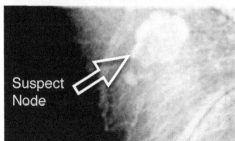

Male Breast CA

- It's uncommon in men, and very uncommon in younger men (average age is around 70).

- BRCA 2 is the more common than BRCA 1 in men

- It's always ductal (usually IDC-NOS), it' cannot be lobular because the male breast doesn't have lobules.

- On mammography it looks like a breast cancer, if it was a woman's mammogram you'd BR-5 it. On ultrasound it's the same thing, it looks like a BR-5.

- *Things that make you think it's breast cancer:* Eccentric to Nipple, Unilateral, Abnormal Lymph nodes, Calcifications

1. Which is Which ?
A. "1" is Gynecomastia "2" is Pseudo - Gynecomastia
B. "1" is Gynecomastia "2" is Breast CA
C. "1" is Breast CA "2" is Gynecomastia

2. Which of the following is true?
A. Males who have had gender reassignment (on hormones) should get screening mammograms
B. BRCA 1 is more common than BRCA 2 - in men with breast CA
C. Klinefelter patients have increased risk for Breast CA.
D. Gynecomastia is typically eccentric to the nipple

Case 45 - "Screening" MRI

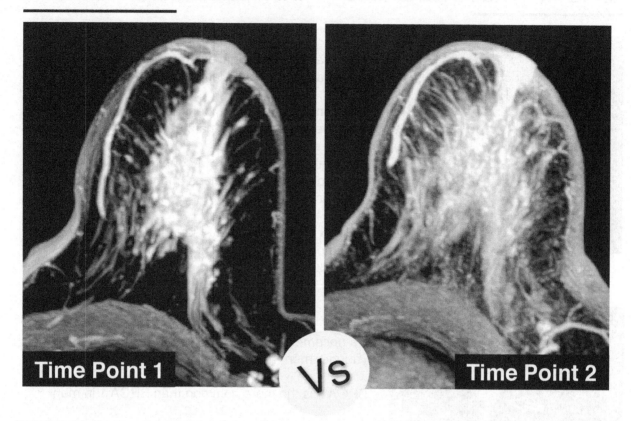

1. Which is Which ?
A. "1" is on Tamoxifen "2" is off Tamoxifen
B. "1" is off Tamoxifen "2" is on Tamoxifen

2. When should you do a screening breast MRI ?
A. Early in the menstrual cycle (day 7-20)
B. Late in the menstrual cycle (day 15-30)
C. Timing of cycle doesn't matter

3. What is the exception to the "T2 Bright things are benign" in the breast rule ?
A. IDC
B. Radial Scar
C. Colloid Cancer

Case 45 - "Screening" MRI

Background Parenchyma Enhancement (BPE):

- *Is it normal?* – Yes

- *Where is it most common?* – Posterior Breast in the upper outer quadrant

- *Why that location?* It's all based on vascular supply to the breast. Enhancement occurs peripheral to central (retro-areolar area enhances last). This is called **"picture framing."** Although enhancement of the nipple is still considered normal - *a common trick is to try and get you to call nipple enhancement Paget's Breast... don't fall for that bush-league shit.*

- *How do you reduce it?* – Do the MRI during the first part of the menstrual cycle (day 7-20). – **Optimal is around week 2.** They say background uptake is highest weeks 1 and 4.

- *What does Tamoxifen do?* – Tamoxifen will decrease background parenchyma uptake. Then **it causes a rebound.**

1. Which is Which?
A. **"1" is on Tamoxifen "2" is off Tamoxifen** *** Rebound Effect***
B. "1" is off Tamoxifen "2" is on Tamoxifen

2. When should you do a screening breast MRI?
A. Early in the menstrual cycle (day 7-20)
B. Late in the menstrual cycle (day 15-30)
C. Timing of cycle doesn't matter

3. What is the exception to the "T2 Bright things are benign" in the breast rule?
A. IDC
B. Radial Scar
C. Colloid Cancer *** also called mucinous.***

Case 46 - Family Medicine Heard a Neck Bruit

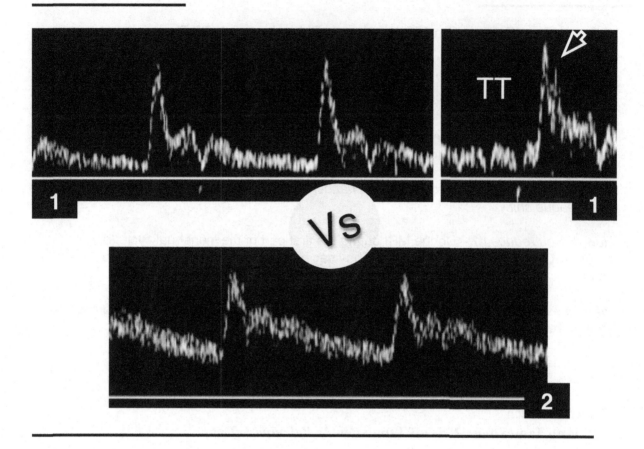

1. Which is Which ?
A. "1" is the internal carotid, "2" is the external carotid
B. "1" is the external carotid "2" is the internal carotid

2. Which is true ?
A. In the internal carotid the diastolic velocity NEVER returns to baseline
B. In the external carotid color flow is continuous through the cardiac cycle
C. In the internal carotid there should be maintained high resistance
D. The internal carotid can be identified by looking for branching vessels

3. What does the "TT" stand for on "1" ?
A. It's the Sonographers initials
B. It describes a confirmatory maneuver for this vessel
C. Patient has had tetanus toxoid
D. Patient has elevated thrombin time

Case 46 - Carotid Ultrasound - Internal vs External

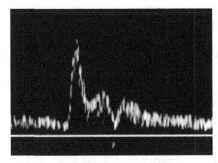

External Carotid

- Flow to muscles of the face is optional (doesn't need to be on). Therefore you can have:

- High Resistance
- High Systolic Velocity
- Diastolic velocity approaches zero baseline
- Color flow is **intermittent** during the cardiac cycle

- **Temporal Tap** – This is a point of trivia, that I guess one can perform. It is a technique Sonographers use to tell the external carotid from the internal carotid. You tap the temporal artery on the forehead and you see ripples in the spectrum.

- **Branches** - Looking for branches is another confirmation test to tell internal vs external.

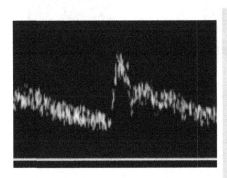

Internal Carotid

- The brain is always on. Therefore you need:

- Low Resistance
- Low Systolic Velocity
- Diastolic velocity NEVER approaches zero baseline (unless the patient is brain dead)
- Color flow is **continuous** during the cardiac cycle

1. Which is Which ?
A. "1" is the internal carotid, "2" is the external carotid
B. "1" is the external carotid "2" is the internal carotid

2. Which is true ?
A. In the internal carotid the diastolic velocity NEVER returns to baseline
B. In the external carotid color flow is continuous through the cardiac cycle
C. In the internal carotid there should be maintained high resistance
D. The internal carotid can be identified by looking for branching vessels

3. What does the "TT" stand for on "1" ?
A. It's the Sonographers initials
B. It describes a confirmatory maneuver for this vessel * temporal tap
C. Patient has had tetanus toxoid
D. Patient has elevated thrombin time

Case 47 - Family History of Aneurysm

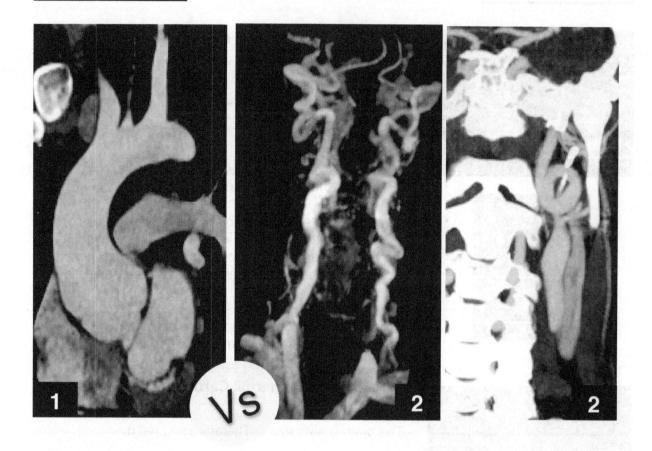

1. Which is Which ?
A. "1" is Marfans, "2" is Loeys-Dietz
B. "1" is Loeys-Dietz "2" is Marfans

2. Which is true ?
A. "2" often presents with a dislocated lens (ectopia lentis)
B. Of the two, "1" has the greater risk of rupture (occurs at smaller diameter)
C. "2" often has a birth history of cleft palate
D. "1" Classically spares the aortic sinus

3. What is the buzzword used to describe #1's aorta ?
A. Tulip Bulb
B. Flower Pot
C. The "Abraham Lincoln"
D. Dropping Lilly

Case 47 - Connective Tissue Disorders
Marfans vs Loeys-Dietz

Marfans

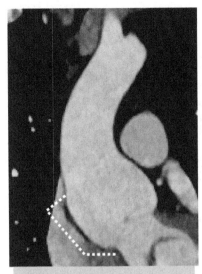
Dilation Favors the Root

- Inherited (AD) Connective tissue disorder
- Caused by retarded Fibrillin (micro-fibrils)

- Think About Marfans With:
  - **"Annulo-Aortic-Aneurysm"** - with dilation starting in the aortic sinus progressing into the sinotubular junction then the annulus — **Tulip Bulb** Appearance
  - This style of dilation leads to **aortic valve regurg**
  - Aneurysms occur early in life (classic before age 50)
  - Calcification of the mitral annulus before age 40
  - Dilation of the main PA before age 40
  - Also, these are tall goofy looking dudes with ugly pectus deformities

Loeys-Dietz

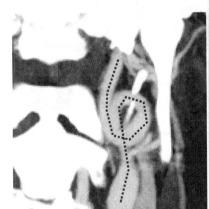
Roller Coaster Loop

- Inherited (AD) Connective tissue disorder
- Caused by retarded Cell Signaling (TGF-β)

- Think About Loeys-Dietz With:
  - **Crazy looking tangled vertebral arteries**
  - "Roller Coaster Loops" in the vessels of the neck
  - Classic Triad: Aneurysms, Hypertelorism ("Crazy Eyes") and a Cleft Palate (sometimes Bifid Uvula).

- Trivia: Unlike Marfans does NOT have an association with lens dislocation (ectopia lentis)
- Trivia: Will **rupture / dissect earlier than Marfans**. *Think about this as the bad ass cousin of Marfans.*

1. Which is Which ?
A. **"1" is Marfans, "2" is Loeys-Dietz**
B. "1" is Loeys-Dietz "2" is Marfans

2. Which is true ?
A. "2" often presents with a dislocated lens (ectopia lentis)
B. Of the two, "1" has the greater risk of rupture (occurs at smaller diameter)
C. **"2" often has a birth history of cleft palate**
D. "1" Classically spares the aortic sinus

3. What is the buzzword used to describe #1's aorta ?
A. **Tulip Bulb**
B. Flower Pot
C. The "Abraham Lincoln"
D. Dropping Lilly

This vs That 96

Case 48 - Hypertension

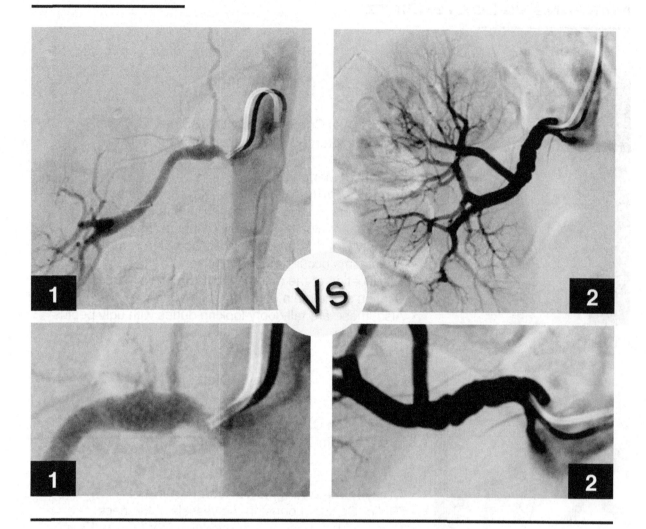

1. Which is Which ?
A. "1" is FMD "2" is Atherosclerosis
B. "1" is Atherosclerosis "2" is FMD

2. Which is the preferred treatment for each ?
A. "1" Gets Angioplasty + Stent, "2" Gets Angioplasty but no stent
B. "1" Gets Angioplasty but no Stent, "2" Gets Angioplasty + Stent
C. They both get Angioplasty + Stent
D. I'm not doing IR! I hate procedures! Why do you think I went into Radiology !?

3. The disease process in "2" is <u>most likely</u> to involve what other vessels ?
A. The Aortic Root
B. The Iliacs
C. The Subclavian
D. The Femoral Artery

This vs That 97

Case 48 - Renal Artery - Atherosclerosis vs FMD

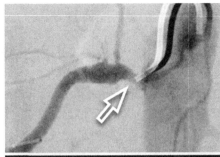

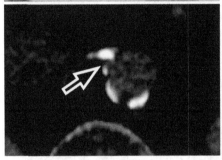

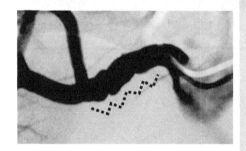

Atherosclerosis

- This is actual disease of the aorta that involves the ostia of the renal arteries. This is why the disease is very proximal (close to the aorta).

- The patient is gonna be old (or a fat diabetic smoker who strongly believes he's entitled to free treatment).

- It's somewhat controversial, but lets just say if you have a significant pressure gradient most people believe that **Angioplasty + Stent** is the right answer.

Fibromuscular Dysplasia

- Nonatherosclerotic vascular disease, primarily affecting the renal arteries of young white women.

- Tends to involve the middle part of the vessel (not proximal like athero).

- Has a "string of beads" appearance.

- Renal arteries are the most commonly involved (carotid #2, iliac #3)

- They are predisposed to spontaneous dissection

- Treatment = Angioplasty WITHOUT stenting.

1. Which is Which ?
A. "1" is FMD "2" is Atherosclerosis
B. "1" is Atherosclerosis "2" is FMD

2. Which is the preferred treatment for each ?
A. "1" Gets Angioplasty + Stent, "2" Gets Angioplasty but no stent
B. "1" Gets Angioplasty but no Stent, "2" Gets Angioplasty + Stent
C. They both get Angioplasty + Stent
D. I'm not doing IR! I hate procedures! Why do you think I went into Radiology !?

3. The disease process in "2" is <u>most likely</u> to involve what other vessels ?
A. The Aortic Root
B. The Iliacs
C. The Subclavian
D. The Femoral Artery

Case 49 - Arthrogram Time

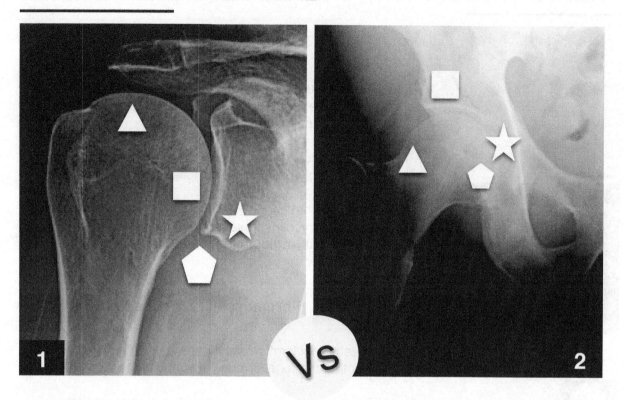

1. Where is the ideal puncture site for an arthrogram on "1" ?
A. Triangle
B. Square
C. Hexagon
D. Star

2. Where is the ideal puncture site for an arthrogram on "2" ?
A. Triangle
B. Square
C. Hexagon
D. Star

3. What is the correct mix to put in shoulder ?
A. 12 total cc (4cc Lidocaine, 7cc Visipaque, and only about 1cc Gd).
B. 12 total cc (4cc Lidocaine, 8cc Visipaque, and only about 0.1cc Gd).
C. 6 total cc (2cc Lidocaine, 4cc Visipaque, and only about 0.1cc Gd).
D. 30 total cc (5cc Lidocaine, 15cc Visipaque, and only about 10cc Gd).

Case 49 - Arthrogram Time

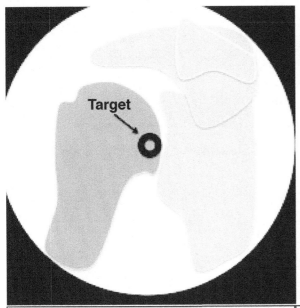
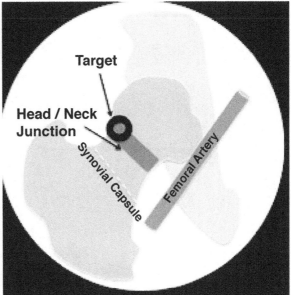

Target: Junction between the middle and inferior thirds of the humeral head - 2mm inside the cortex **Cocktail:** Around 12cc total (4cc Lidocaine, 8cc Visipaque, and only about 0.1cc Gd).	**Target:** Lateral Femoral Head Neck Junction **Cocktail:** Around 14cc total (4cc Lidocaine, 10cc Visipaque, and only about 0.1cc Gd).

1. Where is the ideal puncture site for an arthrogram on "1" ?
A. Triangle
B. Square
C. Hexagon
D. Star

2. Where is the ideal puncture site for an arthrogram on "2" ?
A. Triangle
B. Square
C. Hexagon
D. Star

3. What is the correct mix to put in shoulder ?
A. 12 total cc (4cc Lidocaine, 7cc Visipaque, and only about 1cc Gd).
B. 12 total cc (4cc Lidocaine, 8cc Visipaque, and only about 0.1cc Gd).
C. 6 total cc (2cc Lidocaine, 4cc Visipaque, and only about 0.1cc Gd).
D. 30 total cc (5cc Lidocaine, 15cc Visipaque, and only about 10cc Gd).

Case 50 - Some Fat Diabetic with a 100 Pack Years has a Cold Leg.... IR to the Rescue

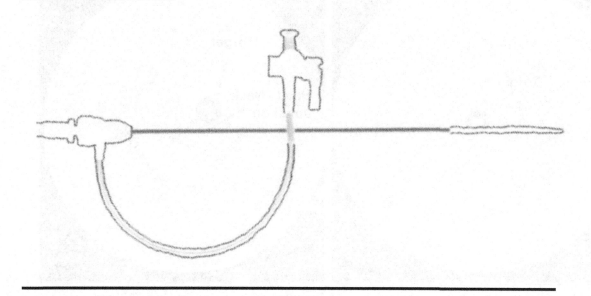

1. What is a "French"?
A. 1 mm
B. 3 mm
C. 0.3 mm
D. A cowardly rude European

2. What sized guide wire will fit in a 5F Catheter?
A. 3 F
B. 4 F
C. 5 F
D. 6 F

3. Which is true?
A. "French" refers to the inner diameter of a sheath, not a catheter
B. "French" refers to the inner diameter of a catheter, not a sheath
C. "French" is a "French" - always means the inner diameter, regardless of catheter or sheath

4. How many French is a standard 0.038 wire?
A. 3 F
B. 4 F
C. 5 F

Case 50 - Angio Sizing Basics

Basic Trivia:

- 3 French = 1mm, so 1 French is 1/3 of a mm or 0.3mm.
- Guidewire terminology "0.038, 0.035... etc..." are actually given in INCHES
- 0.038 (inches) is about 3 French

Catheters:

- The "French Size" refers to the **OUTER** diameter.
- The wall of the device is about 1-2 French
- An 0.038 Wire (3F) will fit in most 5F catheters.

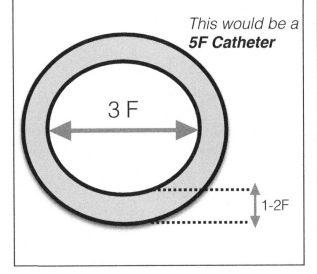

This would be a 5F Catheter

Sheath:

- The "French Size" refers to the **INNER** diameter.
- A 5F introducer (sheath) can accept a 5F Catheter
- The wall of the device is about 1-2 French
- Therefore a 5F introducer (sheath) makes a 6-7F sized hole (about 2mm) hole in the patient's skin

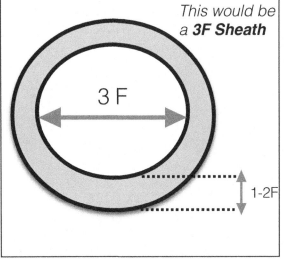

This would be a 3F Sheath

1. What is a "French"?
A. 1 mm
B. 3 mm
C. 0.3 mm
D. A cowardly rude European

2. What sized guide wire will fit in a 5F Catheter?
A. 3 F
B. 4 F
C. 5 F
D. 6 F

3. Which is true?
A. "French" refers to the inner diameter of a sheath, not a catheter
B. "French" refers to the inner diameter of a catheter, not a sheath
C. "French" is a "French" - always means the inner diameter, regardless of catheter or sheath

4. How many French is a standard 0.038 wire?
A. 3 F
B. 4 F
C. 5 F

This vs That 102

This vs That 103

Anatomy Quiz

What is that?
What attaches there?
What goes through that?

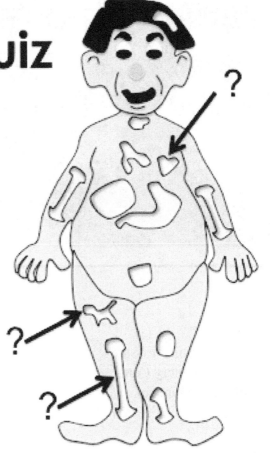

Case 1 - The Skull Base (part 1)

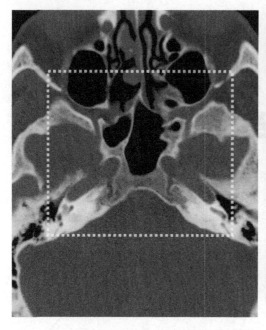
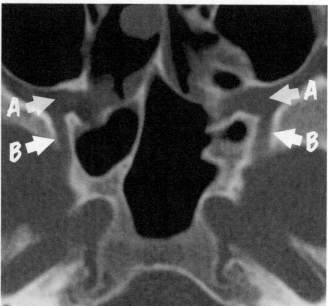

1. What is "A" ?
A. Superior Orbital Fissure
B. Internal Auditory Canal
C. Foramen Rotundum
D. Pterygopalatine Fossa (PPF)

2. What is "B" ?
A. Inferior Orbital Fissure
B. Foramen Ovale
C. Foramen Rotundum
D. Pterygopalatine Fossa (PPF)

3. What passes through "B"?
A. CN V1
B. CN V2
C. CN V3
D. CN 6
E. CN 4

Case 1 - The Skull Base (part 1)

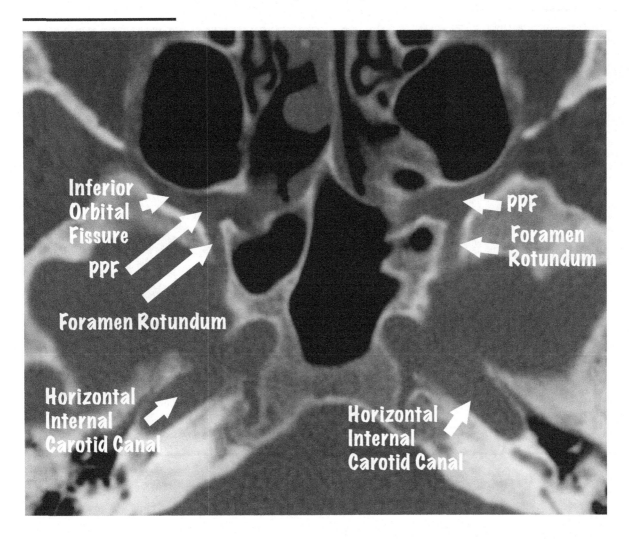

1. What is "A"?
A. Superior Orbital Fissure
B. Internal Auditory Canal
C. Foramen Rotundum
D. Pterygopalatine Fossa (PPF)

2. What is "B"?
A. Inferior Orbital Fissure
B. Foramen Ovale
C. Foramen Rotundum
D. Pterygopalatine Fossa (PPF)

3. What passes through "B"?
A. CN V1
B. CN V2
C. CN V3
D. CN 6
E. CN 4

Anatomy 3

Case 2 - The Skull Base (part 2)

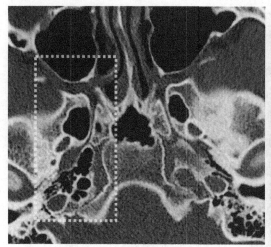
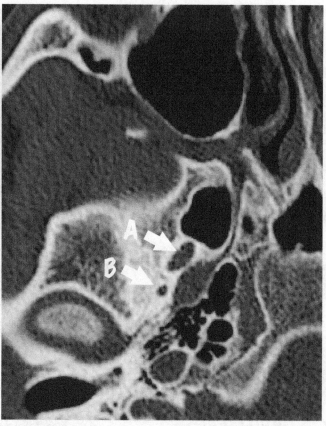

1. What is "A" ?
A. Foramen Spinosum
B. Foramen Ovale
C. Foramen Rotundum
D. Foramen Lacerum

2. What is "B" ?
A. Forament Spinosum
B. Foramen Ovale
C. Foramen Rotundum
D. Foramen Lacerum

3. What passes through "A"?
A. CN V1
B. CN V2
C. CN V3
D. CN 6
E. CN 4

4. What passes through "B"?
A. CN V1
B. CN V2
C. CN V3
D. Middle Meningeal Artery
E. Nothing

Anatomy 4

Case 2 - The Skull Base (part 2)

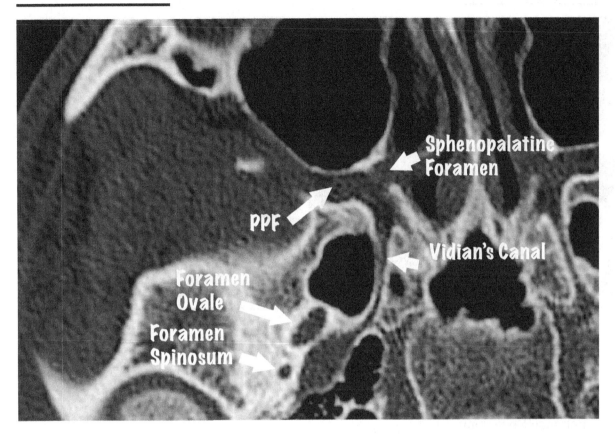

1. What is "A"?
A. Foramen Spinosum
B. Foramen Ovale
C. Foramen Rotundum
D. Foramen Lacerum

2. What is "B"?
A. Forament Spinosum
B. Foramen Ovale
C. Foramen Rotundum
D. Foramen Lacerum

3. What passes through "A"?
A. CN V1
B. CN V2
C. CN V3
D. CN 6
E. CN 4

4. What passes through "B"?
A. CN V1
B. CN V2
C. CN V3
D. Middle Meningeal Artery

Foramen	Contents
Foramen Ovale	CN V3, and Accessory Meningeal Artery
Foramen Rotundum	CN V2 ("**R2V2**"),
Superior Orbital Fissure	CN 3, CN 4, CN V1, CN6
Inferior Orbital Fissure	CN V2
Foramen Spinosum	Middle Meningeal Artery
Jugular Foramen	Jugular Vein, CN 9, CN 10, CN 11
Hypoglossal Canal	CN12
Optic Canal	CN 2, and Opthalmic Artery

Case 3 - The Skull Base (part 3)

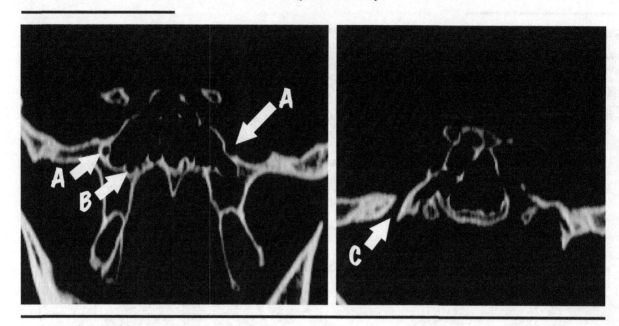

1. What is "A"?
A. Superior Orbital Fissure
B. Internal Auditory Canal
C. Foramen Rotundum
D. Pterygopalatine Fossa (PPF)

2. What is "B"?
A. Inferior Orbital Fissure
B. Vidian Canal
C. Foramen Rotundum
D. Pterygopalatine Fossa (PPF)

3. What is "C"?
A. Forament Ovale
B. Vidian Canal
C. Foramen Rotundum
D. Pterygopalatine Fossa (PPF)

4. All 3 Le Fort Fractures involve fracture of the?
A. Pterygoid Plate
B. Lateral Orbital Wall
C. Zygoma
D. Inferior Orbital Wall

Case 3 - The Skull Base (part 3)

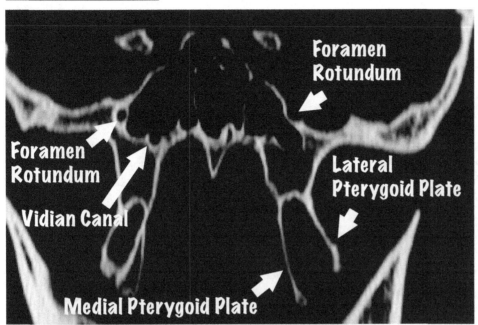

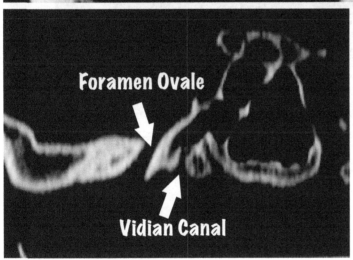

High Yield Point:

Notice that Ovale Runs up and down (vertical)

Where as Rotundum runs in a more horizontal plane.

1. What is "A"?
A. Superior Orbital Fissure
B. Internal Auditory Canal
C. Foramen Rotundum
D. Pterygopalatine Fossa (PPF)

2. What is "B"?
A. Inferior Orbital Fissure
B. Vidian Canal
C. Foramen Rotundum
D. Pterygopalatine Fossa (PPF)

3. What is "C"?
A. Forament Ovale
B. Vidian Canal
C. Foramen Rotundum
D. Pterygopalatine Fossa (PPF)

4. All 3 Le Fort Fractures involve fracture of the?
A. Pterygoid Plate
B. Lateral Orbital Wall
C. Zygoma
D. Inferior Orbital Wall

Case 4 - The Skull Base (part 4)

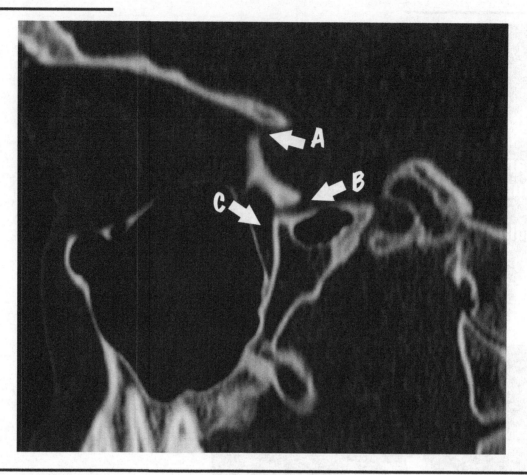

1. What is "A"?
A. Superior Orbital Fissure
B. Foramen Ovale
C. Foramen Rotundum
D. Pterygopalatine Fossa (PPF)

2. What is "B"?
A. Inferior Orbital Fissure
B. Vidian Canal
C. Foramen Rotundum
D. Pterygopalatine Fossa (PPF)

3. What is "C"?
A. Forament Ovale
B. Vidian Canal
C. Foramen Rotundum
D. Pterygopalatine Fossa (PPF)

Case 4 - The Skull Base (part 4)

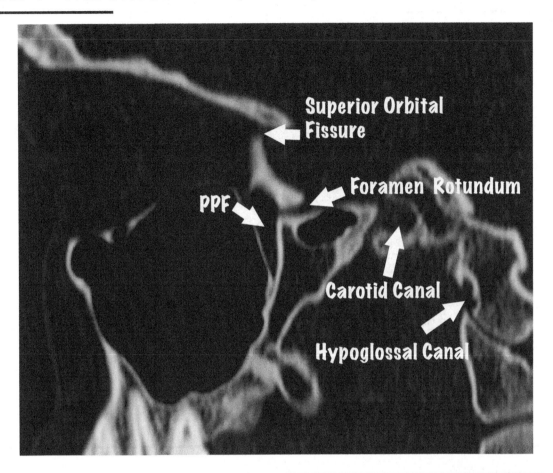

1. What is "A" ?
A. **Superior Orbital Fissure**
B. Foramen Ovale
C. Foramen Rotundum
D. Pterygopalatine Fossa (PPF)

2. What is "B" ?
A. Inferior Orbital Fissure
B. Vidian Canal
C. **Foramen Rotundum**
D. Pterygopalatine Fossa (PPF)

3. What is "C" ?
A. Forament Ovale
B. Vidian Canal
C. Foramen Rotundum
D. **Pterygopalatine Fossa (PPF)**

Pterygopalatine Fossa (PPF)

This is a 3 dimensional box that acts as a gateway, or intersection between the nasal cavity, infra temporal fossa, pharynx, orbit and middle cranial fossa through multiple passages.

*Don't try and memorize all the stuff that goes in and out of it, just realize a bunch of stuff does and be able to recognize the big ones (*Rotundum, Orbital Fissures, Sphenopalatine, & Vidian*).

Case 5 - The Skull Base (part 5)

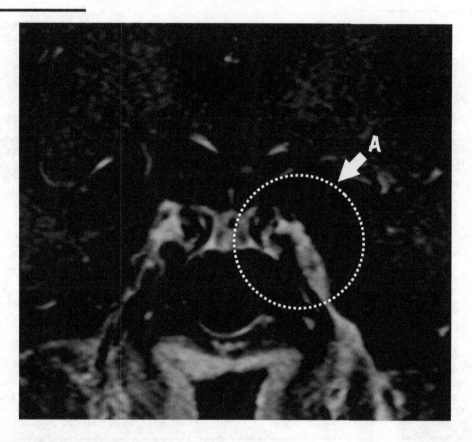

1. What is "A" ?
A. Superior Orbital Fissure
B. The Cavernous Sinus
C. The Pituitary Fossa
D. Pterygopalatine Fossa (PPF)

2. What does NOT run through the Cavernous Sinus?
A. CN 3
B. CN 4
C. CN V1
D. CN V2
E. CN V3

3. What cranial nerve in the Cavernous Sinus does NOT run along the wall
A. CN 3
B. CN 4
C. CN V3
D. CN 6

Case 5 - The Skull Base (part 5)

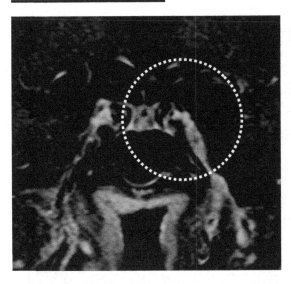
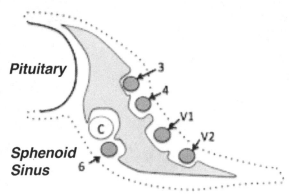

1. What is "A" ?
A. Superior Orbital Fissure
B. The Cavernous Sinus
C. The Pituitary Fossa
D. Pterygopalatine Fossa (PPF)

2. What does NOT run through the Cavernous Sinus?
A. CN 3
B. CN 4
C. CN V1
D. CN V2
E. CN V3

3. What cranial nerve in the Cavernous Sinus does NOT run along the wall
A. CN 3
B. CN 4
C. CN V3
D. CN 6

Cavernous Sinus:

The question is going to be, what's in it (probably asked as what is NOT in it). CN3, 4, CN V1, CNV2, CN6, and the carotid. **CN2 and CN V3 do NOT run through it**.

The only other anatomy trivia I can think of is that CN6 runs next to the carotid, the rest of the nerves are along the wall. This is why you can get lateral rectus palsy earlier with cavernous sinus pathologies.

Case 6 - The Skull Sutures

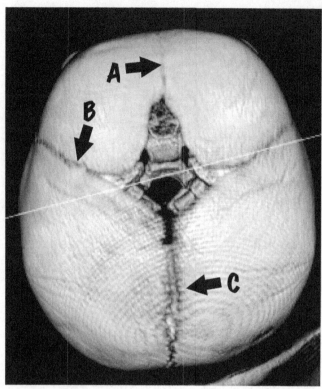
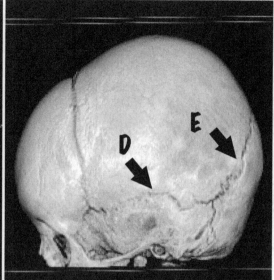

1. What is "A" ?
A. Metopic
B. Coronal
C. Sagittal
D. Lambdoid

2. Premature closure of "B" results in?
A. Brachycephaly (with a Harlequin Eye)
B. Turricephaly
C. Trigonocephaly
D. Dolichocephaly

3. Premature closure of "?" is the most common form of Craniosynostosis?
A. A
B. B
C. C
D. D
E. E

Anatomy 12

Case 6 - The Skull Sutures

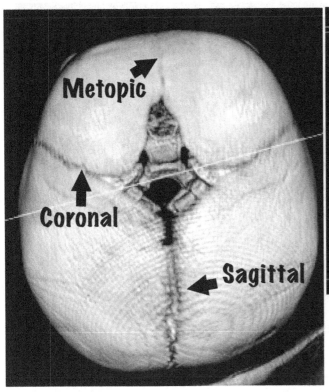
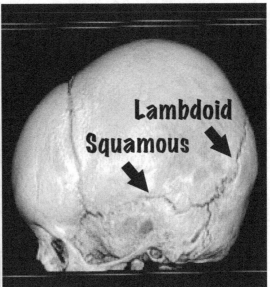

1. What is "A"?
A. Metopic
B. Coronal
C. Sagittal
D. Lambdoid

2. Premature closure of "B" results in?
A. Brachycephaly (with a Harlequin Eye)
B. Turricephaly
C. Trigonocephaly
D. Dolichocephaly

3. Premature closure of "?" is the most common form of Craniosynostosis?
A. A
B. B
C. C (sagittal)
D. D
E. E

Premature Suture Closure	
Sagittal	Dolichocephaly (long and skinny). *most common*
Metopic	Trigonocephaly (pointed forehead)
Coronal	Brachycephaly (also gets orbit issues "harlequin-eye"). Often with associated syndromes.
Unilateral Lambdoid	Plagiocephaly
Bilateral Lambdoid	Turricephaly

Anatomy 13

Case 7 - The Sagittal Brain

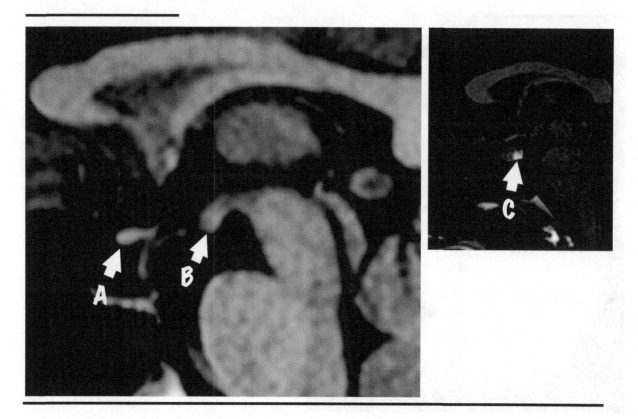

1. What is "A" ?
A. Pituitary
B. Mammillary Body
C. Optic Chiasm
D. Hypothalamus

2. What is "B" ?
A. Pituitary
B. Mammillary Body
C. Optic Chiasm
D. Hypothalamus

3. Is it ever normal for the anterior pituitary to be bright?
A. Nope
B. It should always be bright
C. Yup, it's supposed to be bright in babies.

4. What is "C" ?
A. Neurohypophysis
B. Adenohypophysis

Case 7 - The Sagittal Brain

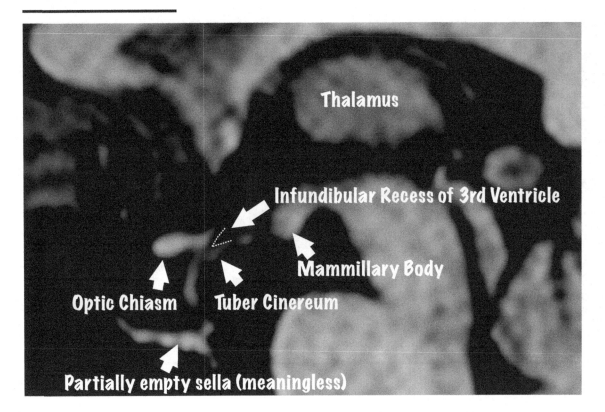

1. What is "A" ?
A. Pituitary
B. Mammillary Body
C. Optic Chiasm
D. Hypothalamus

2. What is "B" ?
A. Pituitary
B. Mammillary Body
C. Optic Chiasm
D. Hypothalamus

3. Is it ever normal for the anterior pituitary to be bright?
A. Nope
B. It should always be bright
C. Yup, it's supposed to be bright in babies. *under the age of 2, it can be*

4. What is "C" ?
A. Neurohypophysis *The posterior pituitary*
B. Adenohypophysis

Case 8 - Temporal Bone (part 1)

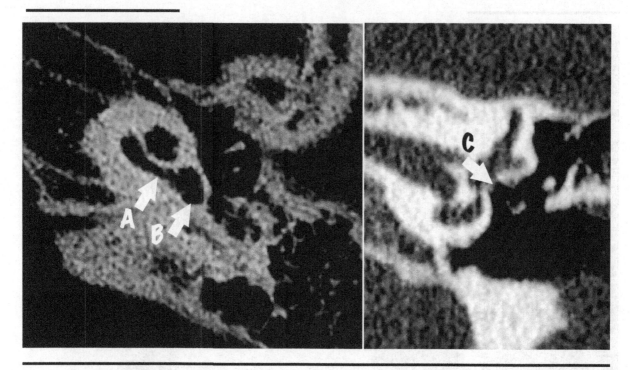

1. What is "A" ?
A. Superior Turn Semicircular Canal
B. Basal Turn of the Cochlea
C. Middle Turn of the Cochlea
D. The Vestibular Aqueduct

2. What is "B" ?
A. The Oval Window
B. The Round Window
C. The Vestibular Aqueduct
D. The Facial Nerve

3. What is "C" ?
A. The Oval Window
B. The Round Window
C. The Vestibular Aqueduct
D. The Facial Nerve

4. What attaches to the oval window?
A. The Malleus
B. The Incus
C. The Stapes

Case 8 - Temporal Bone (part 1)

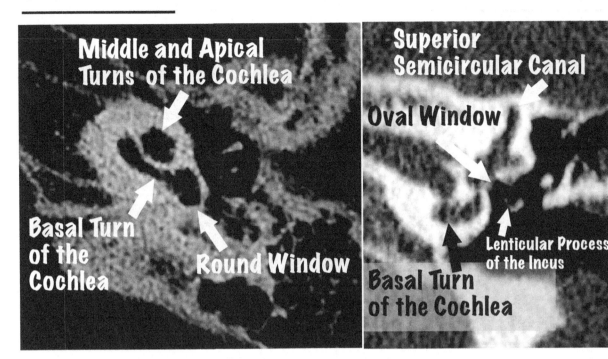

1. What is "A" ?
A. Superior Turn Semicircular Canal
B. Basal Turn of the Cochlea
C. Middle Turn of the Cochlea
D. The Vestibular Aqueduct

2. What is "B" ?
A. The Oval Window
B. The Round Window
C. The Vestibular Aqueduct
D. The Facial Nerve

3. What is "C" ?
A. The Oval Window
B. The Round Window
C. The Vestibular Aqueduct
D. The Facial Nerve

4. What attaches to the oval window?
A. The Malleus
B. The Incus
C. The Stapes

Round Window and Oval Window

I used to get these mixed up all the time when I was in training.

The way I remember which is which, is that the foot print of the stapes is oval, and the *stapes attaches to the oval window*. I find the easiest way to find the stapes is to look for the "elbow" appearance of the Lenticular process of the incus (on coronal), which will hook up to the stapes.

The *Round Window* is at the base of the basal turn of the cochlea (the thing that looks like a smiley face on axials).

Just remember one - and know that the other one is the other one.

Anatomy 17

Case 9 - Temporal Bone (part 2)

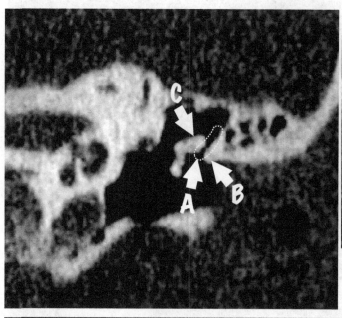
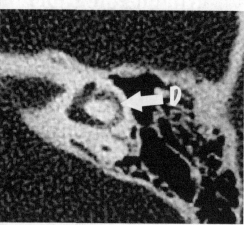

1. What is "A" ?
A. Prussak's Space
B. Pyramidal Eminence
C. Aditus Ad Antrum
D. The Vestibular Aqueduct

2. What is "B" ?
A. Pyramidal Eminence
B. Cochlear Promontory
C. Modiolus
D. Scutum

3. What is "C" ?
A. The Incus
B. The Malleus
C. The Stapes

4. What is "D" ?
A. Horizontal / Lateral Semicircular Canal
B. The Vestibule
C. Middle Turn of the Cochlea

Case 9 - Temporal Bone (part 2)

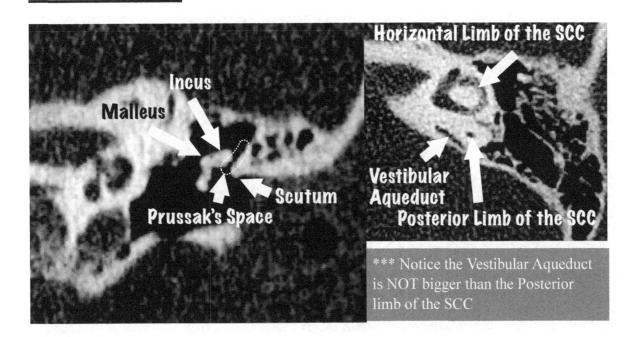

*** Notice the Vestibular Aqueduct is NOT bigger than the Posterior limb of the SCC

1. What is "A" ?
A. **Prussak's Space**
B. Pyramidal Eminence
C. Aditus Ad Antrum
D. The Vestibular Aqueduct

2. What is "B" ?
A. Pyramidal Eminence
B. Cochlear Promontory
C. Modiolus
D. **Scutum**

3. What is "C" ?
A. **The Incu**
B. The Malleus
C. The Stapes

4. What is "D" ?
A. **Horizontal / Lateral Semicircular Canal**
B. The Vestibule
C. Middle Turn of the Cochlea

Relevant Anatomy for the Acquired Cholesteatoma

Acquired Cholesteatoma is a bunch of exfoliated skin debris growing in the wrong place. It creates a big inflammation ball which wrecks the temporal bone and the ossicles.

You have two parts to the ear drum, a flimsy wimpy part "Pars Flaccida", and a tougher part "Pars Tensa." The flimsy Flaccida is at the top, and the tensa is at the bottom. If you "acquire" a hole with some inflammation / infection involving the pars flaccida you can end up with this ball of epithelial crap growing and causing inflammation in the wrong place (typically Prussak's space)..

The first thing it erodes is the scutum. Then you have erosion and displacement of the adjacent ossicles (incus and malleus). Eventually, you can have involvement of the semi-circular canal (most commonly at the lateral / horizontal portion).

Case 10 - Temporal Bone (part 3)

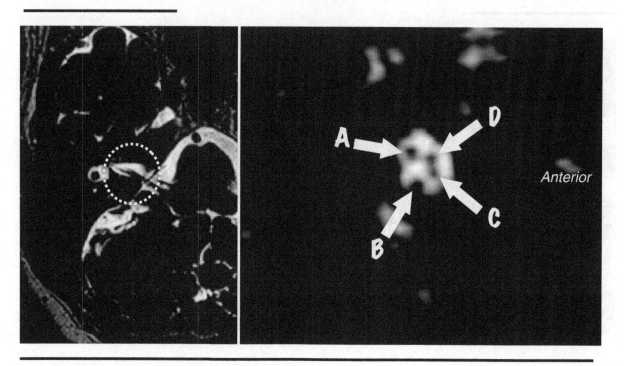

1. What is "A"?
A. Facial Nerve (CN 7)
B. Cochlear Nerve
C. Superior Vestibular Nerve
D. Inferior Vestibular Nerve

2. What is "B"?
A. Facial Nerve (CN 7)
B. Cochlear Nerve
C. Superior Vestibular Nerve
D. Inferior Vestibular Nerve

3. What is "C"?
A. Facial Nerve (CN 7)
B. Cochlear Nerve
C. Superior Vestibular Nerve
D. Inferior Vestibular Nerve

4. What is "D"?
A. Facial Nerve (CN 7)
B. Cochlear Nerve
C. Superior Vestibular Nerve
D. Inferior Vestibular Nerve

Case 10 - Temporal Bone (part 3)

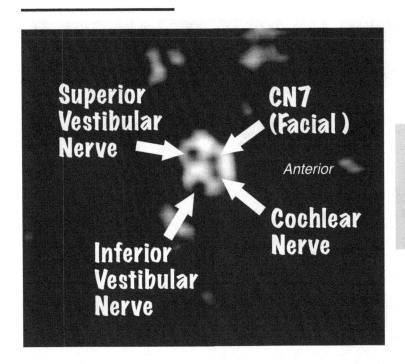

The Mnemonic is *"7up, Coke Down"* - to remember that the Facial Nerve (Cn7) is superior to the Cochlear Nerve

1. What is "A" ?
A. Facial Nerve (CN 7)
B. Cochlear Nerve
C. Superior Vestibular Nerve
D. Inferior Vestibular Nerve

2. What is "B" ?
A. Facial Nerve (CN 7)
B. Cochlear Nerve
C. Superior Vestibular Nerve
D. Inferior Vestibular Nervc

3. What is "C" ?
A. Facial Nerve (CN 7)
B. Cochlear Nerve
C. Superior Vestibular Nerve
D. Inferior Vestibular Nerve

4. What is "D" ?
A. Facial Nerve (CN 7)
B. Cochlear Nerve
C. Superior Vestibular Nerve
D. Inferior Vestibular Nerve

Case 11 - Cervical Lymph Nodes

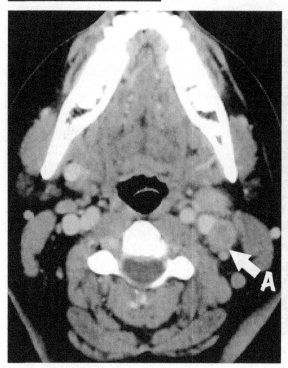
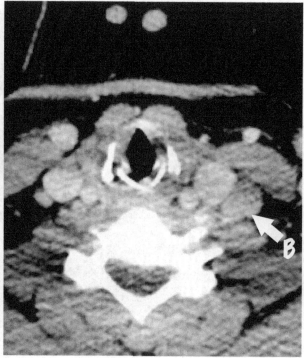

1. What Level is "A"?
A. Level 2
B. Level 3
C. Level 4
D. Level 5

2. What level is "B"?
A. Level 2
B. Level 3
C. Level 4
D. Level 5

3. What land mark distinguishes between a Level 2 and Level 3?
A. Lower Border of the Hyoid
B. Lower Border of the Cricoid
C. The Sternocleidomastoid (SCM)
D. The Posterior Border of the Submandibular Gland

Case 11 - Cervical Lymph Nodes

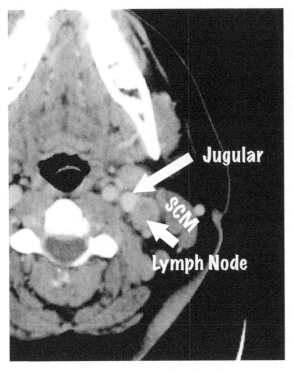
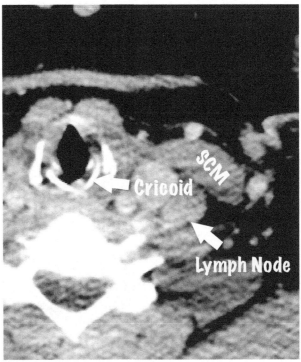

1. What Level is "A" ?
A. **Level 2** *Probably a 2B because its behind the jugular vein*
B. Level 3
C. Level 4
D. Level 5

2. What level is "B" ?
A. Level 2
B. **Level 3** *you can still see Cricoid*
C. Level 4
D. Level 5

3. What land mark distinguishes between a Level 2 and Level 3?
A. **Lower Border of the Hyoid**
B. Lower Border of the Cricoid
C. The Sternocleidomastoid (SCM)
D. The Posterior Border of the Submandibular Gland

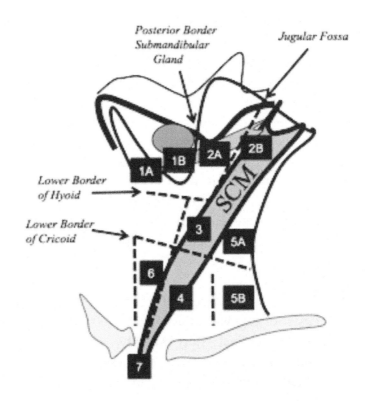

Anatomy 23

Case 12 - Vascular (CNS - Part 1)

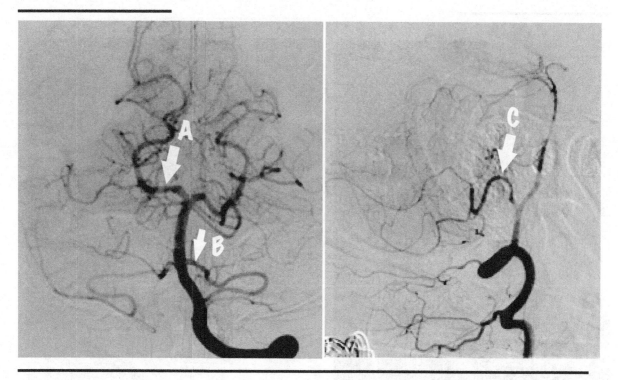

1. What is "A" ?
A. Posterior Inferior Cerebellar Artery (PICA)
B. Posterior Cerebral Artery (PCA)
C. Middle Cerebral Artery (MCA)
D. Superior Cerebellar Artery (SCA)
E. Pontine Artery

2. What is "B" ?
A. Posterior Inferior Cerebellar Artery (PICA)
B. Posterior Cerebral Artery (PCA)
C. Middle Cerebral Artery (MCA)
D. Superior Cerebellar Artery (SCA)
E. Anterior Inferior Cerebellar Artery (AICA)

3. What is "C"
A. Posterior Inferior Cerebellar Artery (PICA)
B. Posterior Cerebral Artery (PCA)
C. Middle Cerebral Artery (MCA)
D. Superior Cerebellar Artery (SCA)
E. Anterior Inferior Cerebellar Artery (AICA)

Case 12 - Vascular (CNS - Part 1)

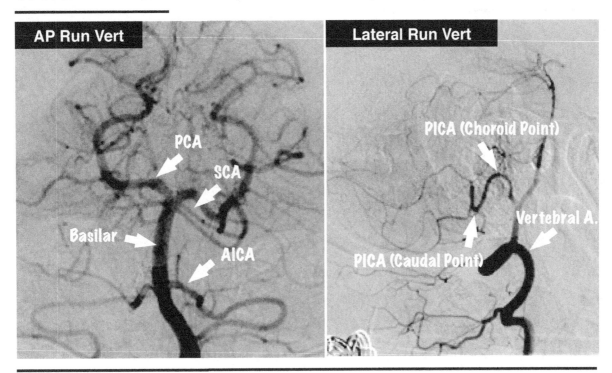

1. What is "A" ?
A. Posterior Inferior Cerebellar Artery (PICA)
B. Posterior Cerebral Artery (PCA)
C. Middle Cerebral Artery (MCA)
D. Superior Cerebellar Artery (SCA)
E. Pontine Artery

2. What is "B" ?
A. PICA
B. PCA
C. MCA
D. SCA
E. Anterior Inferior Cerebellar Artery (AICA)

3. What is "C"
A. PICA
B. PCA
C. MCA
D. SCA
E. AICA

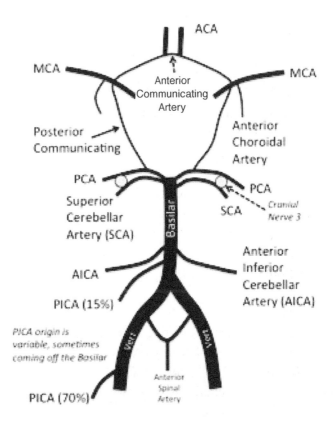

Anatomy 25

Case 13 - Vascular (CNS - Part 2)

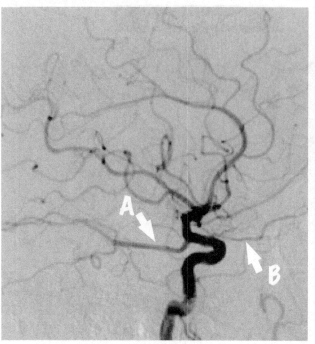
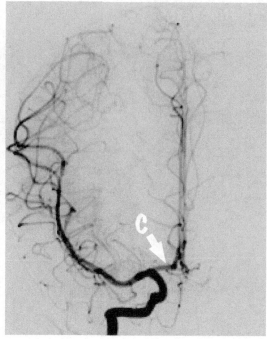

1. What is "A" ?
A. Posterior Communicating Artery (PCOM)
B. Anterior Cerebral Artery (ACA)
C. Middle Cerebral Artery (MCA)
D. Superior Cerebellar Artery (SCA)
E. Ophthalmic Artery

2. What is "B" ?
A. Posterior Communicating Artery (PCOM)
B. Anterior Cerebral Artery (ACA)
C. Middle Cerebral Artery (MCA)
D. Superior Cerebellar Artery (SCA)
E. Ophthalmic Artery

3. What is "C"
A. Posterior Communicating Artery (PCOM)
B. Anterior Cerebral Artery (ACA)
C. Middle Cerebral Artery (MCA)
D. Superior Cerebellar Artery (SCA)
E. Ophthalmic Artery

Case 13 - Vascular (CNS - Part 2)

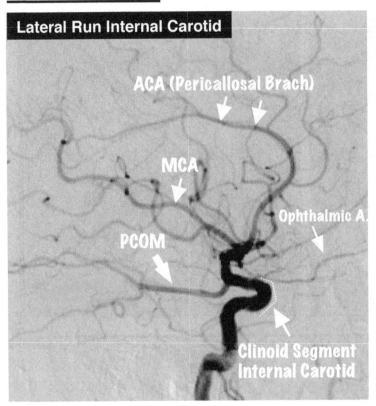
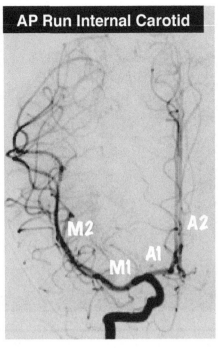

1. What is "A"?
A. Posterior Communicating Artery (PCOM)
B. Anterior Cerebral Artery (ACA)
C. Middle Cerebral Artery (MCA)
D. Superior Cerebellar Artery (SCA)
E. Ophthalmic Artery

2. What is "B"?
A. Posterior Communicating Artery (PCOM)
B. Anterior Cerebral Artery (ACA)
C. Middle Cerebral Artery (MCA)
D. Superior Cerebellar Artery (SCA)
E. Ophthalmic Artery

3. What is "C"
A. Posterior Communicating Artery (PCOM)
B. Anterior Cerebral Artery (ACA) - *A1*
C. Middle Cerebral Artery (MCA)
D. Superior Cerebellar Artery (SCA)
E. Ophthalmic Artery

Ophthalmic Artery - Arises right above the Clinoid Segment (C5) of the internal carotid - *just above that bump thingy*. It is the first intracranial vessel heading in the anterior direction (which makes it testable). "Just above the dural ring" is a buzzword.

The Posterior Communicating (PCOM) - is the vessel heading posterior at about the level of the ophthalmic.

The so called **"Fetal PCOM"** occurs when the PCOM is larger than the PCA. This becomes clinically relevant when you see an anterior circulation stroke that also seems to involve the posterior circulation.

Anatomy 27

Case 14 - Vascular (CNS - Part 3)

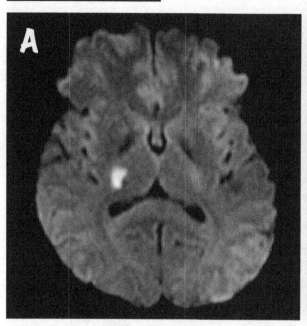
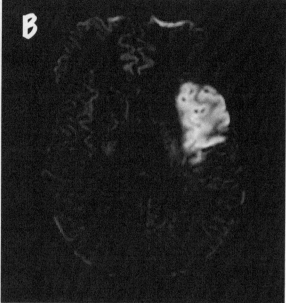

1. What territory is the stroke in "A"?
A. Posterior Communicating Artery (PCOM)
B. Anterior Choroidal Artery
C. Middle Cerebral Artery (MCA)
D. Anterior Cerebral Artery (ACA)
E. Artery of Percheron

2. What territory is the stroke in "B"?
A. Posterior Communicating Artery (PCOM)
B. Anterior Choroidal Artery
C. Middle Cerebral Artery (MCA)
D. Anterior Cerebral Artery (ACA)
E. Artery of Percheron

3. How old (roughly) is a stroke that restricts diffusion, but is NOT bright on FLAIR?
A. 0-6 hours
B. 6-24 hours
C. 24 hours -1 week

Case 14 - Vascular (CNS - Part 3)

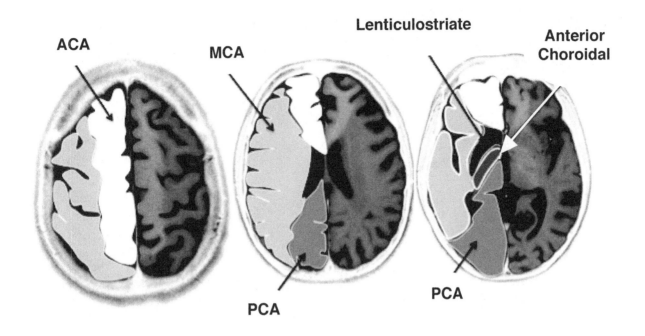

1. What territory is the stroke in "A"?
A. Posterior Communicating Artery (PCOM)
B. Anterior Choroidal Artery
   originates off the ICA (usually)
C. Middle Cerebral Artery (MCA)
D. Anterior Cerebral Artery (ACA)
E. Artery of Percheron

2. What territory is the stroke in "B"?
A. Posterior Communicating Artery (PCOM)
B. Anterior Choroidal Artery
C. Middle Cerebral Artery (MCA)
D. Anterior Cerebral Artery (ACA)
E. Artery of Percheron

3. How old (roughly) is a stroke that restricts diffusion, but is NOT bright on FLAIR?
A. 0-6 hours
B. 6-24 hours
C. 24 hours -1 week

Findings on MRI do change with the age of the stroke. Diffusion restricts early, and lasts, but the key to tell if the stroke is acute is the absence of FLAIR signal. This doesn't always hold up in the real world, but for the purpose of multiple choice - no FLAIR is always acute.

	0-6 hours	6-24 hours	24 hours -1 week
Diffusion	Bright	Bright	Bright
FLAIR	**NOT BRIGHT**	Bright	Bright
T1	Iso	Dark	Dark, with Bright Cortical Necrosis
T2	Iso	Bright	Bright

Anatomy 29

Case 15 - Vascular (Celiac Axis)

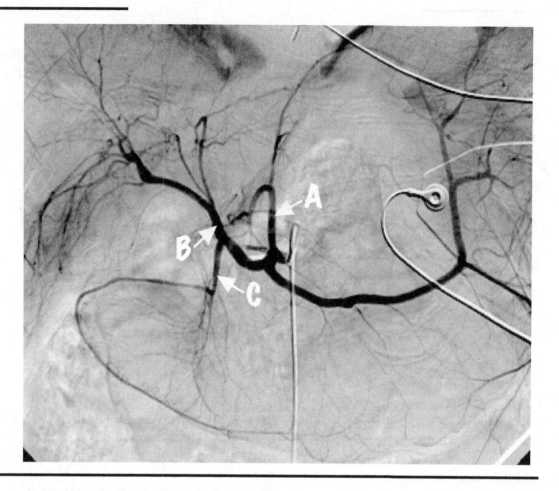

1. What is "A" ?
A. Right Gastric Artery
B. Left Gastric Artery
C. Phrenic Artery
D. Celiac Trunk

2. What is "B" ?
A. Proper Hepatic Artery
B. Common Hepatic Artery
C. Right Gastric Artery
D. Gastroduodenal Artery (GDA)

3. What is "C" ?
A. Superior Pancreaticoduodenal
B. Gastroepiploic Artery
C. Common Hepatic
D. Gastroduodenal Artery (GDA)

Case 15 - Vascular (Celiac Axis)

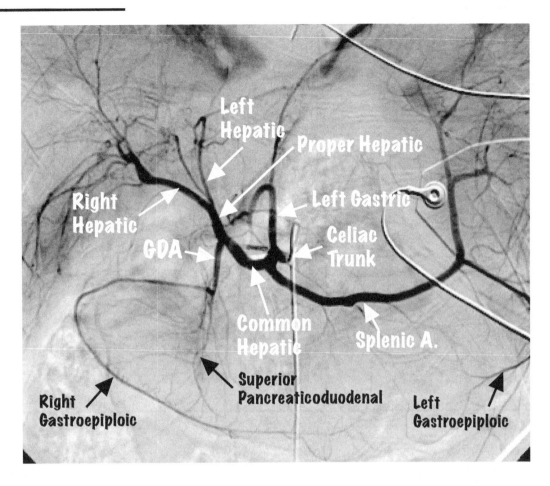

1. What is "A" ?
A. Right Gastric Artery
B. Left Gastric Artery
C. Phrenic Artery
D. Celiac Trunk

2. What is "B" ?
A. Proper Hepatic Artery
B. Common Hepatic Artery
C. Right Gastric Artery
D. Gastroduodenal Artery (GDA)

3. What is "C" ?
A. Superior Pancreaticoduodenal
B. Gastroepiploic Artery
C. Common Hepatic
D. Gastroduodenal Artery (GDA)

Anatomy 31

Case 16 - Vascular (SMA)

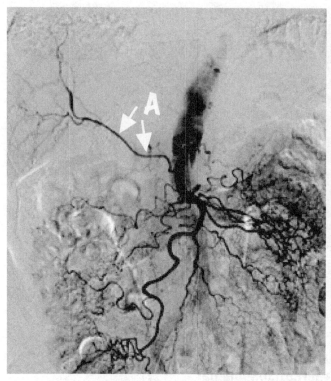
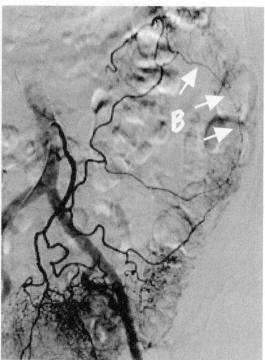

1. What is "A" ?
A. Right Gastric Artery
B. Inferior Pancreaticoduodenal
C. Replaced Hepatic Artery
D. Right Colic Artery

2. What is "B" ?
A. Marginal Artery of Drummond
B. Arc of Riolan
C. Arc of Buhler
D. Pancreatic-Duodenal Arcade

3. The Arc of Riolan is a collateral pathway from?
A. Right Colic of the SMA to the Left Colic of the IMA
B. Middle Colic of the SMA to the Left Colic of the IMA
C. Superior Pancreatic Duodenal to the Inferior Pancreatic Duodenal
D. Superior Rectal of the IMA to the Internal Pudendal (Internal Iliac)

Case 16 - Vascular (SMA)

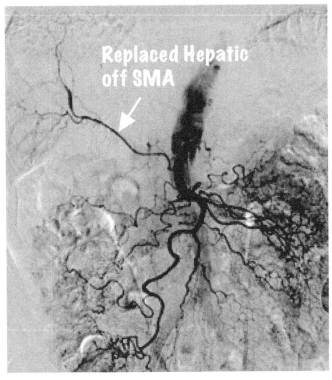
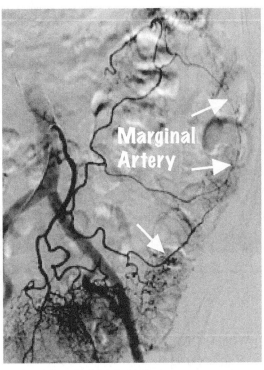

1. What is "A"?
A. Right Gastric Artery
B. Inferior Pancreaticoduodenal
C. Replaced Hepatic Artery
D. Right Colic Artery

2. What is "B"?
A. Marginal Artery of Drummond
B. Arc of Riolan
C. Arc of Buhler
D. Pancreatic-Duodenal Arcade

3. The Arc of Riolan is a collateral pathway from?
A. Right Colic of the SMA to the Left Colic of the IMA
B. Middle Colic of the SMA to the Left Colic of the IMA
C. Superior Pancreatic Duodenal to the Inferior Pancreatic Duodenal
D. Superior Rectal of the IMA to the Internal Pudendal (Internal Iliac).

SMA Trivia

The **Right Hepatic Artery** arising from the SMA - "**replaced**" - is the most common variant of the hepatic arterial anatomy, occurring at 10-15% of the time.

The **Arc of Riolan** is an important collateral between the SMA and IMA — occurring via the middle colic (SMA) and the left colic (IMA).

The **Marginal Artery of Drummond** is another important SMA to IMA collateral. The anastomosis of the terminal branches of the ileocolic, right colic and middle colic arteries of the SMA, and of the left colic and sigmoid branches of the IMA, form a continuous arterial circle or arcade along the inner border of the colon.

Case 17 - Vascular (Upper Extremity)

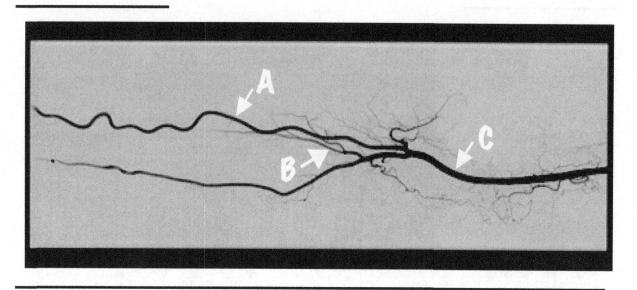

1. What is "A"?
A. Radial Artery
B. Ulnar Artery
C. Interosseous Artery
D. Brachial Artery

2. What is "B"?
A. Radial Artery
B. Ulnar Artery
C. Interosseous Artery
D. Brachial Artery

3. What is "C"?
A. Radial Artery
B. Ulnar Artery
C. Interosseous Artery
D. Brachial Artery

Case 17 - Vascular (Upper Extremity)

1. What is "A" ?
A. Radial Artery
B. Ulnar Artery
C. Interosseous Artery
D. Brachial Artery

2. What is "B" ?
A. Radial Artery
B. Ulnar Artery
C. Interosseous Artery
D. Brachial Artery

3. What is "C" ?
A. Radial Artery
B. Ulnar Artery
C. Interosseous Artery
D. Brachial Artery

Upper Extremity Trivia

- The Axillary Artery becomes of the brachial artery at the lateral margin of the teres major.

- Usually, the ulnar artery is larger than the radial and gives off the common interosseous – which then splits off to form anterior and posterior branches.

- The superficial palmar arch is from the ulna A.

- The deep palmar arch is from the radial A.

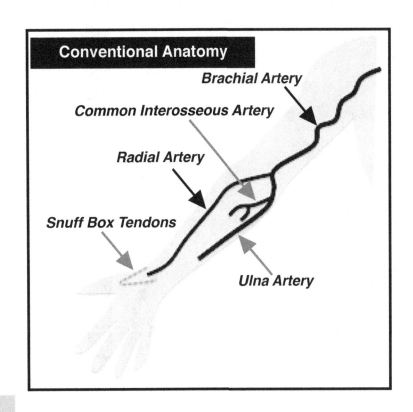

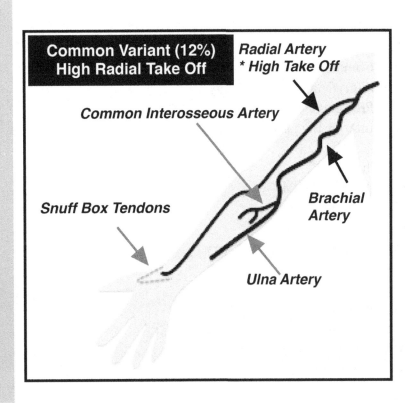

Case 18 - Vascular (Lower Extremity)

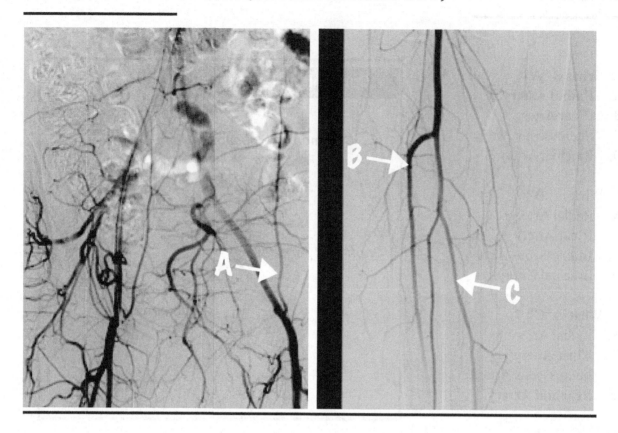

1. What is "A"?
A. Common Femoral Artery
B. Superficial Femoral Artery
C. Profunda Femoris
D. Inferior Epigastric Artery

2. What is "B"?
A. Anterior Tibial
B. Posterior Tibial
C. Peroneal Artery
D. Tibioperoneal Trunk Artery

3. What is "C"?
A. Anterior Tibial
B. Posterior Tibial
C. Peroneal Artery
D. Tibioperoneal Trunk Artery

Anatomy 36

Case 18 - Vascular (Lower Extremity)

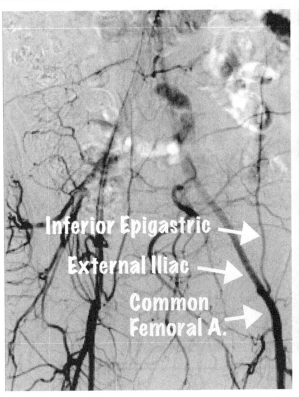
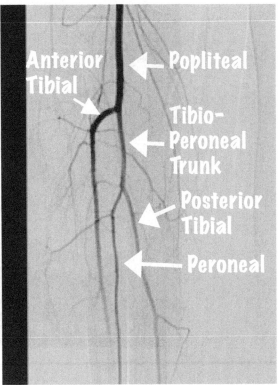

1. What is "A"?
   A. Common Femoral Artery
   B. Superficial Femoral Artery
   C. Profunda Femoris
   D. Inferior Epigastric Artery

2. What is "B"?
   A. Anterior Tibial
   B. Posterior Tibial
   C. Peroneal Artery
   D. Tibioperoneal Trunk Artery

3. What is "C"?
   A. Anterior Tibial
   B. Posterior Tibial
   C. Peroneal Artery
   D. Tibioperoneal Trunk Artery

Lower Extremity Trivia

- Once the inferior epigastric comes off (level of the inguinal ligament) you are dealing with the common femoral artery (CFA).

- The superficial femoral becomes the popliteal when the vessel emerges from Hunter's (ADDuctor) canal.

- The first branch off of the popliteal artery is the anterior tibial.

- The anterior tibial courses anterior and lateral, then it transverses the interosseous membrane, terminating as the dorsalis pedis.

- The most medial artery in the leg is the posterior tibial (felt at the medial malleolus).

Anatomy 37

Case 19 - Vascular (Femoral Access)

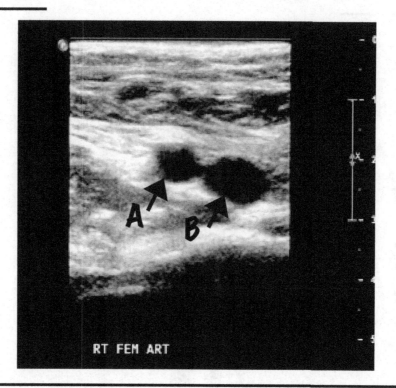

1. Which one is the Femoral Artery?
A. A.
B. B.

2. When treating a femoral artery pseudo aneurysm with thrombin, it is important to " ? "
A. Aspirate blood first into the syringe before injecting the thrombin
B. Confirm the cavity size is less than 1cm before injecting the thrombin
C. Give no more than 100 units
D. Give between 500 and 1000 units

3. A "High Stick" above the inguinal ligament classically carries a risk of?
A. Retroperitoneal Bleed
B. AV Fistula
C. Occluding branching vessels with your sheath
D. Fascial compartment syndrome

4. A "Low Stick" close to or at the femoral bifurcation classically carries a risk of?
A. Retroperitoneal Bleed
B. AV Fistula
C. Fascial compartment syndrome
D. Post thrombotic syndrome

Case 19 - Vascular (Femoral Access)

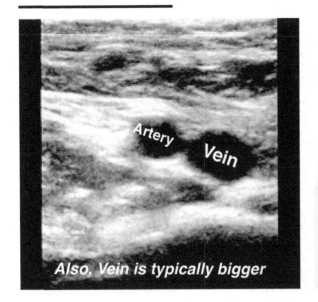

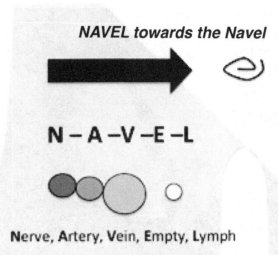

1. Which one is the Femoral Artery?
   A. **A.**
   B. B.

2. When treating a femoral artery pseudo aneurysm with thrombin, it is important to " ? "
   A. Aspirate blood first into the syringe before injecting the thrombin ** *never do this - it will clot in the syringe*
   B. Confirm the cavity size is less than 1cm before injecting the thrombin
   C. Give no more than 100 units
   D. Give between 500 and 1000 units

3. A "High Stick" above the inguinal ligament classically carries a risk of?
   A. Retroperitoneal Bleed
   B. AV Fistula
   C. Occluding branching vessels with your sheath
   D. Fascial compartment syndrome

4. A "Low Stick" close to or at the femoral bifurcation classically carries a risk of?
   A. Retroperitoneal Bleed
   B. AV Fistula
   C. Fascial compartment syndrome
   D. Post thrombotic syndrome

Femoral Access Trivia

- The ideal location is over the femoral head (which gives you something to compress against), distal to the inguinal ligament / epigastric artery and proximal to the common femoral bifurcation.

- If you stick too high (above inguinal ligament): You risk retroperitoneal bleed

- If you stick too low, you risk AV Fistula

- If you stick at the bifurcation: You risk occluding branching vessels with your sheath.

Pseudoaneurysm Treatment

- A lot of the time, small (<3cm) will undergo spontaneous thrombosis.

- The Thrombin Dose is between 500-1000 units, injected into the apex of the cavity.

- Contraindications would include: infected skin, distal ischemia, a large neck (risk of propagation), and a small sac size (< 1cm)

Case 20 - Cardiac (Part 1)

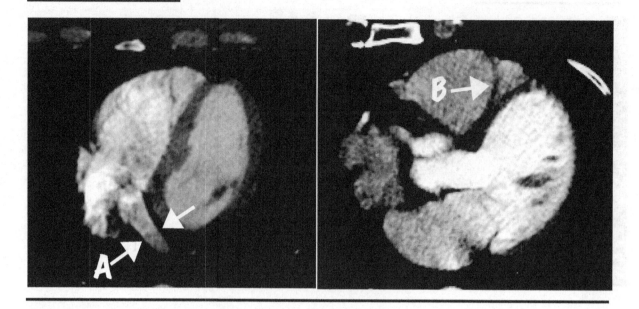

1. What is "A" ?
A. Pulmonary Vein
B. Pulmonary Artery
C. IVC
D. Coronary Sinus

2. What is "B" ?
A. Crista Terminalis
B. Papillary Muscle
C. Moderator Band
D. Tricuspid Valve

3. The Morphologic Right Atrium is Defined by?
A. The absence of a draining pulmonary vein
B. The absence of an emerging pulmonary artery
C. The moderator band
D. The attachment of the IVC

4. The Morphologic Right Ventricle is Defined by?
A. The absence of a draining pulmonary vein
B. The absence of an emerging pulmonary artery
C. The moderator band
D. The attachment of the IVC

Case 20 - Cardiac (Part 1)

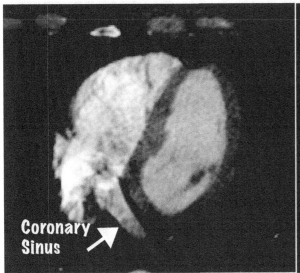 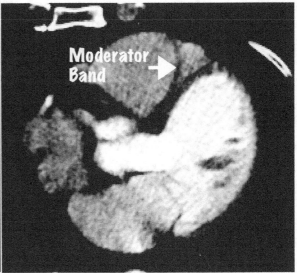

1. What is "A"?
A. Pulmonary Vein
B. Pulmonary Artery
C. IVC
D. Coronary Sinus

2. What is "B"?
A. Crista Terminalis
B. Papillary Muscle
C. Moderator Band
D. Tricuspid Valve

3. The Morphologic Right Atrium is Defined by?
A. The absence of a draining pulmonary vein
B. The absence of an emerging pulmonary artery
C. The moderator band
D. The attachment of the IVC

4. The Morphologic Right Ventricle is Defined by?
A. The absence of a draining pulmonary vein
B. The absence of an emerging pulmonary artery
C. The moderator band
D. The attachment of the IVC

Coronary Sinus

- The main draining vein of the myocardium. It runs in the AV groove on the posterior surface of the heart and enters the right atrium near the tricuspid valve

- The persistent left SVC classically drains into the coronary sinus

Trivia

- The Right Atrium is defined by the IVC

- The Right Ventricle is defined by the moderator band.

- The moderator band is a muscular band that extends from the ventricular septum to the anterior papillary muscle. It carries with it the right bundle branch of

Case 21 - Cardiac (Part 2)

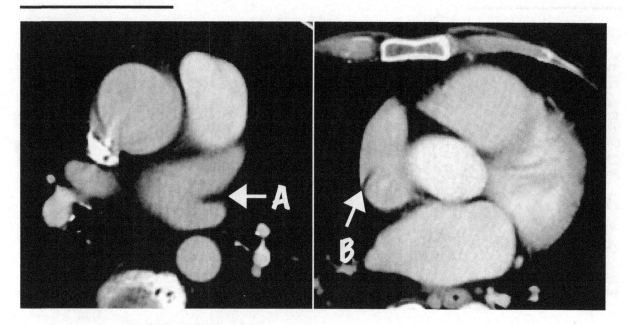

1. What is "A" ?
A. A clot
B. A tumor - probably a myxoma
C. A tumor - probably an elastofibroma
D. Coumadin Ridge

2. What is "B" ?
A. A clot
B. Papillary Muscle
C. Crista Terminalis
D. Chiari Network

3. The papillary muscles of the mitral valve inserts on the "?", and the papillary muscles of the tricuspid valve insert on the "?"
A. MV = Septum, TV = Lateral and Posterior Walls
B. MV = Lateral and Posterior Walls, TV = Septum
C. MV = Septum, TV = Septum
D. MV = Lateral Walls, TV = Lateral Walls

Case 21 - Cardiac (Part 2)

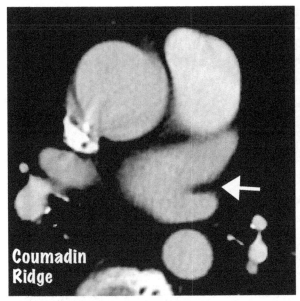
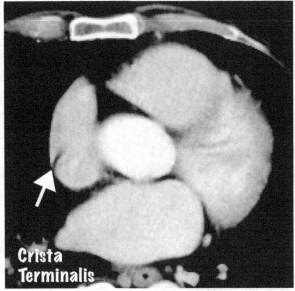

1. What is "A" ?
   A. A clot
   B. A tumor - probably a myxoma
   C. A tumor - probably an elastofibroma
   D. Coumadin Ridge

2. What is "B" ?
   A. A clot
   B. Papillary Muscle
   C. Crista Terminalis
   D. Chiari Network

3. The papillary muscles of the mitral valve inserts on the "?", and the papillary muscles of the tricuspid valve insert on the "?"
   A. MV = Septum, TV = Lateral and Posterior Walls
   B. MV = Lateral and Posterior Walls, TV = Septum
   C. MV = Septum, TV = Septum
   D. MV = Lateral Walls, TV = Lateral Walls

Coumadin Ridge

- The ridge of atrial tissue separating the left atrial appendage from the left upper pulmonary vein.

- This structure is often mistaken for thrombus and resulted in patient being prescribed anticoagulation therapy with warfarin (Coumadin).

Crista Terminalis

- A frequently tested normal structure (it's not a clot or a tumor).

- It is a muscular ridge that runs from the entrance of the superior- to that of the inferior vena cava.

Trivia

- The tricuspid papillary muscles insert on the septum

- The mitral valve papillary muscles insert into the lateral and posterior walls as well as the apex of the left ventricle (not the septum).

Case 22 - Abdominal Ultrasound

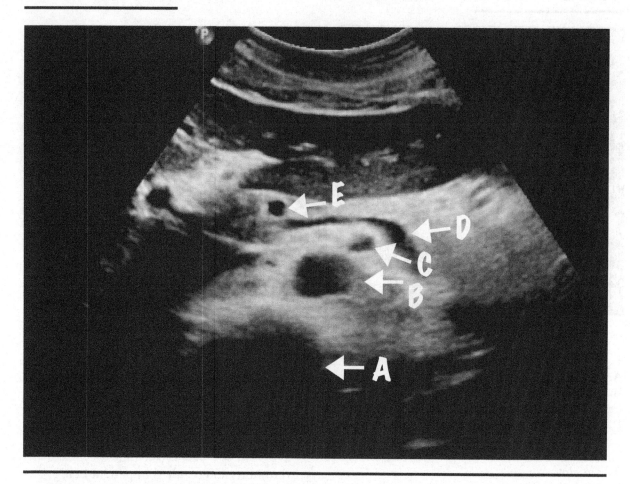

1. What is "A"?
A. IVC
B. Aorta
C. Celiac Artery
D. Vertebral Body

2. What is "B"?
A. IVC
B. Aorta
C. Celiac Artery
D. SMA

3. What is "C"?
A. IVC
B. Aorta
C. Right Renal Artery
D. SMA

4. What is "D"?
A. Left Renal Vein
B. Right Renal Vein
C. Splenic Vein
D. Splenic Artery

5. What is "E"?
A. Hepatic Artery
B. Hepatic Vein
C. Portal Vein
D. Common Bile Duct

Case 22 - Abdominal Ultrasound

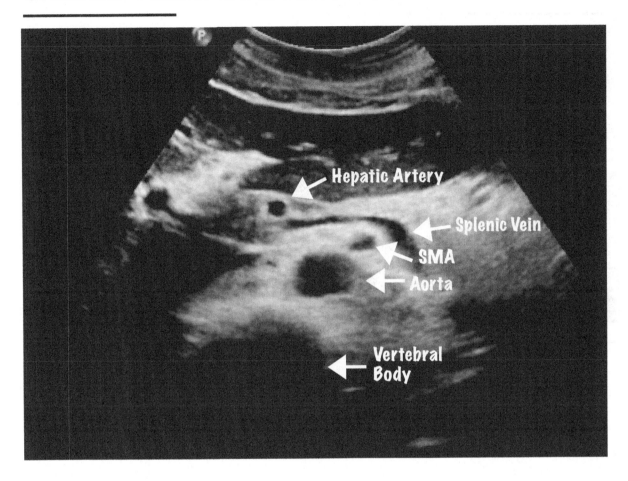

1. What is "A"?
A. IVC
B. Aorta
C. Celiac Artery
D. Vertebral Body

2. What is "B"?
A. IVC
B. Aorta
C. Celiac Artery
D. SMA

3. What is "C"?
A. IVC
B. Aorta
C. Right Renal Artery
D. SMA

4. What is "D"?
A. Left Renal Vein
B. Right Renal Vein
C. Splenic Vein
D. Splenic Artery

5. What is "E"?
A. Hepatic Artery
B. Hepatic Vein
C. Portal Vein
D. Common Bile Duct

Case 23 - The Prostate

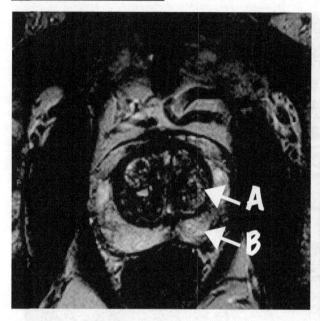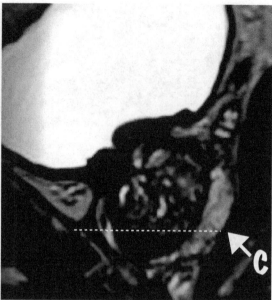

1. What is "A"?
A. Central Gland
B. Peripheral Zone
C. Bright Zone
D. Fibromuscular Zone

2. What is "B"?
A. Central Gland
B. Peripheral Zone
C. Bright Zone
D. Fibromuscular Zone

3. What is "C"?
A. The Apex
B. The Base

4. Prostate Cancer is typically "?", and found in the "?"
A. T2 Dark - in the Central Gland
B. T2 Dark - in the Central Zone
C. T2 Bright - in the Peripheral Zone
D. T2 Dark - in the Peripheral Zone

Anatomy 46

Case 23 - The Prostate

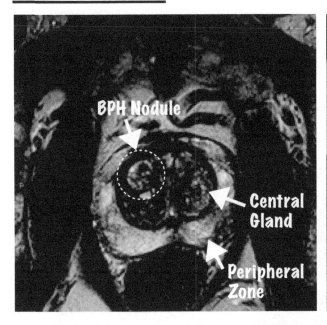
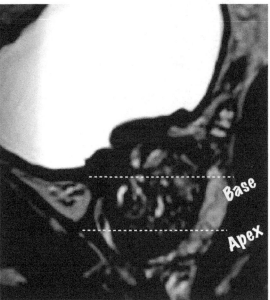

1. What is "A" ?
A. **Central Gland**
B. Peripheral Zone
C. Bright Zone
D. Fibromuscular Zone

2. What is "B" ?
A. Central Gland
B. **Peripheral Zone**
C. Bright Zone
D. Fibromuscular Zone

3. What is "C" ?
A. **The Apex**
B. The Base

4. Prostate Cancer is typically "?", and found in the "?"
A. T2 Dark - in the Central Gland
B. T2 Dark - in the Central Zone
C. T2 Bright - in the Peripheral Zone
D. **T2 Dark - in the Peripheral Zone**

Trivia

- The terms "central *gland*" and "central *zone*" can be used as distractors. There is a difference, so be careful.

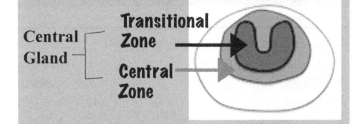

- Central **GLAND** = Central Zone + the Transitional Zone

- Central Gland is where is the BPH nodules live.

- Peripheral Zone is where the Cancer lives (usually). It is typically T2 dark, enhances, restricts diffusion, and has rapid wash out kinetics.

- The Rare Central Gland Cancer is supposed to look like *"Smudged Charcoal"* on T2

Anatomy 47

Case 24 - MSK (The Pelvis)

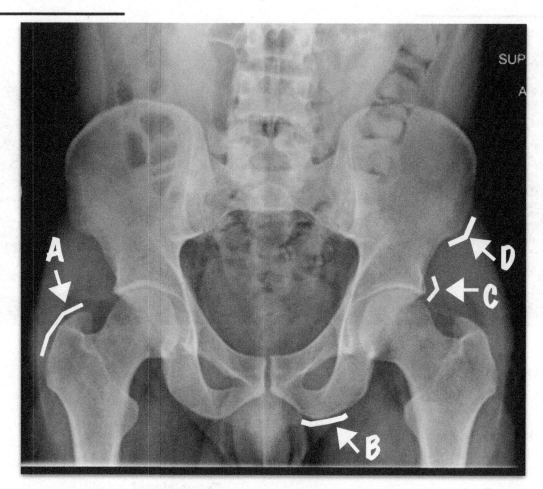

1. What attaches at "A"?
A. ADDuctors
B. Iliopsoas
C. Gluteal Muscles
D. Tensor Fascia Lata

2. What attaches at "B"?
A. ADDuctors
B. Hamstrings
C. Sartorius
D. Abdominal Muscles

3. What attaches at "C"?
A. Sartorius
B. Rectus Femoris
C. ADDuctors
D. Iliopsoas

4. What attaches at "D"?
A. Sartorius
B. Rectus Femoris
C. ADDuctors
D. Iliopsoas

Case 24 - MSK (The Pelvis)

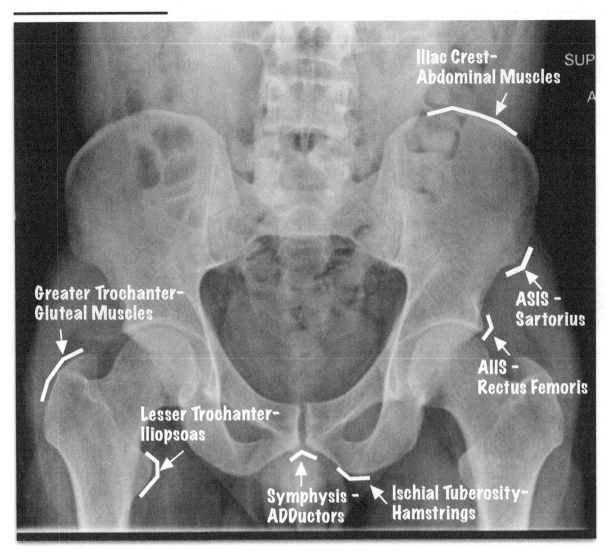

1. What attaches at "A" ?
A. ADDuctors
B. Iliopsoas
C. Gluteal Muscles
D. Tensor Fascia Lata

2. What attaches at "B" ?
A. ADDuctors
B. Hamstrings
C. Sartorius
D. Abdominal Muscles

3. What attaches at "C" ?
A. Sartorius
B. Rectus Femoris
C. ADDuctors
D. Iliopsoas

4. What attaches at "D" ?
A. Sartorius
B. Rectus Femoris
C. ADDuctors
D. Iliopsoas

Anatomy 49

Case 25 - MSK (The Shoulder)

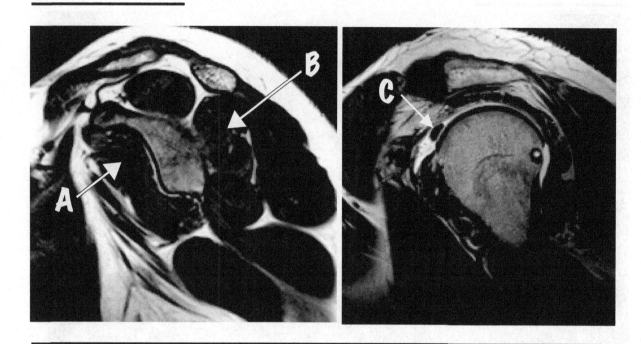

1. What is "A"?
A. Supraspinatous (SS)
B. Infraspinatous (IS)
C. Teres Minor (TM)
D. Subscapularis (Sub S)

2. What is "B"?
A. Supraspinatous (SS)
B. Infraspinatous (IS)
C. Teres Minor (TM)
D. Subscapularis (Sub S)

3. What is "C"?
A. The Subscapularis Tendon
B. Labral Fragment
C. Middle Glenohumeral Ligament
D. Long Head of Biceps Tendon

4. If the long head of the biceps attaches to the glenoid at 12 o'clock, what attaches at 6 o'clock?
A. The Short Head of the Biceps
B. The Triceps

Anatomy 50

Case 25 - MSK (The Shoulder)

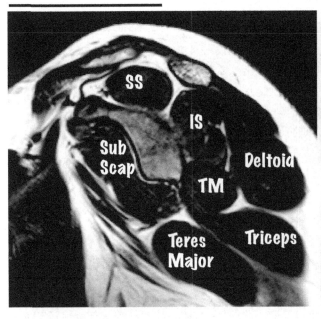
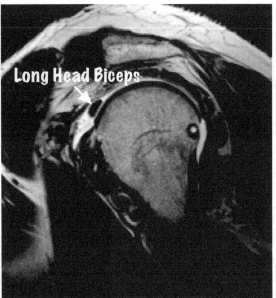

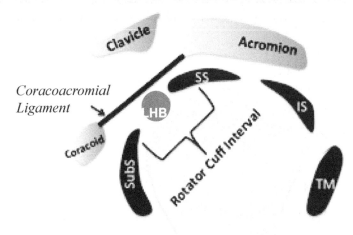

1. What is "A" ?
A. Supraspinatous (SS)
B. Infraspinatous (IS)
C. Teres Minor (TM)
D. Subscapularis (Sub S)

2. What is "B" ?
A. Supraspinatous (SS)
B. Infraspinatous (IS)
C. Teres Minor (TM)
D. Subscapularis (Sub S)

3. What is "C" ?
A. The Subscapularis Tendon
B. Labral Fragment
C. Middle Glenohumeral Ligament
D. Long Head of Biceps Tendon

4. If the long head of the biceps attaches to the glenoid at 12 o'clock, what attaches at 6 o'clock?
A. The Short Head of the Biceps
B. The Triceps

Case 26 - MSK (The Wrist)

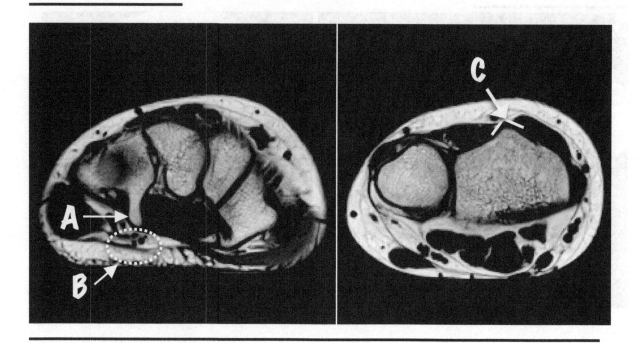

1. What is "A" ?
A. Scaphoid
B. Capitate
C. Hamate
D. Trapezoid

2. What is "B" ?
A. Radial Nerve
B. Ulnar Nerve
C. Median Nerve
D. Musculocutaneous Nerve

3. What is "C" ?
A. Listers Tubercle
B. Radial Styloid
C. Ulnar Tubercle
D. Os Styloideum

4. Which of the following does NOT pass through the carpal tunnel
A. Flexor Dig. Profundus
B. Flexor Dig. Superficialis
C. Flexor Pollicis Longus
D. Flexor Carpi Ulnaris

Case 26 - MSK (The Wrist)

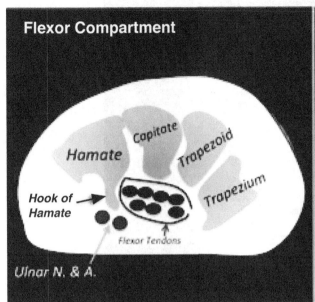
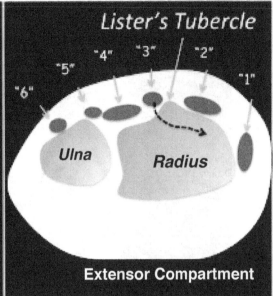

1. What is "A"?
A. Scaphoid
B. Capitate
C. Hamate
D. Trapezoid

2. What is "B"?
A. Radial Nerve
B. Ulnar Nerve
C. Median Nerve
D. Musculocutaneous Nerve

3. What is "C"?
A. Listers Tubercle
B. Radial Styloid
C. Ulnar Tubercle
D. Os Styloideum

4. Which of the following does NOT pass through the carpal tunnel
A. Flexor Dig. Profundus
B. Flexor Dig. Superficialis
C. Flexor Pollicis Longus
D. Flexor Carpi Ulnaris

Trivia

- The hook of the hamate is right next to the ulnar nerve / artery. Therefore fracture or repetitive trauma can cause adjacent injury (ulnar nerve palsy or pseudo-aneurysm). This is sometimes seen in bike riders - the so called *"handle bar palsy"*, where the ulnar nerve is compressed between the handle bar and the hamate hook within *"Guyon's Canal."*

- The 3rd Extensor compartment "Extensor Pollicis Longus" - wraps around "Lister's Tubercle" on it's way to the thumb.

- Flexor tendons and the median nerve go through the carpal tunnel. The **ones that don't are: Flexor Carpi Ulnaris, Flexor Carpi Radialis, Palmaris Longus** *(if you have one)*.

Anatomy 53

Case 27 - MSK (The Ankle)

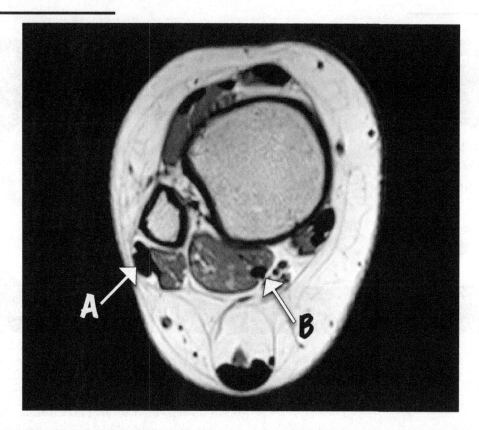

1. What is "A" ?
A. Flexor Digitorum Longus
B. Flexor Hallucis Longus
C. Peroneus Brevis
D. Peroneus Longus

2. What is "B" ?
A. Flexor Digitorum Longus
B. Flexor Hallucis Longus
C. Peroneus Brevis
D. Peroneus Longus

3. What is "Henry's Knot" ?
A. Crossing of Flexor Hallucis over Flexor Digitorum
B. Crossing of Flexor Hallucis over The Posterior Tibial
C. Crossing of the Flexor Digitorium Longus over Flexor Digitorium Brevis
D. None of the Above

4. Is it ever normal for the Flexor Hallucis Longus to have extra fluid in the sheath?
A. Nope
B. Yup

Case 27 - MSK (The Ankle)

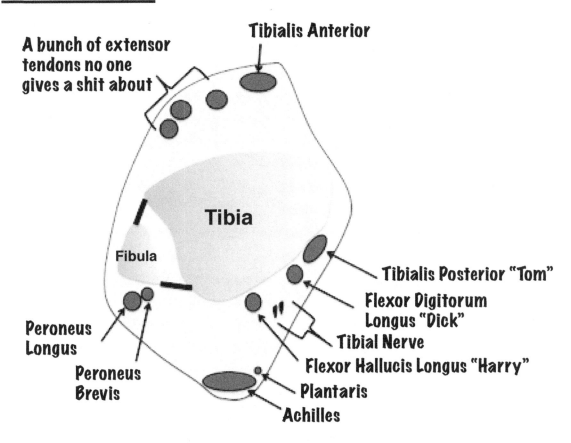

1. What is "A" ?
A. Flexor Digitorum Longus
B. Flexor Hallucis Longus
C. Peroneus Brevis
D. Peroneus Longus

2. What is "B" ?
A. Flexor Digitorum Longus
B. Flexor Hallucis Longus
C. Peroneus Brevis
D. Peroneus Longus

3. What is "Henry's Knot" ?
A. Crossing of Flexor Hallucis over Flexor Digitorum
B. Crossing of Flexor Hallucis over The Posterior Tibial
C. Crossing of the Flexor Digitorium Longus over Flexor Digitorium Brevis
D. None of the Above

4. Is it ever normal for the Flexor Hallucis Longus to have extra fluid in the sheath?
A. Nope
B. Yup

Ankle Trivia

- Achilles Tendon has NO tendon Sheath

- It may be possible to plantar flex with a torn Achilles, assuming your plantaris is still intact

- *Henry's Knot is a "Harry Dick"* - refers to the cross of Hallucis over Digitorum

- Flexor Hallucis Longus has a communication with the ankle joint 20% of the time, so an effusion in the tendon sheath can be normal

Anatomy 55

Case 28 - Nukes (Mystery Whole Body Scan 1)

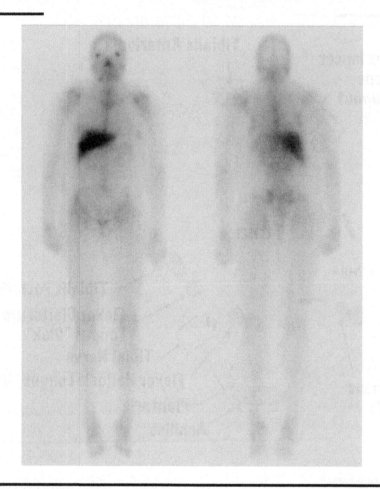

1. What scan is it?
A. Gallium
B. Indium - WBC
C. MIBG
D. I would ask the tech what tracer they injected. If they said "I don't know", I would fire them on the spot, and have security remove them from the hospital immediately.

2. This tracer mimics the physiologic behavior of?
A. Iron
B. WBC
C. Potassium (Na/K pump)
D. Calcium

3. What is the half life of this tracer?
A. 74 Hours
B. 72 Hours
C. 78 Hours

Case 28 - Nukes (Gallium Scan)

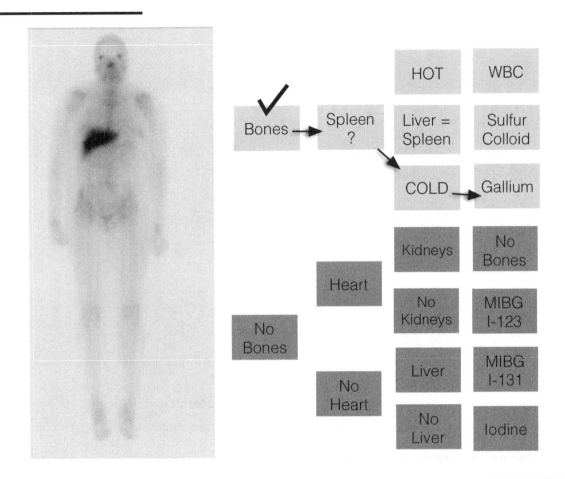

1. What scan is it?
A. Gallium
B. Indium - WBC
C. MIBG
D. I would ask the tech what tracer they injected. If they said "I don't know", I would fire them on the spot, and have security remove them from the hospital immediately.

2. This tracer mimics the physiologic behavior of?
A. Iron
B. WBC
C. Potassium (Na/K pump)
D. Calcium

3. What is the half life of this tracer?
A. 74 Hours
B. 72 Hours
C. 78 Hours

Gallium Trivia

- Handled by the body like Fe^{+3} - which gets bound (via lactoferrin) and concentrated in areas of inflammation and infection.

- It's the "poor mans bone scan."

- The classic use is for spinal osteomyelitis (it's way better than In-WBC in the spine).

- Renal uptake can be normal up to 24 hours, after than - think about interstitial nephritis

- Has 4 photo peaks (roughly 100, 200, 300, 400).

- Made via electron capture (GIIT).

Anatomy 57

Case 29 - Nukes (Mystery Whole Body Scan 2)

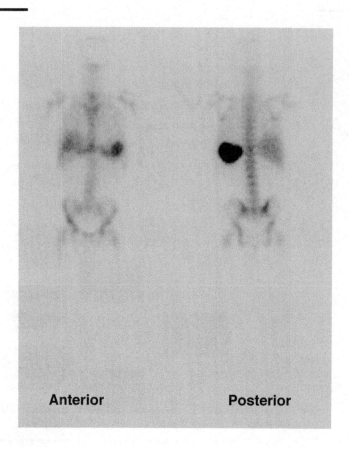

1. What scan is it?
A. Gallium
B. Indium - WBC
C. MIBG
D. I would ask the tech what tracer they injected. If they said "I don't know", I would fire them on the spot, and have security remove them from the hospital immediately.

2. What are the photon peaks of this tracer?
A. Single Peak at 81
B. Four Peaks at 93, 184, 300, & 393
C. Two Peaks at 173 & 247
D. Single Peak at 365

3. What is the half life of this tracer?
A. 67 Hours
B. 73 Hours
C. 8 Days

Case 29 - Nukes (Indium-WBC)

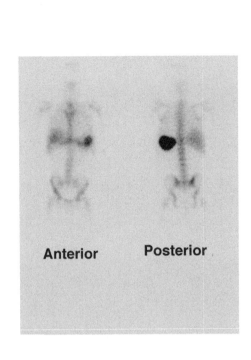

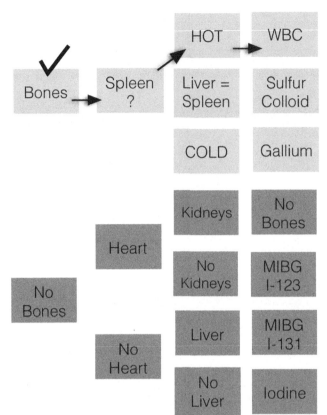

1. What scan is it?
A. Gallium
B. Indium - WBC
C. MIBG
D. I would ask the tech what tracer they injected. If they said "I don't know", I would fire them on the spot, and have security remove them from the hospital immediately.

2. What are the photon peaks of this tracer?
A. Single Peak at 81
B. Four Peaks at 93, 184, 300, & 393
C. Two Peaks at 173 & 247
D. Single Peak at 365

3. What is the half life of this tracer?
A. 67 Hours
B. 73 Hours
C. 8 Days

Indium Trivia

- Tagged onto a Neutrophil - they travel to areas of infection / inflammation and the RES (why the spleen is HOT)

- Indium can actually be hooked onto lots of stuff (Octreotide, DTPA, etc...)

- You can also do WBC scanning be using Tc (instead on Indium). Both will have hot spleens but the Tc study looks cleaner and because of its higher counts.

- Tc -WBC labeling is preferred for small parts (hands and feet) and small people (kids).

- In-WBC is gonna be way better for bowel pathology (inflammatory or infected), as Tc has normal bowel uptake (Indium does not).

Case 30 - Nukes (Mystery Whole Body Scan 3)

1. What scan is it?
A. Sulfur Colloid
B. MIBG
C. Iodine 131
D. I would ask the tech what tracer they injected. If they said "I don't know", I would fire them on the spot, and have security remove them from the hospital immediately.

3. What is the half life of this tracer?
A. 13 Hours
B. 13 Days
C. 8 Hours
D. 8 Days

3. Which is true regarding breast feeding?
A. You can resume breast feeding 24 hours after I-131
B. You can resume breast feeding 3 days after I-123
C. You can resume breast feeding immediately after Tc-99m

Anatomy 60

Case 30 - Nukes (Iodine -131)

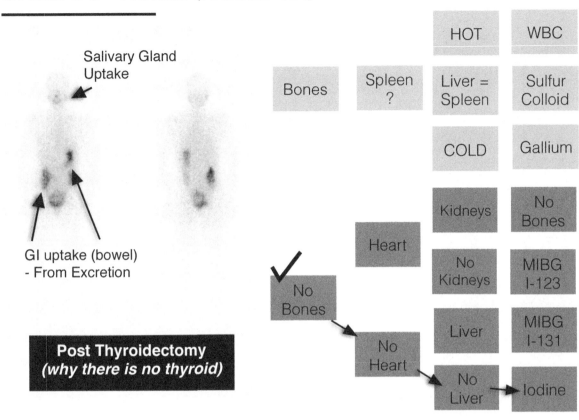

1. What scan is it?
A. Sulfur Colloid
B. MIBG
C. Iodine 131
D. I would ask the tech what tracer they injected. If they said "I don't know", I would fire them on the spot, and have security remove them from the hospital immediately.

3. What is the half life of this tracer?
A. 13 Hours
B. 13 Days
C. 8 Hours
D. 8 Days

3. Which is true regarding breast feeding?
A. You can resume breast feeding 24 hours after I-131
B. You can resume breast feeding 3 days after I-123
C. You can resume breast feeding immediately after Tc-99m

Iodine Trivia

- I-131 is cheap but has a longer half life (8 days), and is high energy (364)

- I-123 is more expensive, but has a shorter half life (13 hours), and a more ideal energy (159)

- Tc99m can also be used to image the thyroid, but is not organified, so it just diffuses in and out of the thyroid - this causes more background uptake.

- Any bone uptake should be considered a met with I-123 and I-131.

- The shadow of the heart on a grey lung, should make you think lung mets.

- Uptake in the liver can be seen post I-131 ablation treatment.

Anatomy 61

Case Index

Aunt Minnie's

1) CADASIL
2) Agenesis of the corpus callosum (ACC)
3) Jouberts
4) Central Pontine Myelinolysis
5) Hypothalamic Hamartoma
6) Artery of Percheron Infarct
7) Superficial siderosis (SS)
8) Skull Base Fibrous Dysplasia
9) NF-2
10) Esthesioneuroblastoma
11) Inverting Papiloma
12) Labyrinthitis Ossificans
13) Endolymphatic Sac Tumor
14) Large Vestibular Aqueduct Syndrome (LVAS)
15) Superior Canal Dehiscence (SCD)
16) Otospongiosis
17) Retinoblastoma
18) Spinal Ependymoma
19) Tethered Cord with Lipoma
20) De Quervain's tenosynovitis
21) Kohlers
22) Juvenile Rheumatoid Arthritis
23) Psoriasis Arthritis
24) Gout
25) Erosive OA
26) Systemic Lupus Erythematosus Arthritis
27) Osteochondral Lesion
28) Synovial Osteochondromatosis
29) Pagets
30) Particle Disease
31) Polyethylene Wear
32) Partial UCL Tear – T Sign
33) Aneurysmal bone cysts (ABC)
34) Bucket Hand Meniscal Tear - Double PCL sign
35) Discoid Meniscus
36) Split Brevis
37) Posterior Tibial Tendon Tear
38) Adhesive Capsulitis
39) Buford Complex
40) Calcific Tendonitis
41) Anisotropy - Ultrasound Artifact
42) SLAC wrist
43) Displaced medial humeral epicondyle fracture
44) Arrhythmogenic right ventricular cardiomyopathy (ARVC)
45) Cor Triatriatum Sinistrum
46) Coronary Artery Aneurysm
47) Non-compaction cardiomyopathy (NCC)

48) Ischemia on Cardiac MRI
49) Myocarditis
50) Sinus of Valsalva Aneurysm
51) Ebsteins Anomaly
52) Tetralogy of Fallot
53) Total anomalous pulmonary venous return (TAPVR)
54) UIP
55) NSIP
56) Fibrosing Mediastinitis
57) Kaposi Sarcoma
58) Pulmonary Alveolar Proteinosis (PAP)
59) Tracheobronchopathia Osteochondroplastica (TBO)
60) HOT Quadrate Syndrome
61) Bud Chiari
62) Duodenal Hematoma
63) CF Pancreas (SDS)
64) Gamma Gandy Bodies
65) Rectal CA – T3 staging
66) Appendix Mucocele
67) Biliary Cystadenoma
68) Shock Bowel
69) Typhlitis
70) Pheochromocytoma
71) Xanthogranulomatous Pyelonephritis (XGPN)
72) Autosomal Dominant Polycystic Kidney Disease (ADPCKD)
73) Multilocular Cystic Nephroma
74) HIV Associated Nephropathy (HIVAN)
75) Urachal Carcinoma
76) Tamoxifen Uterus
77) Adenomyosis
78) Theca Lutein Cysts
79) Cervical Cancer
80) MIBG with Breast CA
81) Gallium Pneumonia (PCP)
82) FDG Brain Alzheimers
83) Normal pressure hydrocephalus
84) Duodenal Atresia
85) Choroid Plexus Cyst
86) Mid Gut Herniation
87) Cystic Rhombencephalon
88) Aqueductal Stenosis Congenital Hydrocephalus
89) Choanal Atresia
90) Mesenchymal Hamartoma
91) Septate Uterus
92) Bicornuate Uterus
93) Pyloric Stenosis
94) Posterior Urethral Valve (PUV)
95) Neonatal Pneumomediastinum and the Spinnaker-Sail Sign
96) Osteosarcoma

97) Prostaglandin Therapy
98) Blount's disease
99) Rickets
100) Malrotation
101) Breast Hamartoma
102) NMLE (DCIS) on MRI
103) Sternalis Muscle
104) Type B Aortic Dissection
105) Stent Graft Endoleak
106) May–Thurner syndrome
107) Popliteal Artery Aneurysm
108) Giant cell arteritis
109) MRI Artifact 1 - Pulsation
110) MRI Artifact 2 – Magnetic Susceptibility
111) MRI Artifact 3 – Cs -1
112) MRI Artifact 4 – CS -2
113) MRI Artifact 5 – Fat inhomogeneity
114) MRI Artifact 6 – Coil Flair
115) MRI Artifact 7 – Gibbs
116) MRI Artifact 8 – Dielectric Artifact
117) MRI Artifact 9 – Zipper
118) MRI Artifact 10 – Magic Angle
119) Star Artifact
120) NM colloid clump VQ
121) Beam Hardening Artifact
122) Ring Artifact
123) Ultrasound QC – Focal Zone Wrong
124) Ultrasound Artifact – Mirror Image
125) Ultrasound Artifact – Comet Tail
126) Non-Interpretive Skills - Medication Labeling and Blood
127) Non-Interpretive Skills - Time Out / Site Marking
128) Non-Interpretive Skills - BIER 7 and Radiation Risk
129) Non-Interpretive Skills - Just Culture and Human Reliability
130) Non-Interpretive Skills - LEAN

This vs That

1) Acoustic Schwannoma vs Meningioma vs Epidermoid
2) Holoprosencephaly Spectrum
3) Schizencephaly vs Porencephalic Cyst
4) Herpes Encephalitis vs Limbic Encephalitis
5) Intracranial Hypotension vs Intracranial Hypertension
6) HIV Encephalitis vs PML
7) CMV calcifications vs Toxoplasma calcifications
8) JPA vs Hemangioblastoma
9) Thyroglossal Duct Cyst vs Brachial Cleft Cyst
10) Cholesteatoma vs Cholesterol Granuloma
11) Vocal Cord Paralysis vs Tumor
12) Glomus vs Giant-cell tumor of the tendon sheath (GCT-TS)
13) Infraspinatus vs Quadrilateral Space Atrophy
14) Perthes vs GLAD
15) Monteggia Fx vs Galeazzi Fx
16) HALO vs Reverse Halo Sign
17) LAM vs LCH
18) Upper vs Lower Lobe Predominant
19) Pulmonary Nodule Patterns
20) Hemochromatosis vs Fatty liver
21) Primary vs secondary hemochromatosis
22) Dysplastic Nodule vs HCC
23) Pancreatic serous cystadenoma vs Mucinous Cystadenoma (MCN)
24) Crohns vs Ulcerative Colitis
25) Endometrioma vs Dermoid on MRI
26) Traction vs Pulsion Diverticulum
27) T sign vs Twin Peak Sign
28) Pre vs Post ECMO
29) UAC vs UVC
30) Polysplenia vs Asplenia
31) SCFE vs Perthes
32) Wilms vs Neuroblastoma
33) Hirschsprung's disease (HD) vs Meconium Ileus
34) VQ anatomy Projections
35) Renal Transplant Rejection vs ATN - on MAG 3
36) Super Scans - Metabolic vs Mets
37) Geiger Muller Counter vs Ionization Chamber
38) Yellow 1 vs Yellow 2
39) Major Spill vs Minor Spill
40) Radiochemical Purity vs Chemical Purity
41) Decay Line Diagrams
42) PET corrected vs uncorrected
43) Breast Implants on MRI - Radial Folds vs Intracapsular Rupture
44) Male Gynecomastia vs Male Breast CA
45) Breast MRI - Tamoxifen on Vs Tamoxifen Off — Rebound Effect
46) Carotid Doppler - Internal Carotid vs External Carotid
47) Marfans vs Loeys–Dietz syndrome
48) Renal Artery Angiograms: Atherosclerosis vs FMD
49) Arthrogram - Shoulder vs hip
50) Catheter Basics - Inner vs Outer Diameter (Sheath vs Catheter)

Anatomy

1) Skull Base - Part 1
2) Skull Base - Part 2
3) Skull Base - Part 3
4) Skull Base - Part 4
5) Skull Base - Part 5 (Cavernous Sinus)
6) Skull Sutures
7) Sagittal Brain MRI -
8) Temporal Bone - Part 1 (CT)
9) Temporal Bone - Part 2 (CT)
10) Temporal Bone - Part 3 (MRI)
11) Cervical Lymph Nodes
12) Vascular (CNS - Part 1)
13) Vascular (CNS - Part 2)
14) Vascular (CNS - Part 3)
15) Vascular (Celiac Axis)
16) Vascular (SMA)
17) Vascular (Upper Extremity)
18) Vascular (Lower Extremity)
19) Vascular (Femoral Access)
20) Cardiac (Part 1)
21) Cardiac (Part 2)
22) Abdominal Ultrasound
23) Prostate MRI
24) MSK - Pelvis
25) MSK - Shoulder
26) MSK - Wrist
27) MSK - Ankle
28) Nukes Mystery Whole Body Scan 1
29) Nukes Mystery Whole Body Scan 2
30) Nukes Mystery Whole Body Scan 3

Blank on Purpose For Note Writing:

Blank on Purpose For Note Writing:

Blank on Purpose For Note Writing:

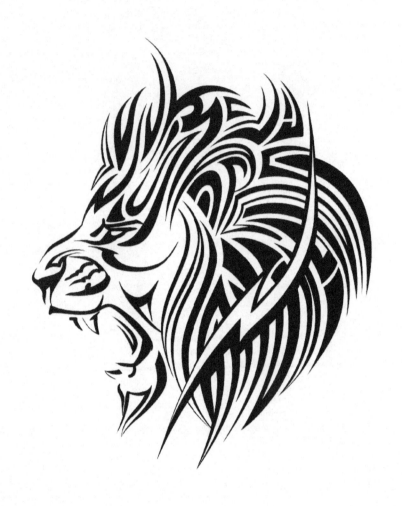

RISE AND GRIND

Made in the USA
Las Vegas, NV
28 January 2024

85032024R00256